OXFORD MEDICAL PUBLICATIONS

Wounds:
Biology and Management

Wounds: Biology and Management

Edited by

D. J. Leaper

Professor of Surgery,
University of Newcastle
Professorial Unit of Surgery,
North Tees General Hospital,
Stockton-on-Tees, Cleveland

and

K. G. Harding

Professor of Rehabilitation
Medicine (Wound Healing) and
Director, Wound Healing Research
Unit, University Department of
Surgery, University of Wales
College of Medicine

OXFORD   NEW YORK   TOKYO
OXFORD UNIVERSITY PRESS
1998

Oxford University Press, Great Clarendon Street, Oxford ox2 6dp

Oxford New York
Athens Auckland Bangkok Bogota Bombay
Buenos Aires Calcutta Cape Town Dar es Salaam
Delhi Florence Hong Kong Istanbul Karachi
Kuala Lumpur Madras Madrid Melbourne
Mexico City Nairobi Paris Singapore
Taipei Tokyo Toronto Warsaw
and associated companies in
Berlin Ibadan

Oxford is a trade mark of Oxford University Press

Published in the United States
by Oxford University Press, Inc., New York

© D. J. Leaper and K. G. Harding, 1998

A catalogue record for this book is available from the British Library

Library of Congress Cataloging in Publication Data
(Data applied for)

ISBN 0 19 262332 X (Hbk)

Typeset by Best-set Typesetter Ltd., Hong Kong

Printed in Hong Kong

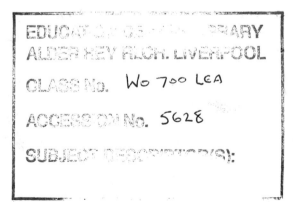

Foreword

by PROFESSOR THOMAS K. HUNT

Another book on wound healing! How many do we need? They are not exactly common, but the old average, one a decade, has suddenly risen to one a year, and the pace of new insights has made it not only possible but necessary. This book, however, is not the usual wound healing book. It is a practical book, designed for the multidisciplinary team involved in wound management. The new theory is here set into practical terms, and books like this come along a lot less often.

Why, though, would anyone want to spend time and money on a rehash of healing when it isn't a problem? The fact is, healing is a problem. Wound problems are, together with transplantation immunity, the major limitations on the horizons of surgical, medical, and nursing capacities. Perhaps my surgical unit is somewhat unusual, but a quarter to a third of our patients at any given time are there because of some failure of wound healing, and we don't just collect chronic wounds. We also collect failed operations, fistulas, bowel obstructions, peritonitis from anastomotic leaks, bile duct strictures, failed intestinal pouches and dehisced mediastinums.

'You see what you look for and you look for what you know.' Consider this dialogue: 'Vascular grafts still commonly fail.' 'Really? Mine are almost always successful. 'When did you last do one in a 2 mm vessel?' 'Oh, well, those don't usually work.' My question is whether they can't work or surgeons just don't ('didn't', to be exact) know how to make them work. The same goes for operations done in the presence of infection. If there is stool from a perforated colon in the peritoneal cavity, anastomoses often fail. True, but is that a law of nature or a failing of surgical knowledge and skill? More and more, we are learning that our limitations reflect that there is a failure of medical knowledge and skill.

We wound managers have been remarkably obtuse about these things. If most surgeons were asked to sew up a cut on a hand that was contaminated with stool, they would back away in horror. Yet, most sew up haemorrhoid wounds. Why the difference? I often ask that question, and few surgeons have an answer. If I prod, however, they will often say that hands may have less blood supply than the anus, and that is a better answer, but still it doesn't achieve full points. Actually, normal hands have a rich anatomical set of blood vessels. The difference is not the capacity of the vessels. The difference is in the way blood flow is regulated in the hand where blood vessels are richly supplied with adrenergic receptors and hence obey the rules of the sympathetic nervous system. Hands vasoconstrict as anyone who has a clammy handshake is painfully aware. Could adrenergic blocking agents be useful

wound healing agents? Of course they could, but have you ever used one? If you have, you may not need this book.

The lore of wound healing has a rich tradition going back centuries. Tradition can be a wonderful thing, but in the clinical management of wounds, it has been a serious problem that bothers us as much today as it bothered Ambroise Paré when he tried almost 500 years ago, and largely failed, to introduce into other surgeons' practices a rudimentary degree of consideration for wounded tissue. James Lind was no more successful when, after he did the first prospective trial in the history of medicine, he tried to introduce some nutritional considerations into the every day routine of the British Navy 300 years ago. Nor was Joseph Lister a smashing success with his antiseptic concept. Today, it seems, we ride on the shoulders of these giants and still assume, as Paré's, Lind's, and Lister's contemporaries did, that wounds can do no better than we see now and that there is no need to do better. The greatest enemy of progress is still the illusion of knowledge.

My revered professor, J. E. Dunphy, rode on the shoulders of Halstead. He made me close abdominal incisions with tiny sutures of fine silk, and blamed my technique when they fell open. I hid it from him when I did 'mass closures' of abdominal incisions as we all do now. He once published, 'Surgeons have long sought means to hasten the healing of wounds, but in the end they have made no improvement on nature's normal period.' No matter that we could not then, nor can we now, define 'nature's normal period.' It varies, of course, from tissue to tissue and probably from hour to hour. Every time I look, it becomes shorter.

On the other hand, our forebears taught us that healing is somehow related to blood flow, that tension on suture lines is unhealthy, that cleanliness keeps one from having to report wound infections to one's morbidity conferences. What they did not know, and what we still may not appreciate, is how powerfully these observations can be developed and refined.

Consider, for instance, the subject of blood flow and healing, one close to my heart. As I noted above, surgeons have 'always' known that poorly perfused tissues heal poorly. Keeping that in mind, can I ask whether giving more blood is the right way to cope with anaemia, or is vascular surgery the only way to heal wounds in ischaemic tissues? By exploration of the mechanisms of healing, we now know that the major item delivered by blood to wounds is oxygen, and that we can make up for considerable lack of anatomical vascularity by providing oxygen at high partial pressures. In a related question, anaemia still ranks high in many surgeons' minds as a cause of inadequate healing despite repeated demonstrations to the contrary. Only recently has the obvious been demonstrated that a high flow or perfusion rate compensates nicely for anaemia especially in tissues that use only small amounts of oxygen, as wounds do. Controlled anaemia may be part of the solutions to wound problems in some patients! These developments will be discussed in detail in the rest of the book.

In this book you will be exposed to the concept of growth factors, one of the two most important conceptual advances in this field in this century. At this moment, no matter how conceptually important, growth factors are still in search of a practical application. It will come. You will be forced to look anew at chronic wounds, mentally to take off the bandages and look beneath at the tissues lacking oxygen and angiogenesis, and you will see a challenge to restore oxygenation to these starving tissues, even if there is no obvious ischaemia or venous disease. If you do learn to look further, if you learn to see, you will find both venous and arterial disease, and poorly vascularized scar as well. You may be challenged to drop the 'wet-to-dry' wound care in favour of a moist environment, and that might take some courage.

Resistance to infections is an integral part of wound healing. In this book you will be asked to look for physiological reasons for wound infections, not just technical or disciplinary ones. There will be simple clinical directions for nutritional care of wounded patients, and some new ideas on staplers and sutures.

Not all that is new is both good and reliable. Surgeons and dermatologists are already being exposed to claims of magical cures for chronic wounds and burns, I am almost daily asked to accept anecdotes about some new remedy together with superb pictures before and after. Some have substance, some do not, and I cannot always decide which is which. All of us need to develop some sales resistance, and this is the time.

I wonder where it will all stop, or will it never stop. Some day will we arrange for our patients to regenerate their feet and lungs? Then, perhaps, we will heal by a beam of intelligent healing energy as they do now in television's versions of outer space. This is not entirely fanciful. Electromagnetic waves are today accelerating healing in bone. And why not in soft tissue? Why not?

I suppose I am one of the few people alive who would pick up a book like this and find an adventure story in it. Remember, though, I was taught to close abdominal incisions with small silk sutures. I have seen a lot of wounds fall open, and a lot of water flow under the bridge since that time, and I feel some pride in having been part of the current. Have a nice swim. Take a good leap at it. You might find it refreshing.

Acknowledgements

The Publishers wish to acknowledge the generosity of Smith and Nephew in the production of this book, in particular Mr J. Dick. The authors wish to thank their secretaries, Mrs Leigh Morgan and Miss Susan Taylor for their constant patience in the writing and editing of this book.

Dedication

To our wives Fran and Sue.

Contents

The colour plates fall between pages 116 and 117

Contributors

Major contributors:

Ehrlich, H. P. Division of Paediatric Surgery, Pennsylvania State University College of Medicine, USA

Gottrup, F. Copenhagen Wound Healing Center, Bispebjerg University Hospital, Copenhagen, Denmark

Harding, K. G. Director, Wound Healing Research Unit, University of Wales College of Medicine, Cardiff

Leaper, D. J. Professorial Unit of Surgery, North Tees General Hospital, Cleveland

Mulder, G. D. Director, Wound Healing Institute, Aurora, Colorado, USA

Other contributors:

Agren, M. S. Associate Professor, Department of Pathology, Faculty of Health Sciences, Sweden

Baragwanath, P. Director, Wound Healing Research Unit, University of Wales College of Medicine, Cardiff

Boyce, D. E. Director, Wound Healing Research Unit, University of Wales College of Medicine, Cardiff

Brazinsky, B. A. Regional Burns Center, University of California, Department of Surgery, San Diego, California, USA

Faria, D. Department of Dermatology Henry Ford Hospital, Lorton, Virginia, USA

Feneley, R. C. L. Consultant Urologist, Southmead Hospital, Bristol

Iocono, J. A. Division of Paediatric Surgery, Pennsylvania State University College of Medicine, USA

Irvin, T. T. Consultant Surgeon, Royal Devon and Exeter Hospital

Lane, I. F. Cardiff Vascular Unit, University Hospital of Wales, Cardiff

Leigh, I. M. Professor of Dermatology, Royal London Hospital

Moorehead, R. J. Professor and Consultant Surgeon, North Down and Ards Hospital Trust, Co. Down

Robson, M. C. Professor, Department of Surgery, University of South Florida, USA

Rodriguez, J. L. Associate Professor of Surgery, University of Michigan Medical Center, Ann Arbor, USA

Salaman, J. Director, Wound Healing Research Unit, University of Wales College of Medicine, Cardiff

Salaman, R. Director, Wound Healing Research Unit, University of Wales College of Medicine, Cardiff

Sampson, J. A. G. Plastic Surgeon, Michigan, USA

Smith, E. J. Consultant Senior Lecturer, Department of Orthopaedic Surgery, University of Bristol

Thomas, S. Director, Surgical Materials Testing Laboratory, Bridgend General Hospital

Vickery, C. J. Surgical Registrar, Frenchay Hospital, Bristol

Wainwright, A. M. Department of Orthopaedic Surgery, Avon Orthopaedic Centre, Southmead Hospital

Whiston, R. J. Cardiff Vascular Unit, University Hospital of Wales, Cardiff

Whiteside, M. C. R. Senior Registrar in Surgery, Institute of Clinical Science, Belfast

Williams, N. A. University of Bristol, Department of Pathology and Microbiology, Bristol

1

Wounds: the extent of the burden

K. G. HARDING and D. E. BOYCE

The epidemiology of wounds is too vast a topic to be considered in one chapter when looking at the great variation in wound aetiology. Wound types can vary from burns, chronic, and non-surgical wounds through to surgical, incisional, or excisional wounds. Surgical wound types vary from area to area, even within one hospital, depending on the practice of individual surgeons. Take, for example, the pilonidal sinus – many surgeons within the United Kingdom treat this condition by excision with open treatment and formation of granulation tissue (secondary infention), whereas in the United States, more patients are treated by primary suture.

With respect to accidental traumatic wounds, of the 11 million patients attending Accident and Emergency Departments in England and Wales each year, approximately 25 per cent present with wounds of one sort or another, i.e. 3 million traumatic wounds per year (1). These have a variety of aetiologies ranging from accidental incised wounds and lacerations to bites, crush wounds, abrasions, and burns. This obviously weighs heavily on the purse strings of any health service, but most heal without complication. The problem arises when they do not, and this is what is considered in this chapter: the epidemiology of chronic, non-healing wounds.

'Ulcers . . . form a very extensive and important class of disease . . . the treatment of such cases is generally looked upon as an inferior branch of practise; an unpleasant and inglorious task where much labour must be bestowed and little honour gained.' This quote comes not from a modern text but one published in 1805 (2) – little appears to have changed in the last 190 years! Non-healing wounds still present a huge challenge to modern society, despite recent advances in most aspects of health care. Pressure sores alone affect 6.7–11 per cent of the adult population of the UK, mainly the elderly or disabled, at an estimated cost of £60–300 million per year, and this does not even include the cost of personal suffering (3). However, the true cost of pressure sore prevention and management is unknown and this is mainly due to a lack of consensus in obtaining the data required from hospitals and the community. In a recent study of over 3000 hospitalized elderly people, 18.8 per cent were found to have pressure damage (4). Little research has been published which has assessed the cost of pressure sores to the health services, but recently the Department of Health (UK) estimated that £40 million was spent in the community alone each year. Other estimates have included figures as high as £300 million (5).

One difficulty in trying to assess the aetiology of pressure ulcers is first of all defining what they are in the first place. The consensus of opinion is that they are localized areas of tissue necrosis which tend to develop when soft tissue is compressed between a bony prominence and an external surface for a prolonged period (6). Non-blanchable or even blanchable erythema may sometimes be regarded as early pressure ulceration, and a variety of classifications exist (7–10), but the most manageable system was that advocated by Shea (11). Stage I includes non-blanchable erythema, with or without an epithelial defect; stage II, a full thickness skin ulcer extending into subcutaneous fat; stage III, a full thickness skin ulcer extending deeply into fat but limited by deep fascia; stage IV, penetration of deep fascia with extensive soft tissue spread, which may include bone and joint involvement.

The past few years have seen an increase in awareness of the sequels following the development of pressure ulceration. Its epidemiology mirrors that of immobility, and it is therefore at its highest level in the disabled and those in hospital or long term care environments. Its incidence has been reported to range from 3 to 18.8 per cent (4, 9–14). At least 60 per cent of those who develop ulcers do so in the hospital environment; 18 per cent develop them in the home, and 18 per cent within a nursing home (15). In the acute hospital environment, an overall prevalence between 1 and 5 per cent has been reported (9). Most develop early, 70 per cent within the first two weeks of hospitalization (16). The highest levels of ulceration are found in longer term care environments and, in particular, those with spinal injury suffer an incidence of 20–30 per cent at 1–5 years after injury (17). In the United States a third national pressure ulcer survey of 177 hospitals was carried out in 1993 (18). It is of concern that the overall prevalence was 11 per cent, which was an increase on the figure of 9.2 per cent which had been reported four years earlier (19). This compared favourably with the UK, but not with some other European countries, as shown in Fig. 1.1 (20). The variation in incidence between each country may in fact be due to differences in age of the hospital population: in Holland and the UK 57 per cent of patients are over the age of 65 years compared with only 44 per cent in Italy and Germany. The ulcers were largely hospital acquired in all four countries (Fig. 1.2).

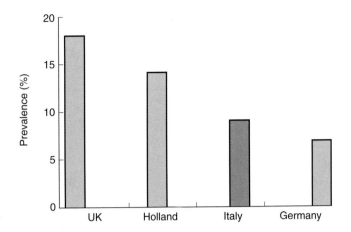

Fig. 1.1 Overall hospital prevalence of pressure ulceration in four European countries.

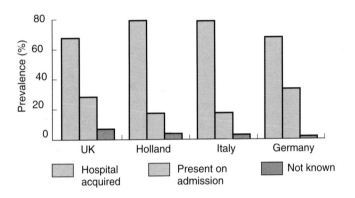

Fig. 1.2 Source of pressure damage as a percentage of the total.

Table 1.1 Ulcer aetiology amongst patients attending a hospital-based wound clinic (29)

Aetiology	Number	Percentage
Venous	285	58
Arterial	44	9
Mixed	40	8
Trauma	37	8
Pressure	20	4
Vasculitic	18	4
Diabetic	12	2
Post-surgical	10	2
Lymphoedema	5	1
Neuropathic	4	1
Unclear	15	3

From the data shown, it can be seen that pressure sores are a major problem on both sides of the Atlantic. However, one of the most interesting findings is the large variation in incidence between two European countries: Germany with an incidence of 7 per cent and the UK with an incidence of 18.6 per cent. This could in part be explained by differences in terminology, and by recognizing stage I, non-blanching erythema, as pressure damage. It again illustrates the importance of a universal classification system such as the four stage method described above.

Another chronic wound, which presents a huge burden to patients and health services alike, is the chronic leg ulcer. The frequent lack of specialist clinical assessment in the community has led to long periods of ineffective and often inappropriate treatment. This not only applies to graduated compression in ulcers of venous aetiology, but also delays in potentially limb-salvaging procedures for those of arterial cause. The first modern study of leg ulcer prevalence and aetiology was performed about 30 years ago (21). This reported a leg ulcer prevalence of 1 per cent, with 80% being due to venous disease. A similar study a decade later by Widmer (22) found comparable results. In a British population study of 198 900 during 1986, 356 patients with 424 ulcerated legs

were reported, giving an overall point prevalence of 0.18 per cent (23). The prevalence in the population aged 40 years or more was 0.38 per cent. This epidemiology seems to have changed little in the past ten years: a more recent study published in 1996 showed a prevalence of 0.11 per cent (24). This is consistent with findings of other population-based questionnaire studies in various countries and communities (22, 25–28). These have reduced the current estimate of leg ulcer prevalence to 0.1–0.3 per cent of the general population rising to 2 per cent in the population aged 80 years or more. With respect to aetiology, those ulcers secondary to venous disease account for 67 per cent (27) to 76 per cent (29), whereas those due to arterial disease account for 9 per cent (23) to 28 per cent (26) of cases. In a different environment, a recent study, looking at patients attending a dedicated hospital-based wound clinic in Cardiff (29), found a lower incidence of ulcers of purely venous aetiology (Table 1.1), and a wider range of alternative pathologies. However, this probably reflects the fact that many of the ulcers were tertiary referrals which were refractory to conventional management.

Another major pathology causing chronic ulceration of the lower limb is that of microangiopathy secondary to diabetes mellitus. This syndrome, characterized by chronic hyperglycaemia affects approximately 14 per 100 000 population in the UK and ranges from 1 to 29 per 100 000 worldwide (30). Approximately 25 per cent of diabetic patients at some point present at a specialist clinic suffering from foot ulcers and 10–15 per cent require surgical treatment. The diabetic foot causes more hospitalization of diabetic patients than any other diabetes-associated complication (31). Admissions resulting from this condition are increasing in both type I and type II diabetes, and represent 2.5 per cent of all hospital admissions. Epidemiological research is extremely limited with regard to the diabetic foot and mainly deals with the frequency of angiopathy, neuropathy, ulcers, and amputations in specified populations. The prevalence of diabetes in patients undergoing major amputations has been estimated at between 40 and 70 per cent (32–34). Only a quarter of ulcers are caused by arterial insufficiency: the majority are caused by other factors such as infection and neuropathy (35). Much interest has been generated recently in trying to reduce the complications of such diabetic foot disease. Specialist clinics in preventative care have been set up, with individuals trained in orthotics and podiatry as well as medical and nursing staff. These have resulted in a reduction in major amputations of 78 per cent in some centres (36). This improvement is encouraging bearing in mind that between 41 and 70 per cent of diabetics who have a leg amputation do not survive for more than five years after their surgery (32, 37, 38), although they obviously also suffer from other complications more commonly found in this group.

Any chapter describing the epidemiology of wounds would be incomplete without mentioning burn injuries. Worldwide there are huge differences in burn aetiology and epidemiology in association with differences in culture and urbanization of individual countries. For example, one would not expect many hot kettle burns in deepest India, whereas in the UK tea making and drinking accounts for a substantial proportion of childhood scalds (39). In fact, the commonest burn profile in Western India is that of a 15–19 year old girl with flame burns as a result of her sari catching fire while learning to cook on a makeshift stove (40). This international perspective can be further typified by the fact that in Scandinavia, scalds in sauna rooms can constitute the largest groups of injuries (41).

Detailed epidemiological studies of burn injuries have only been made since World War II, and even these are relatively limited in that apart from mortality data, national estimates of burns and scalds are very approximate and give little information on causation in relation to the nature of the injury. One of the most extensive studies on the epidemiology of burn injuries was published by the Royal Society for the Prevention of Accidents in 1990 (42). This documented a very large number of burns occurring in the West Midlands region of the UK, representing a population of 5 million (1 million of whom live in the City of Birmingham) over an eight year period. In essence, the highest incidence of burns and scalds was found to be in the very young: burns in children accounted for 45 per cent of the work of the burns unit. Scalds were a particularly common cause, accounting for 79 per cent of the under five year olds admitted. In general, 14 per cent of burn injury patients sustained their injury at work, whereas 95 per cent of 'non-industrial' thermal injuries occurred in the home. Burns comprised 91 per cent of industrial admissions, whereas the non-industrial cases were almost equally divided between burns and scalds. Males accounted for 65 per cent of all admissions with 93 per cent of accidents at work. When looking at scald injuries alone, 79 per cent were children, 15 per cent adults of working age, with the remainder occurring in persons over the age of 65 years. In elderly people, 61 per cent of burn injuries were to women.

The epidemiology of chronic wounds encountered in modern medical or surgical practise has been outlined. Information has been kept concise, partly due to great variations in wound aetiology and the sparsity of available data. Although most wound categories exist globally, there remain international variations in epidemiology depending on the culture, customs, and development of the individual society. What is obvious, however, is that problems with wound healing still exist worldwide, throughout all cultures and nationalities, maintaining a heavy burden on all societies. In this respect,

surprisingly little appears to have changed in the last two centuries (2).

The range and extent of wound problems make them common and challenging clinical problems. The need to have an awareness of the basic pathophysiological process is an important prerequisite for delivering optimal clinical care. Understanding the biology of wounds and developing optimal treatments for them are essential components of an important, but still evolving, area of clinical care.

References

1. Holborn, C. J. and Lester, R. (1994). Setting standards in traumatic wound care. In *Proceedings of the 4th European Conference on Advances in Wound Management*, pp. 14–16. MacMillan Magazines, London.
2. Louden, I. S. L. (1981). Leg ulcers in the 18th and 19th centuries. *J. R. Coll. Gen. Pract.*, **31**, 263–73.
3. Department of Health (1992). *The Health of the Nation: a strategy for health in England*. HMSO, London.
4. O'Dea, K. (1993). Prevalence of pressure damage in hospital patients in the UK. *J. Wound Care*, **2**, 221–5.
5. Waterlow, J. (1988). Prevention is better than cure. *Nursing Times*, **84**, 69–70.
6. The National Pressure Ulcer Advisory Panel (1989). Pressure ulcers: prevalence, cost and risk assessment statement. *Decubitus*, **2**, 24–8.
7. Yarkony, G. M., Kirk, P. M., Carlson, C., *et al.* (1990). Classification of pressure ulcers. *Arch. Dermatol.*, **126**, 1218–19.
8. Manley, M. T. (1978). Incidence, contributory factors and costs of pressure sores. *S. Afr. Med. J.*, **53**, 217–22.
9. Barbenel, J. C., Forbes, C. D., and Lowe, G. D. O. (1983). *Pressure sores*. Pitman Press, Bath.
10. Allman, R. M., Laprade, C. A., Noel, L. B. *et al.* (1986). Pressure sores among hospitalised patients. *Ann. Intern. Med.*, **105**, 337–43.
11. Shea, J. D. (1975). Pressure sores: classification and management. *Clin. Orthop.*, **112**, 89–100.
12. Anderson, K. E. and Kvorning, S. A. (1982). Medical aspects of the decubitus ulcer. *Int. J. Dermatol.*, **21**, 265–70.
13. Moody, B. L., Fanale, J. E., Thompson, M., Vaillancourt, D. *et al.* (1988). Impact of staff education and pressure sore development in elderly hospitalised patients. *Arch. Intern. Med.*, **148**, 2241–3.
14. Barbanel, J. C., Jordan, M. M., Nicol, S. M., and Clark, M. O. (1977). Incidence of pressure sores in the Greater Glasgow Health Board Area. *Lancet*, **ii**, 548–50.
15. Phillips, T. J. (1994). Chronic cutaneous ulcers: etiology and epidemiology. *J. Invest. Dermatol.*, **102**, 38S–41S.
16. Norton, D., McLaren, R., and Exton-Smith, A. N. (1975). *An investigation of geriatric nursing problems in hospital*, pp. 193–236. Churchill Livingstone, Edinburgh.
17. Young, J. S., Burns, P. E., Bowen, A. M., and McCutchen, R. (eds) (1982). *Spinal cord injury statistics: experience of the regional spinal cord injury systems*, pp. 95–6. National Spinal Cord Injury Data Research Centre, Phoenix.
18. Meehan, M. (1994). National pressure ulcer prevalence survey. *Advances in Wound Care*, **7**, 27–30.
19. Meehan, M. M. (1990). Multi-site pressure ulcer prevalence survey. *Decubitus*, **3**, 14–17.
20. O'Dea, K. (1995). The prevalence of pressure sores in four European countries. *J. Wound Care*, **4**, 192–5.
21. Bobek, K., Cajzl, L., Cepelak, V., Slaisova, V., Opatzny, K., and Barcal, R. (1966). Etude de la frequence des maladies

phlebologiques et de l'influence de quelques facteurs etiologiques. *Phlebologie*, **19**, 217–30.

22. Widmer, L. K. (1978). *Peripheral venous disorders: prevalence and sociomedical importance.* Hans Huber, Berne.

23. Cornwall, J. V., Dore, C. J., and Lewis, J. D. (1986). Leg ulcers: epidemiology and aetiology. *Br. J. Surg.*, **73**, 693–6.

24. Freak, L., Simon, D., Kinsella, A., McCollum, C., Walsh, J., and Lane, C. (1996). Leg ulcer care: an audit of cost-effectiveness. *Health Trends*, **27**, 133–6.

25. Callam, M. J., Ruckley, C. V., Harper, D. R., and Dale, J. J. (1985). Chronic ulceration of the leg: extent of the problem and provision of care. *Br. Med. J.*, **290**, 1855–6.

26. Nelzen, O., Bergqvist, D., and Lindhagen, A. (1991). Leg ulcer aetiology: a cross-sectional population study. *J. Vasc. Surg.*, **14**, 557–64.

27. Baker, S. R., Stacy, M. C., Singh, G., Hoskin, S. E., and Thompson, P. J. (1992). Aetiology of chronic leg ulcers. *Eur. J. Vasc. Surg.*, **6**, 245–51.

28. Ruckley, C. V., Dale, J. J., Callam, M. J., and Harper, D. R. (1982). Causes of chronic leg ulcers. *Lancet*, **ii**, 615–16.

29. Salaman, R. A. and Harding, K. G. (1994). Aetiology and prognosis of chronic leg ulcers. In *Proceedings of the 4th European Conference on Advances in Wound Management*, pp. 149–51.

30. Bodansky, J. (1994). *Diabetes*, (2nd edn). Wolfe, London.

31. Hatz, R. A., Niedner, R., Vanscheidt, W., and Westerhof, W. (1994). *Wound healing and wound management.* Springer, Berlin.

32. Silverstein, M. J. (1973). A study of amputations of the lower extremity. *Surg. Gynecol. Obstet.* **137**, 579–80.

33. Levin, M. E. (1977). *The diabetic foot.* C. V. Mosby, St Louis.

34. Most, R. S. and Sinnock, P. (1983). The epidemiology of lower extremity amputations in diabetic individuals. *Diabetes Care*, **6**, 87–91.

35. Lithner, F. and Tornblom, B. (1980). Gangrene localised to the lower limbs in diabetics. *Acta Med. Scand.*, **208**, 315–20.

36. Lithner, F. (1994). Centralisation of diabetic foot care: the impact on the number of major amputations. In *Proceedings of the 4th European Conference on Advances in Wound Management*, pp. 167–71.

37. Cameron, H. C., Lennard-Jones, J. E., and Robinson, M. D. (1964). Amputations in the diabetic: outcome and survival. *Lancet*, **ii**, 605–7.

38. Haimovici, H. (1970). Peripheral arterial disease in diabetes mellitus. In *Diabetes mellitus: theory and practice*, (ed. M. Ellenberg and H. Rifkin), pp. 890–911. McGraw-Hill, New York.

39. Lawrence, J. C. (1995). Some aspects of burns and burns research at Birmingham Accident Hospital 1994–93. A.B. Wallace Memorial Lecture, 1994. *Burns*, **21**, 403–13.

40. Kumar, P., Sharma, M., and Chadha, A. (1993). Epidemiological determinants of burns in paediatric and adolescent patients from a centre in Western India. *Burns*, **20**, 236–40.

41. Zeitlin, R., Somppi, E., and Jarnberg, J. (1993). Paediatric burns in central Finland between the 1960s and 1980s. *Burns*, **19**, 418–22.

42. Ro., S. P. A. (1990). *Home safety topic briefing: burn and scald injuries.* The Royal Society for the Prevention of Accidents, Cannon House, Birmingham.

2

History of wound healing

D. J. LEAPER

Background
Methods for primary closure of wounds
Infection and healing

Background

The history of wound management throughout the development of human society is a fascinating topic, often based on 'full stops' of misconception (with disastrous results) but punctuated by remarkable advances made all the more impressive by the lack of scientific background. In the Neolithic period it is known that wounds were inflicted by the early hominids and australopithecines on each other during the hunt for food, or self-preservation. This is clear from the fossil records and from skull trephination that was undertaken, perhaps for some unknown ritual, and which was followed by healing (Fig. 2.1) (1).

The first recorded management of wounds documented the control, or lack of control, of infection. The history of man and wound in the ancient world has been superbly explored by Guido Majno (2). The physiological understanding of wound healing could not be unravelled without a microscope or a laboratory and we have many instances of confusion between the inflammation which precedes healing and the inflammation which is prolonged and modified as a response to invasive organisms. The Roman scholar Celsus described the cardinal signs of inflammation – calor, rubor, dolor, and tumor (Fig. 2.2 – to which may be added *functio laesa*: if it hurts the inflamed part is not used) but he understood that inflammation was not always related to infection (3). John Hunter, well over 1500 years later, still distinguished 'adhesive' inflammation, which he recognized was the basis for healing and allowed the surgeon to practise his art, from 'suppurative' inflammation, which he regarded as an aberration related to infection and pus formation (4). We would not distinguish between these end results of inflammation today in quite the same way, but the mechanisms and pathways have many similarities. The understanding of the biology of wound healing is a new science, less than 100 years old, and developments continue apace.

The earliest texts of wound management stem from Assyria and ancient Egypt. The Assyrian cuneiform scripts define laws for practising wound healers who, like the Egyptians, were definitive in their teaching of the need to drain pus.

Probably independently, succeeding wound managers throughout history have made the same assertion. Hippocrates taught that cleanliness and, to some extent, aseptic technique was important. He realized that wounds could heal primarily but also practised wound irrigation with antiseptics such as vinegar and wine, in preparation for delayed primary or secondary closure (5). The covering of wounds has always been popular, it seems, perhaps to keep out invisible 'ill humours'. Interestingly, there is relatively recent evidence that the prolonged covering of open contaminated wounds and compound fractures sustained in humans can result in successful healing without the risk of lethal spreading infection (6).

Methods for primary closure of wounds

Modern materials used for wound closure incorporate a thread which is swaged (crimped) on to a needle, thereby obviating the need for an 'eye'. The passage of the needle's eye and its looped thread had the potential to traumatize tissues as it was passed through. However, needles and threads, together with adhesive strips and clips, have been in use for millennia. The future for tissue closure may lie in the development of the cyanoacrylates and fibrin glues and their applicability in all circumstances, but they are comparatively expensive.

The first methods used for primary wound closure involved the ingenious use of thorns and, later, in the bronze and iron ages, metal pins. The Egyptians used thorns but the use of bronze had to wait until Grecian medicine was established, and copper until Celsus (3). The thorn or a pin was placed through the lips of the wound and held under tension using a thread or a metal clip device, rather like a cleat (Fig. 2.3). Celsus would have called this a fibula and similar devices have been noted to be still in use amongst the Masai (7). The embalmer's sutures, used years before in the late Egyptian dynasties, must have employed a more modern type of needle. In early Hindu and Arabic surgery, and later European military surgery, the use of metal needles was widespread.

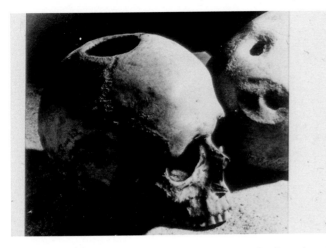

Fig. 2.1 Trephined skull of the Neolithic period. There is evidence of healing in some fossil skulls which suggests the 'patient' survived the procedure.

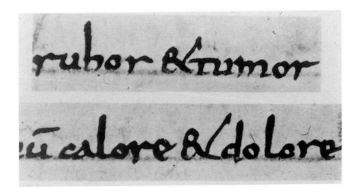

Fig. 2.2 *Rubor et tumor cum calor et dolor.* From a 10th century Celsian manuscript.

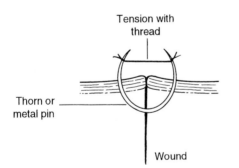

Fig. 2.3 Simple fibula for wound closure (after Celsus). A thorn or pin is passed through the lips of the wound and held together by a fibre or metal clip.

Modern needles do not have an eye to mount a thread but have the thread swaged into the end of a hollow needle. Drag through tissues is thereby minimized as the needle and its thread are passed through.

The first fibres were not used as sutures, but to hold in place

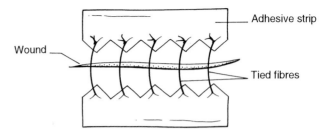

Fig. 2.4 Strips of linen are glued adjacent to the edge of the wound and approximated using fibres tied to the strips.

the thorn or metal pin closing the wound (8). Primary sutures did exist in Egypt (the YDR) but a technique of securing strips of linen together, which had been adhered to skin adjacent to the wound, was also in use (the AWY – Fig. 2.4). The adhesive was probably resin. Many fibres have been used for wound suture (9). The Indian practitioner, Susruta, used cotton, silk, hemp, and linen (10), whereas Celsus favoured the hair of a woman (3) and Galen used a primitive type of catgut (11). Catgut is now made from twisted dried animal intestine and has enjoyed widespread use. Lord Lister prolonged the integrity of catgut in tissues by immersing it in chromic acid (12). Catgut causes a marked tissue reaction and is being replaced by modern synthetic absorbable polymers which are much more predictable, albeit more expensive. Suture techniques were also well practised at an early stage in the development of wound management (3). Susruta, who described many plastic surgical techniques, also advocated that young surgeons practised suturing on animal hide (10); perhaps the first workshops in wound management were organized in his time. The Samhita (a collection of Susruta) was a huge collection of medical and surgical practice used over hundreds of years, although its precise origin and time of writing is not entirely clear. Suture materials were used principally for the suture of skin, and silk was favoured in early European practice by Arnold de Villanova (13) and Guy De Chauliac (14). Galen advocated suturing muscle but the more advanced techniques, of vascular suture for example (15), came much later in development.

Bandages have always been popular to bind wounds together loosely and are an alternative to suturing injured tissues together. Theodoric of Cervia had recognized that primary healing could proceed without suppuration, although he seemed loath to undertake suture (16). In the early 19th century Young actually decried the use of sutures (17). Adhesive strips were a more manageable alternative to closure of wounds with bandages (Fig. 2.5). The Egyptians were aware of this in their much earlier attempts at wound closure. It is now universally recognized that adhesive strip closure of wounds gives a good cosmetic result and renders the wound less prone to infection, particularly if it is only a few hours old, as there is some associated contamination of the wound edges.

The use of clips to hold the edges of a wound together is also not novel. The use of ants' heads was described in the Susruta Samhita (10), and there is reliable evidence of this still being used in this century in South America (18). The formidable mandibles of the leaf-cutter ant or soldier ant are en-

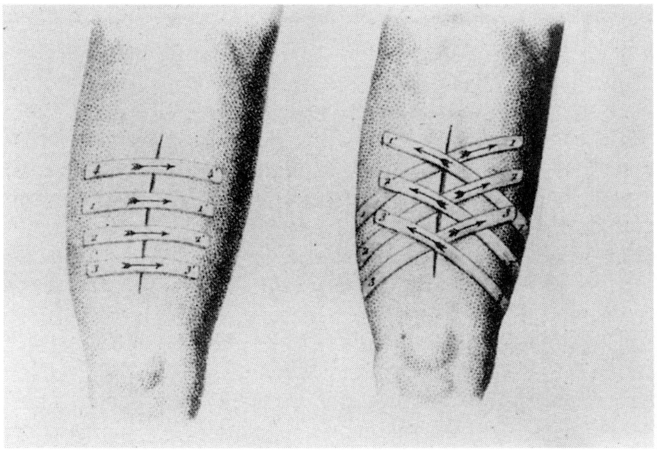

Fig. 2.5 Closure of wounds with adhesive strips (from a 19th century French manual).

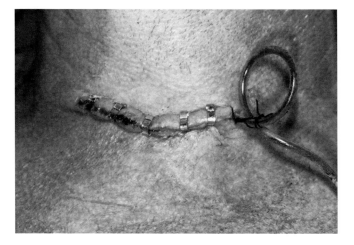

Fig. 2.6 Michel clips to close a collar incision after thyroidectomy. (See plate section.)

couraged to close around a wound edge, the body of the ant is pinched off, and by the time the head and mandibles separate, the wound is healed. Clips, made of stainless steel or titanium, are widely used in modern surgical practice. They can be of modest cost, applied one by one by hand from a loaded rail on tissue forceps (Michel clips), used classically for 'thyroid' collar ulcerations in the neck (Fig. 2.6). Alternatively, they can be used in a disposable dispensing unit, as in stapling devices, for rapid insertion or for use in difficult access surgery. Such instruments are expensive.

Sutures are time honoured for use in wound closure. The marked tissue reaction caused by natural materials such as catgut and silk favours infection and they are being replaced by modern, predictable, monofilament and braided polymers such as polyglactin (Vicryl) and polyamide (Nylon). The future holds promise. Tissue adhesives may become more refined; the cyanoacrylates or 'superglues' have been in use for many years for skin closure and anchoring of skin grafts. Biological fibrin glues have already been established for microvascular and internal closure – their continued development will be an interesting one.

Infection and healing

Infection has always been recognized as a scourge to healing and a history of wound management would be incomplete without another delve into the past. It is clear that the Egyptians recognized that a suppurating wound needed drainage (19). This fundamental act in wound management was restated many times in Assyrian, Greek, Roman, and medieval teaching. Galen followed Hippocratic teaching, but his views were modified and, from being an observant scientist and acclaimed teacher, he increasingly chose a theoretical and dogmatic approach to practice (11). Certainly he recognized that pus needed drainage as Hippocrates had taught before him (5). Galen realized that when infection was localized in a wound, then healing might follow the drainage or discharge of pus ('*pus bonum et laudabile*' – laudable pus). Overwhelming

spreading infection in gladiatorial wounds must have killed many of Galen's patients. A misinterpretation followed that healing could only follow the development of suppuration and discharge of pus, which was dogmatically and unquestioningly practised for over the next 1500 years. Many substances were introduced into wounds to encourage suppuration which could only have added to the risks of spreading infection and mortality – Galen's use of dung is a classic example (how many patients died of tetanus, let alone spreading infection?). The use of wine or vinegar, honey, or milk perhaps had some logic (and even modern adherents), even urine could have served as a readily available sterile irrigant, particularly on the battlefield where wound cleansing fluids were in short supply. Such applications are quoted in several of Shakespeare's plays. Spider webs are more esoteric but were apparently issued to the English soldiers fighting in Crecy in 1346 to help staunch haemorrhage from battle wounds. This seems to have been a backward step when ligatures, styptics, and vasoconstricting applications such as ephedra had been described over 1000 years before (3, 11, 20).

Ignorance persisted in medieval wound management. Even the remarkable differences in appreciation of anatomy can be seen between the contemporary Rembrandt's 'anatomy lesson of Dr Tulp' (Fig. 2.7) and the more recently hackneyed 'wound man' (Fig. 2.8) (21). So there was some light in this dark tunnel and a few practitioners also recognized that wound repair could proceed without infection. Guy de Chauliac, Henri de Mondeville, and Paracelsus were anti-Galenic (7, 14, 22). Ambroise Paré found almost by accident that, when boiling oil ran out, wounds treated with egg yolk fared better (23). His dictum of 'Je le pensay, Dieu le guarist' – I dress it (the wound), God heals it – does seem to be a little defeatist, however. Like De Chauliac he realized the value of gentleness with tissues which was championed in modern surgery by William Halstead (24).

Personal hygiene, the simple act of hand washing, prior to assisting delivery was recognized by Semmelweis to reduce significantly maternal mortality due to puerperal sepsis (25). The Austrian obstetrician was ignored but his concept was all

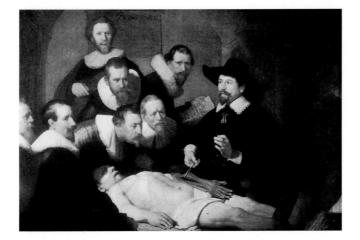

Fig. 2.7 The anatomy lesson of Dr Tulp (Rembrandt). (See plate section.)

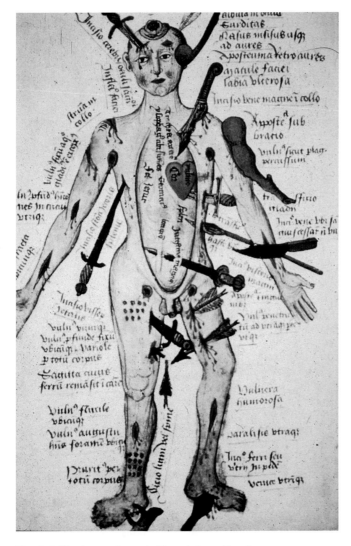

Fig. 2.8 The 'wound man'. (See plate section.)

the more remarkable as microbes and their pathogenic effects had not been described. Lord Lister realized that an antiseptic principle directed against these microbes, recognized by Pasteur a few years before as the cause of 'spoilt wine', would reduce infection (26). However, antiseptic surgery was replaced by aseptic technique at the beginning of this century. The antibiotic era began with penicillin (27–29) and now even contaminated surgical wounds can be closed primarily, with appropriate antibiotic prophylaxis, without a high risk of infection, provided there is no foreign body in the wound, or ischaemia.

The biology and biochemistry of wound healing began with seminal work by Virchow and Metchnikoff (30, 31). We are beginning to realize that hypertrophic and keloid scars, anastomotic stenosis, rheumatic vegetations on heart valves, chronic static wounds, and infection are all aberrations of the healing process. The use of plastic surgical techniques, prophylactic antibiotics, aseptic gentle surgery, and anaesthesia which permits continuous optimal tissue perfusion, allows even abdominal incisions to result in fine acceptable scars. Some caution is needed for indolent, chronic, skin ulcer management; despite the plethora of dressings there is no panacea. There will be no substitute for adequate medical and nursing care which recognizes the cause and institutes the specific treatment for ulceration, together with attention to systemic disease or poor nutrition.

We have come a long way from the concept of 'laudable pus' but there is a long way to go to be able to produce fetal healing without scarring.

References

1. Steinbeck, R. T. (1976). *Paleopathological diagnosis and interpretation* (Bone disease in ancient human populations). C. C. Thomas, Springfield, Illinois.
2. Majno, G. (1975). *The healing hand: man and wound in the ancient world.* Harvard University Press, Cambridge, MA.
3. Celsus, A. C. (25BC–AD50). *De medicina*, Vols I and II, transl. W. G. Spencer. Harvard University Press, Cambridge, MA.
4. Hunter, J. (1835). Lectures on the principles of surgery, Chapters XII–XIV (notes taken, 1786, 1787). *The works of John Hunter FRS with notes.* Vol I. James Palmer. Royal College of Surgeons of England, London.
5. Littre, E. (1839–1861). *Oeuvres completes d'Hippocrate* (10 Vols). Ballivere, Paris.
6. Trueta, J. (1939). Closed treatment of war fractures. *Lancet*, **i**, 1452–5.
7. Haeger, K. (1988). *The illustrated history of surgery.* A. B. Nordbok, Gothenburg.
8. Breasted, J. H. (1930). *The Edwin Smith surgical papyrus.* University of Chicago Press, Chicago.
9. Goldenberg, I. S. (1959). Suture and ligature materia. *Surgery*, **46**, 908–12.
10. *Susruta Samhita* (1963). An English translation of the *Susruta Samhita*, (ed. K. K. Bhishagratna), (2nd edn). Varanasi Chowkamba Sanskrit Series Office.
11. Galen (AD130–200) (1821–1833). *Opera omnia*, (ed. E. M. Curavit and C. G. Kuhn), 20 Vols. Lipsiae C. Cnobloch.
12. Lister, J. (1881). President's Address. *Trans. Clin. Soc. London*, **13**, 43–63.

13. Walsh, J. L. (1920). *Medieval medicine*. R & C Black, London.
14. De Chauliac, Guy (1235–1311) (1923). *On wounds and fractures*, transl. W. A. Brennan. University of Chicago Press, Chicago.
15. Carrel, A. (1912). Ultimate result of aortic transplantation. *J. Exp. Med.*, **15**, 389.
16. Theodoric, Bishop of Cervia (1210–1298) (1955–60). *The surgery of Theodoric*, transl E. Campbell and J. Colton, 2 Vols. Appleton Century Crofts, New York.
17. Young, S. (1808). *An attempt at a systematic reform of the modern practice of adhesion especially in relation to the use and abuse of the thread suture.* Matthews and Leigh, London.
18. Wheeler, W. M. (1910). *Ants, their structure and behaviour.* Columbia University Press, New York.
19. Ebbell, B. (1937). *The Ebers papyrus. The greatest Egyptian medical document.* Oxford University Press, Oxford.
20. Pliny (The elder) (1956–1966). *Natural history*, transl. H. Rackham and W. H. S. Jones. De Eichholr Loeb Classical Library, 10 Vols. Harvard University Press, Cambridge MA.
21. Galen (1563). *Certain works of chirurgerie.* Hall, London.
22. Cumston, C. G. (1903). Henri de Mondeville and his writings. *Buffalo Med. J.*, **11**, 1–50.
23. Paré, A. (1510–1590) (1840–41). *Oeuvres completes D'Ambroise Pare*, (ed. J. F. Malgaigne), 3 Vols. Balliere, Paris.
24. Halstead, W. S. (1913). Ligature and suture material. *J. Am. Med. Ass.*, **60**, 1119–26.
25. Semmelweis, I. F. (1941). *The aetiology, the concept and the prophylaxis of puerperal fever*, transl. F. F. Murphy. Medical Classics, Vol. 5 No 5. R. H. Krieger, Huntington, NY.
26. Lister, J. (1967). Illustrations of the antiseptic treatment in surgery. *Lancet*, **ii**, 668–9.
27. Fleming, A. (1943). Streptococcal meningitis treated with penicillin. *Lancet*, **ii**, 434–8.
28. Fleming, A. (1929). *Br. J. Exp. Pathol.*, **10**, 226–32.
29. Chain, E., Florey, H. W., Gardner, A. D., *et al.* (1940). *Lancet*, **ii**, 226–36.
30. Virchow, R. L. K. (1860). *Cellular pathology as based upon physiological and pathological history*, transl. F. Chance. John Churchill, London.
31. Metchnikoff, E. (1905). *Immunity in infective diseases*, transl. F. G. Binnie. Cambridge University Press, London.

3

The biology of healing

J. A. IOCONO, H. P. EHRLICH, F. GOTTRUP, and D. J. LEAPER

Introduction

Despite great efforts in the study of wound repair, discerning the mechanisms for its control remains far from complete. As late as the early 20th century, poor healing and non-healing wounds were the rule rather than the exception. The additions of aseptic technique, careful observation, and supportive care of wounds markedly improved wound management and outcome. Today, as we prepare to enter the 21st century, clinicians and researchers alike toy with the notions of scarless repair and eradicating the complications of wound healing. Ideas that topical additions or new dressings may close wounds more rapidly and eliminate scarring complications are plentiful. Indeed, much progress has been made into the understanding of the effects of the myriad of growth factors present in wounds, and deciphering the differences between the repair process in the adult and the fetus. However, one needs to look no further than a severely burned child, a keloid resulting from a minor trauma, or a diabetic patient with chronic unhealed wounds to realize that there is still room for improvement. This chapter provides a fundamental overview of the biology of healing. This is not meant to be a comprehensive review of the biology of wound healing, rather it is proposed to provide a framework to help understand some basic principles in the treatment of healing wounds.

Types of repair

Crucial to the survival of living organisms is the capacity to repair and restore function effectively to damaged and lost tissues. Trauma resulting in irreversible tissue loss initiates the repair process. The processes by which haemostasis is attained, invasion by microorganisms repelled, and restoration of normal tissue physiology achieved, are key determinants of patient survival.

If any of these components are deficient, or at the other extreme, too abundant, the risk of morbidity or even mortality rises. For this reason, the clinical aspects of wound healing have been of interest to the physician for many years (see Chapter 2).

In the past decade, however, there has been a new interest in discovering the precise details of the mechanisms involved in tissue repair, with particular interest in the possibilities of intervention in the repair process in order to speed up the rate of healing or to prevent the adverse effects of excessive scarring.

The fundamentals of the host's response to trauma is basic to understanding some of the principles of wound repair. Historically, the wound healing process has been described in a time sequence of three phases: lag (inflammation), proliferative, and remodelling. This teaching, although somewhat simplistic, serves as the framework from which to consider tissue repair in more detail. Although these three phases overlap, each appears as a clearly identifiable event in the wound healing process (Fig. 3.1).

Primary wound repair, healing by primary intention, occurs in immediately sutured closed incisional wounds (Chapter 4). This type of repair requires minor epidermal cell migration to cover the defect and minimal new connective tissue deposition to fill the defect. The cut tissue edges are approximated using staples, sutures, or adhesive strips. A critical issue in the

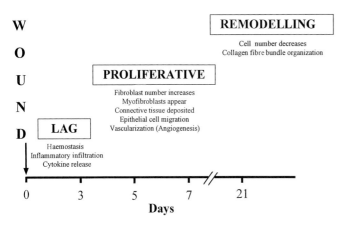

Fig. 3.1 Phases of wound healing.

mechanism for the success of such a repair is the welding of newly deposited bundles of connective tissue fibres by granulation tissue within the defect, with the native dermal fibre bundles residing at the wound edges. Testing wound repair in wounds healing by primary intention utilizes wound breaking strength studies, which measures the force it takes to break open a healed wound. These wounds do not break in the centre of the defect, but rather at its edges. The point of cleavage is at the junction between the newly deposited granulation tissue and the wound edge. The degree of wound remodelling and the maturation of the newly deposited connective tissue matrix as well as its association with adjacent dermal fibres is critical for functional restoration of the strength of an epithelial wound (as in skin, in particular).

Wound repair, by secondary intention, follows when a deep wound is caused, with a defect too large for the wound edges to be approximated. Here, the repair requires both a new epidermal surface and a new connective tissue matrix. The depth of a wound healing by secondary intention will dictate the volume of the scar required to mend the defect, which is directly proportional to the chances of complications of excess scarring. A wound, in skin, whose depth does not eliminate subepidermal appendages like hair follicles and sweat glands will undergo rapid epithelialization, because of the store of epidermal cells residing in the surviving subepidermal structures deep within the defect. From these many loci, epidermal cells migrate out and grow over the denuded area. Since the depth of the dermal connective tissue loss is minimal, the volume of new connective tissue needed is modest.

Typically, defects such as uncomplicated second-degree burns or abrasions are closed within two weeks and produce minimal cosmetic or functional scar problems. With dermal loss involving greater depth, the healing by secondary intention of these wounds requires epithelial cell migration from the wound edges, a greater volume of new connective tissue deposited, and in some cases, the intervention of the wound contraction process. The closure of such wounds is slow, and often leads to scar problems of both a cosmetic

and functional nature due to the excessive deposition of scar.

Delayed primary repair aims to derive the benefits of both primary and secondary closure, where a contaminated or possibly contaminated wound is packed open and in which the dressings are placed to keep the defect remaining open. At three to five days following packing, the wound is unpacked, the tissue edges approximated, and the wound sutured closed as in a primary closure (see Chapter 4). The theory behind this procedure is that the delay in closure allows time for optimizing the inflammatory response, increasing the ingrowth of new vessels at the edges of the wound site and the natural decontamination of the wound. All wounds contain bacteria. However, a wound with a count of bacteria greater than 10^5 organisms per gram of tissue is an infected wound which should not be sealed closed, but allowed to drain. Figure 3.2 depicts the mechanistic differences among these three types of healing (1).

Response to injury

Trauma comes in many forms and degrees of severity. In general, the greater the injury-induced volume of tissue loss and healing burden, the greater the amount of resources needed to close and repair that tissue defect. In addition to the volume of tissue loss, the type of trauma can affect the healing process. Examples are that the healing of a full thickness burn wound is quite different from the closure and healing of a full thickness freeze wound (2). In rats, a liquid nitrogen-induced full-thickness freeze injury will heal in the absence of wound contraction, while an identically sized full-thickness burn injury will heal by wound contraction. The difference between the two types of wounds is that the dermal matrix in the frozen tissue survives and acts as an internal splint, preventing wound contraction. In the full-thickness burn, all the dermis is lost and is replaced with granulation tissue. The wound closes and heals by wound contraction, similar to the wound healing process by secondary intention.

Haemostasis

The disruption of skin leads to the escape of circulating blood elements from the vascular tree. At the injury site, the initial response is to terminate bleeding. Vasoconstriction provides a rapid, but transient, decrease in bleeding, but it seldom lasts more than a few minutes. The combined effects of vasoconstriction along with aggregation of platelets and the initiation and activation of the coagulation cascade achieves haemostasis via the formation of a fibrin-based haemostatic plug. Adherent platelets undergo a morphological change which is related to the triggered release of stored mediators. There are a great number of mediators released that are not limited to, but include, chemoattractants, growth factors, and vasoactive substances. Table 3.1 outlines the major cytokines involved in wound healing and their functions. These released products help initiate as well as amplify the host's inflammatory response. In addition to platelet metabolites, local necrotic tissues release products that also maintain and amplify the inflammatory response (3).

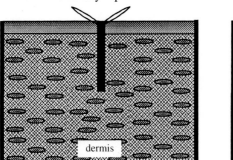
Primary repair

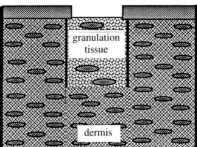
Secondary repair

granulation tissue

dermis

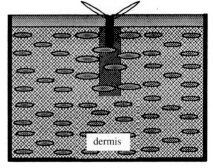
Delayed primary repair

dermis

dermis

Fig. 3.2 Three types of wound healing.

Table 3.1 The principal growth factors, chemoattractants, and vasoactive substances involved in the wound healing process (other than those involved in clotting and complement cascades).

Growth factors	Platelet derived growth factor	PDGF
	Fibroblast growth factor	FGF
	Insulin-like growth factor	IGF-1, JGF-2
	Epidermal growth factor	EGF
	Transforming growth factor	TGFα,β
Arachidonic acid metabolites	12-hydroxyeicosatetranoic acid	12-HETE
	Thromboxanes	TxA$_2$
	Leukotrienes	
	Prostacyclin	PGI$_2$
	Prostaglandin	PGE$_2$, F$_{2α}$, 6-keto F$_{12}$
Cytokines	Tumour necrosis factor	TNFα
	Interleukins	IL-1, IL-6 etc.
	Interferon gamma	IFγ

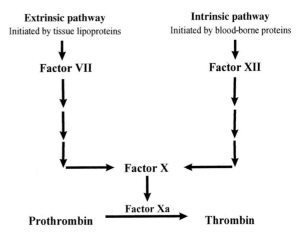

Fig. 3.3 Schematic coagulation pathway showing extrinsic and intrinsic clotting cascades.

Coagulation cascades and complement

The process by which prothrombin is converted into thrombin, which is needed to cleave the fibrinogen molecule to fibrin in order to produce an insoluble fibrin network, produces coagulation. Traditionally, the scheme for the clotting cascade follows two pathways. Simply stated, the intrinsic pathway is initiated by factor XII and involves components normally present in blood, while the extrinsic pathway is initiated by tissue lipoproteins that activate factor VII. These pathways terminate independently with the production of factor X, which itself cleaves prothrombin to form thrombin. Figure 3.3 shows a schematic representation of these two pathways (4).

The generation of complement is another cascade scheme which is initiated by tissue injury and acts as a host-defence mechanism against microbial survival within the wound site (Fig. 3.4). Any one of several events may trigger the complement cascade, including factor XII activation (intrinsic coagulation cascade), necrotic tissue, or thrombin activation. All complement pathways lead to the generation of two powerful anaphylatoxins, C5a and C3a. Whereas C5a is 100 to 1000 times more powerful than C3a, C3a is much more abundant at the wound site. One result of the activation of complement is the promotion of infiltration of neutrophils into the wound site (5).

Fibrinolysis

Fibrinolysis is the process directed at maintaining the patency of blood vessels occluded by the deposition of a fibrin thrombus. This process is initiated concurrently with coagulation, forms the fibrin matrix, and is dependent upon the activation of the proteolytic enzyme, plasmin, which is derived from the zymogen, plasminogen. Plasminogen is produced in the liver, its synthesis is increased following trauma and inflammation, and its active form, plasmin, cleaves a variety of proteins involved in the clotting cascade. The most important function of plasmin is the digestion of fibrin, leading to the removal of thrombi, restoration of vascular patency, as well as the generation of fibrin degradation products (6).

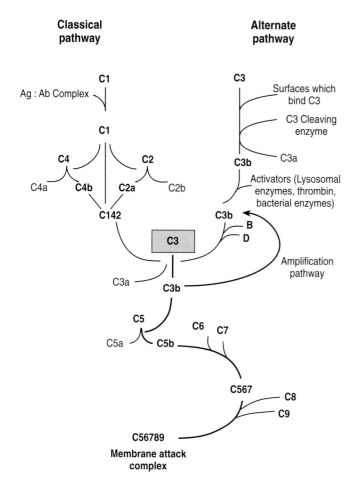

Fig. 3.4 Complement cascade.

response, macrophages and lymphocytes migrate into the wound site. The ultimate goals of these actions are to decontaminate and debride the wound site as well as recruit fibroblasts. Fibroblasts are necessary for the synthesis, deposition, and organization of a new connective tissue matrix, which is needed to restore the integrity of the skin (8).

Cytokines

Platelets initially release a number of substances that contribute to the intensity of the inflammatory response (see Table 3.1). These metabolites (cytokines) are soluble factors which advance tissue repair. Much remains to be learned regarding the spectrum of reactions mediated by any one of these compounds, and they remain a subject of interest to the basic scientist, as well as the clinician seeking tools to better control the wound repair process.

The cytokines may be considered as wound hormones because they are first synthesized, then released, and can affect cell functions distant from their site of secretion. These compounds can be classified broadly on the basis of the cells targeted for their actions. Paracrine cytokines act upon cells that are distant from the cells that produce them. Examples of paracrine cytokines are IL-1 and IL-8. Autocrine cytokines (e.g. IL-1, IL-4, and TNFα) are secreted from the cell and their action is back to that producing cell. Intracrine cytokines (e.g. granulocyte macrophage-colony stimulating factor, GM-CSF) remain inside the cell of production and exert their effects upon that cell without being secreted (9).

Neutrophils

Once the bleeding is controlled, changes in the permeability of the vessel wall adjacent to the injury facilitate the migration of inflammatory cells into the injury site. The initial inflammatory cell population to enter the wound site is the neutrophil, whose major functions are to destroy microbes and release chemoattractants. Neutrophils leave the microvasculature, migrating between the altered endothelial cells. These leucocytes function primarily as a first line of defence, working to both phagocytize and kill microorganisms invading through the breached integument. Neutrophils are often found between surviving tissues and necrotic tissues. In open wounds, they reveal the path that will be followed by the tongue of migrating epidermal cells which re-epithelialize the surface of the defect.

In experimental animal wound healing studies, it has been shown that blocking the invasion of neutrophils into the wound site does not alter the outcome of the repair process (10). However, in human chronic granulomatous disease where an absence of the enzyme NADPH-oxidase occurs, the intracellular killing of bacteria and fungi within neutrophils is compromised. This inability to kill microbes results in chronic infections which retard the repair process, leading to decreased survival of the affected host (11). In burn trauma, there is a delayed tissue necrosis due to secondary vascular occlusion caused by the deposition of thrombi in the vascular bed surrounding the burn wound. By 24h after injury, the lack of blood flow through those vessels results in tissue necrosis and an increase in the healing burden. Preventing the infiltra-

Disturbances of system

Disturbances of haemostatic mechanisms can be divided into two types: congenital and acquired, both of which include disorders of platelets or coagulation factors. The most common congenital diseases of haemostasis include von Willebrand disease, a defect in the platelet receptor responsible for subendothelial adhesion, factor VIII deficiency (classic haemophilia), and factor IX deficiency (Christmas disease). Acquired diseases of haemostasis usually occur as a result of depletion of stores of necessary blood components. Treatment for these deficiencies includes replacement therapy through the introduction of an individual factor or a platelet transfusion (7).

Lag (inflammation) phase

Drawn by the release of chemoattractants from aggregated platelets, necrotic cells, and disrupted tissues, inflammatory leucocytes infiltrate the wound site in a predictable manner. The first inflammatory leucocyte population to enter the wound space is the neutrophil. Later in the inflammatory

tion of neutrophils into the tissue surrounding the burn site by systemic injections of antibody directed to neutrophil surface receptors prevents delayed secondary burn necrosis (12). This demonstrates that neutrophil-released factors such as oxygen radicals can be detrimental to the well-being of the host.

Macrophages

Within 24 h after the invasion of neutrophils, a second wave of inflammatory cells – the monocytes – invade the wound site. Upon exiting the vasculature and entering the wound site, the monocyte becomes a tissue macrophage which has numerous activities that are critical for the continuation and progression of the repair process. Tissue macrophages have the capacity to divide within the wound site, and are responsible for eradicating microbes and clearing non-viable tissue, having ferocious appetites for the ingestion and breakdown of necrotic debris. Another function of the macrophage is the release of growth factors which promote the migration of synthetic cells into the wound site and the production of a new connective tissue matrix. Macrophages synthesize and release growth factors which are important for the initiation of the next phase of the repair process – the proliferative phase. The successful progression through this phase is vital to the subsequent repair process. However, it should be remembered that control of inflammation is important since too much or too little response is detrimental to the repair process (13).

Proliferative phase (granulation tissue)

In response to chemoattractants such as TGFβ, the invasion of fibroblasts into the wound site marks the initiation of the proliferative phase of the repair process. In this phase, all the necessary components of the final repair are synthesized in excess. Fibroblasts are responsible for replacing the fibrin matrix laid down during the lag phase of repair with the collagen-rich granulation tissue characteristic of the proliferative phase. In addition to collagen, fibroblasts also produce and release proteoglycans and glycosaminoglycans (GAGs) which are important components of the extracellular matrix of granulation tissue. Simultaneously, vascular restoration proceeds using this new matrix as a scaffold. In turn, these conduits supply nutrients and building blocks to the cellular components of granulation tissue. While these underlying processes continue, epidermal cells migrate over the surface of the healing defect and restore the epithelial barrier function of the skin (9).

Fibroblasts

Fibroblasts migrate into wounds as early as two days after injury and by day four, they are the major cell type in the developing granulation tissue. Initially, they populate the wound site by migration and increase their numbers by proliferation. Between the first and second week of repair, they reach a very high density. Both the migration and proliferation of fibroblasts are influenced by soluble mediators such as platelet derived growth factor (PDGF), transforming growth factor beta (TGFβ), basic fibroblast growth factor (bFGF), and complement C5a (14). A number of these mediators are produced and released from the resident tissue macrophages.

In addition to soluble mediators, the chemical composition of the matrix on which the fibroblast 'crawls' is important. It is critical to remember that fibroblasts cannot swim; they are limited to crawling and the surface on which they crawl can influence their function, morphology, and behaviour. Early in the repair process, the presence of hyaluronic acid promotes cell migration and proliferation. Later in the repair process, the absence of hyaluronic acid and its replacement with chondroitin sulphate impairs fibroblast migration and proliferation, but promotes fibroblast differentiation and connective tissue synthesis (15).

Fibroblasts residing in normal dermis and fibroblasts participating in the repair process are different. Morphologically, the actin of dermal fibroblasts tends to be minimally polymerized, indicating that these cells are sedentary, are distant from one another, and are at low density. In contrast, fibroblasts in young granulation tissue have their actin in a polymerized state – as required for migrating cells. These cells are in close proximity to one another, and are at high density. When granulation tissue fibroblast populations reach a high density with a great deal of cell–cell contact, their polymerized actin filaments condense into thick cytoplasmic stress fibres that have been demonstrated to contain an isoform of actin, α-smooth muscle actin (16). These differentiated fibroblasts are called myofibroblasts (17).

Myofibroblasts are proposed to be a specialized cell type responsible for wound contraction (18). Based upon the morphological identification of myofibroblasts, their absence *in vivo* in contracting mouse wounds was reported (19) and *in vitro* their non-function in the model of fibroblast-populated collagen lattice contraction has been documented (20). Experimental evidence supports the hypothesis that wound contraction is dependent upon cellular forces generated by fibroblasts (cells having fine actin filaments). The fibroblast packing of collagen fibrils through a cellular mechanism of cell-tractional forces rather than cell contraction is responsible for wound contraction. The myofibroblasts may be a differentiated fibroblast preparing for programmed cell death, apoptosis, rather than the organization of collagen fibrils (21).

Connective tissue

The major protein component of wound connective tissue, granulation tissue, is collagen. The chemical composition of collagen is responsible for its biological function of being the bonding component which holds tissues together. At least fourteen unique gene products or types of collagen have been described (22). The interstitial collagens have a common triple helical structure composed of repeating units of the tripeptide sequence glycine-X-Y, where Y is often hydroxyproline or proline. The abundance of glycine and proline residues are essential for the triple helical structure of collagen. Different types of collagen are found in different tissues; for example, type I collagen is the predominant type of bone and tendon. Type III along with type I collagens are found in more elastic tissues, such as blood vessels and skin. Skin has approximately 80 per cent type I and 20 per cent type III collagens. In contrast, granulation tissue has an increase of approximately 30 per cent type III collagen in it (23).

Collagen synthesis and secretion requires hydroxylation of

proline and lysine residues. Molecular oxygen, ferrous iron, α-ketoglutarate, and vitamin C are cofactors required for collagen hydroxylation reactions. Deficiencies of any one of these cofactors (i.e. hypoxia, vitamin C) results in impaired wound healing. Collagen functions fully when incorporated into fibres. In addition to synthesizing and releasing collagen, the fibroblast also packs collagen into fibres within specialized cellular clefts (24). Fibrillar collagen is made more insoluble by the actions of an interstitial enzyme (lysyl oxidase) which catalyses covalent cross-links between collagen peptides at the non-helical ends of the molecules. At one time, much interest was directed at altering the formation of collagen cross-links and the clinical modulation of wound healing and scar formation (25). β-amino proprionitrile was proposed as a treatment for controlling scarring based upon the hypothesis that cross-links were critical for collagen fibre formation. Because the formation of collagen fibres is independent of the formation of these covalent cross-links, the effectiveness of β-amino proprionitrile or another collagen cross-link inhibitor (D-penicillamine) was found to be clinically ineffective and no longer pursued in modulation of scarring. The organization of collagen fibre bundles within granulation tissue and scar are different from skin. In dermis, the collagen fibre bundles are arranged in a basket weave pattern; in granulation tissue, the collagen fibre bundles are arranged in arrays which are parallel to the skin surface.

Epithelialization

The inflammatory cells provide the initial defence against invasion by microbes passing through the uncovered integument. Eventually, the open wound is closed by the migration of epidermal cells which migrate as a sheet from the wound edges. These tongues of epidermal cells pass between the non-viable scab above and the viable granulation tissue below. When the defect has been resurfaced, the wound is considered to be closed. This process of wound closure does not contribute to a gain in wound breaking strength, which is a process that continues long after the wound has been resurfaced. The early closure of an open wound with a viable epidermis initiates the remodelling process within the underlying granulation tissue. Early wound closure reduces the chances for the development of hypertrophic scar and other related problems of scarring.

Vascularization

Essential to the progression of the repair process and the deposition of a new connective tissue matrix is a supply of nutrients to the cells within that tissue. Early on, there is no vascular supply to the centre of the defect, the presence of new viable tissue is limited to regions which are located at the wound edges and are in continuity with the underlying vasculature. The filling in of the defect with granulation tissue is achieved by outgrowths from beneath and the edges of the wound. The establishment of new blood vessels in the developing granulation tissue occurs by the budding or sprouting of intact vessels within the deep dermis. This arborization process allows for the ingrowth of new vessels in the absence of haemorrhage because the process is a closed system (26). The development of sprouts on vessel walls requires endothelial cell proliferation while contained in a vessel structure. Numerous growth factors play a critical role in the process and the control of these endothelial growth factors may prove to have clinical value (27). In addition, the presence of macrophages in a hypoxic environment is needed for vessel ingrowth (28).

Remodelling phase

Granulation tissue is a transitional tissue which replaces the fibrin clot which initially filled the wound defect, and its maturation produces scar. Granulation tissue is characterized by a high density of blood vessels, capillaries, fibroblasts, myofibroblasts, macrophages, and loosely organized fine collagen fibril bundles. The metabolic activity of this tissue is quite high, supporting cell proliferation, protein synthesis, and CO_2 production. Granulation tissue expands until the defect is completely filled. When the granulation tissue is covered by a viable epidermal surface, it undergoes remodelling whereby the cell density of macrophages, fibroblasts, and myofibroblasts is reduced. The outgrowth of capillaries is halted, blood flow to the area moderates, and the level of metabolic activity declines. The fine collagen fibre bundles of granulation tissue are then consolidated into thicker collagen fibre bundles.

Cellular

The remodelling phase of repair begins at different times and at various regions within the healing wound site. The granulation tissue covered by an epidermis undergoes remodelling earlier than the granulation tissue near the centre of the wound which remains uncovered. The differentiation of fibroblasts into myofibroblasts followed by programmed cell death (apoptosis) of the myofibroblasts are components of granulation tissue remodelling and its maturation into scar (29). It is not clear what process or trigger releases mediators from the epidermis to promote apoptosis in myofibroblasts. During the period of wound remodelling the density of fibroblasts diminishes. With the completion of the repair process, a scar forms with a cell density that is sparse, like that of normal dermis, unlike the cell-dense granulation tissue. The epidermis of a scar differs from that of normal skin because it lacks the rete pegs which are anchored within the underlying connective tissue matrix. The epidermis of scar is thicker compared to normal skin, but not as thick as that of freshly closed wounds. There is no regeneration of lost subepidermal appendages such as hair follicles or sweat glands in scar.

Connective tissue

The remodelling of granulation tissue may prove to be the critical factor in determining problems developing from scarring. It has been demonstrated that in healed burns the development of hypertrophic scar (deposition of excess connective tissue) is not the result of the continuation of the proliferative phase of repair, but rather an alteration of the remodelling phase of repair (30). A major difference between dermis and scar tissue is the arrangement of the organized collagen fibre bundles (Fig. 3.5). Factors which may affect that arrangement include the location of the healed defect, the age of the patient, and inherited factors. The cellular mechanism proposed for scar maturation is the translocation of granulation tissue collagen fibres by fibroblasts. The fibroblast packing of collagen fibres will compact these fibres into thicker bundles. The arrangement of granulation tissue collagen fibre bundles is similar to the arrangement of scar collagen bundles; they are organized in arrays parallel to the skin surface. In dermis, the arranged collagen bundles are in a basket weave pattern. The absence of a connective tissue basket weave pattern in scar contributes to the rigidity of the scar.

The connective tissue composition of granulation tissue differs from scar, where type III collagen drops from 30 per cent to 10 per cent. The quality of scars varies in terms of appearance, volume, and restriction to movement of adjacent structures. In cosmetic surgery, a scar must be invisible; in abdominal surgery, the scar must be strong; and in healed burns, the scar must be flat and pliable. There are clinical complications with repair, associated with too much or too little scarring. Examples are prominent facial scars, abdominal wound dehiscence, healed hypertrophic burn scars, and leg ulcers remaining open for years. If the repair process was better understood and the scar process better controlled, then most problems associated with scarring and repair could be greatly diminished.

Wound contraction/scar contracture

Through the action of fibroblasts packing collagen fibres, a contractile element of cells and matrix is generated within the wound site, producing centripetally directed forces which pull in surrounding skin. The result of such forces is wound contraction which causes a reduction in the wound size by skin rather than scar. Scar contracture is where the compaction of the collagen fibre bundles in established scars located over joints impairs the mobility of those joints. The process of scar contracture renders the joint non-functional. The wound healed by wound contraction renders a defect mostly filled with normal skin rather than scar. In the contracting hypertrophic scar, the forces of contraction are associated with unique structures within the scar: nodules. It appears that collagen which is more organized on the periphery of the nodule is associated with fibroblasts, and less organized collagen within the centre of the nodule is associated with myofibroblasts (31). In human contracting wounds, regions with less organized collagen have fibroblasts, and regions of more organized collagen fibre bundles are associated with myofibroblasts. The evidence presented supports the notion that the mechanism for the organization of collagen in wound contraction is different from the mechanism for collagen organization in scar contracture. Figure 3.5 provides a schematic representation of the differences between wound contraction and scar contracture.

Other considerations

Fetal wound healing

In general, wounds in children are treated according to the principles of adult wound care. There are, however, several physiological and psychological considerations that affect clinical decision making regarding this group of patients. Generally speaking, children demonstrate a reduced amount of subcutaneous adipose tissue, resulting in a decreased potential for contaminated dead space. This difference, coupled with a more efficient circulatory system, allows the closure of some large wounds by primary closure. Wounds, such as the incision made for removal of a ruptured appendix or even the defect remaining following a colostomy takedown, can be considered candidates for primary closure, or at least a loose dermal approximation.

Surgeons have long had an empirical sense that very young patients have an advantage in tissue repair, with a more rapid return to function and a superior cosmetic result in comparison to their adult counterparts. In addition, the concept of fetal tissue repair as an entity distinct from adult repair was discussed in the first half of this century with the observation that embryonic extracts applied topically to wounds in adults promoted a more rapid healing (32). In 1969 Somasundaram and Prathap demonstrated scarless repair in fetal rabbits (33); and in 1971, Burrington demonstrated the scarless healing of linear incisions in fetal lambs (34). In 1979, these observations were extended to humans when Rowlatt reported on the healing of limb amputations, probably caused by amniotic constriction bands, in a still-born 20 week fetus (35). Subsequently, Hallock described *in utero* cleft lip repair, first in mice and then in rhesus monkeys, building a strong case for the ability to turn the unique repair capabilities of the fetus to clinical advantage in the future (36). These seminal observations have promoted research devoted to understanding the mechanisms of fetal tissue repair, resulting in the discovery of a number of key differences in tissue repair between the mid-gestation fetus and the adult. Fetal wounds lack an inflammatory response; hyaluronic acid levels remain elevated; a marked proliferative phase of repair is not observed; and new collagen deposition is markedly reduced.

Excess scarring

Despite the best efforts of surgeons, some patients will experience collagen deposition out of the range of normal, even for a prominent scar. The two types of excessive scar are hypertrophic scars and keloids. Although both have in common the deposition of collagen scar beyond that seen in normal repair, these two entities exhibit distinct clinical properties and this should not be confused. The organization of collagen fibre bundles in scar, hypertrophic scar, and keloid are all different, and each is characteristic of the specific fibrotic defect (21). A scar is a 'patch' which fills a wound defect. The volume of tissue needed to fill that defect should be the same as the tissue replaced, but excess scarring and keloids often develop from minor trauma and can exceed the boundaries of the initial injury. The differences between hypertrophic scar and keloid are that hypertrophic scar remains within the boundaries of the initial injury, and keloid scar exceeds the boundaries of the original injury. Histologically, hypertrophic scars contain nodules and keloids do not. The collagen bundles on the surface of the nodule (hypertrophic scar) are arranged in parallel sheets like that of an onion skin, while the collagen bundles within the centre of

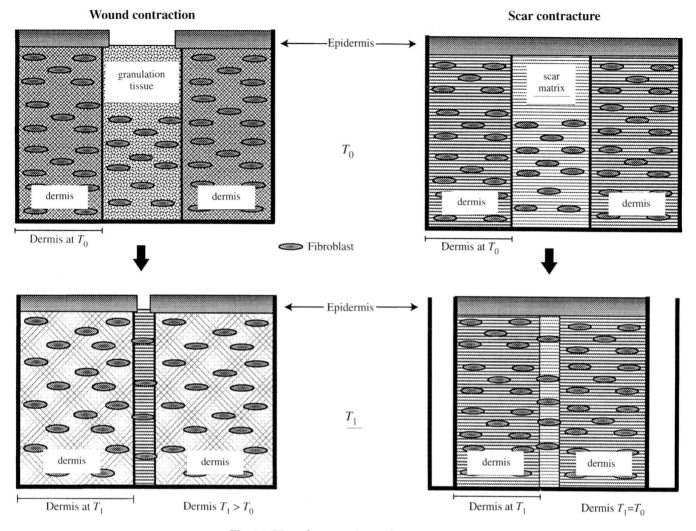

Fig. 3.5 Wound contraction and scar contracture.

the nodule are randomly arranged fibrils. The collagen bundles of keloid are arranged in braided sheets running parallel to each other. Hypertrophic scar can cause scar contractures, keloid scar can not. Keloids can develop from a superficial injury while hypertrophic scars develop and are restricted to full thickness injuries. As a rule, keloids do not regress over time and frequently recur after removal. For this reason, their removal is indicated only for functional impairment or a severe cosmetic deficit.

The topic of burn treatment receives a thorough discussion elsewhere in this text (Chapter 9). The results of the natural pattern of healing in a burn wound often place it into the category of problematic wound healing. This is most often manifested as a hypertrophic scar and/or a scar contracture. Prevention is the best modality of treatment for these conditions, with early skin grafting and aggressive rehabilitation employed to promote scar flattening and maintain joint mobility.

The biology of wound repair centres around cell migra-

tions, cell proliferation, apoptosis, and organization of collagen fibre bundles. If and when the caretaker of the wound can predictably control any one of these parameters, a contribution to better wound care will have been made. The elimination of infection by antimicrobials, the rapid and efficient removal of necrotic wound tissues, the creation of a wound environment that promotes cell movements, the addition of growth factors or mediators that direct cells to function optimally, and physical therapy to promote normal mobility are some of the paths available to improve the outcome of the wound repair process.

Oxygen and healing

Cell function and oxygenation

The wound healing process is dependent on optimal collagen synthesis, neovascularization, epithelalization, and resistance to infection. To obtain these goals the cells in the body require energy to maintain their structure and functional capacities. This energy is acquired primarily by the oxidation of nutrients. For energy to be obtained by aerobic metabolism a substrate, such as carbohydrate, protein, or fat, and molecular oxygen must be present in the cell in adequate concentration. Anaerobic metabolism is much less economic and maintains cell function for a shorter period. For these reasons a principal goal of management is preservation of optimal oxygenation and perfusion.

A fundamental response to tissue injury involves compromise of the nutritional supply to the tissue and development of local hypoxia (37–40). Local hypoxia following tissue injury and vascular damage in surgical wounds is between 0 and 30 mmHg (0–4 kPa) in the wound space (41). Therefore, in some cells, the minimal oxygen partial pressures are less than 1 mmHg (133 Pa) in the region of mitochondria; lower than the so called 'critical mitochondrial oxygen partial pressure' (42). Below this level metabolism cannot continue at a normal rate because of incomplete enzyme function. In many cases, however, measured local tissue oxygen is much higher than the critical mitochondrial oxygen pressure, implying that mitochondrial function, which accounts for 85–90 per cent of the resting whole-body oxygen consumption, will continue unaffected.

Other enzymes important for wound healing and development of infection unfortunately need higher oxygen tensions for optimal function. Collagen synthesis is dependent on prolyl hydroxylase with a K_M (concentration of substrate at which the rate of reaction is 50 per cent of maximal) of approximately 20 mmHg (2.7 kPa) (43) and a V_{max} of 50–100 mmHg (6.5–13.5 kPa) (44). Enzymes important for cross-linking and development of strength of the wound have a similar K_M for oxygen, of more than 20 mmHg (2.7 kPa), and if oxygen tension in the tissue falls below 40 mmHg (5.3 kPa) their maximal function rate start to fall. This function of these enzymes leads to weak, poorly cross-linked collagen and it is possible that hypoxia will have the same effect (45). The synthesis of collagen seems to be limited if collagen-producing fibroblasts exist in an extracellular environment in which oxygen tension is less than 50 mmHg (6.5 kPa) but this will probably not be seen clinically before the range is of 20–30 mmHg (2.5–4.0 kPa) (46).

Collagen accumulation in healing wounds relates to arterial oxygen tension (47). An oxygen tension of 20 mmHg (2.7 kPa) has shown to be a crucial level, beneath which accumulation of collagen is impaired (48, 49). Most primarily closed surgical incisions have an oxygen tension in the tissue which exceeds 20 mmHg. This will, in normal conditions, be followed by sufficient deposition of collagen and cross-linking. Collagen synthesis is dependent on the availability of molecular oxygen and in incised wounds systemic hypoxia suppresses the healing rate, while an increase in ambient oxygen concentration increases tensile strength until breathing 100 per cent oxygen at 101 kPa (1 atm) pressure. This effect of oxygen enhances accumulation of collagen and a smaller increase in cross-linking. This accords with the observation that biomechanical strength of all types of surgical wounds are directly related to collagen deposition and cross-linking (50).

Microenvironments in the wound

Wounds contain a number of microenvironments of which some are conducive to the replication of fibroblasts and endothelial cells (51). To explore the significance of local environment, the rabbit ear chamber is a useful model. A characteristic oxygen tension and lactate concentration profile can be measured in the healing wound by microprobes (48). The relationships of the cells involved in repair are important. By the fourth day after injury the pattern of cellularity normally has developed and persists until the wound is healed. This arrangement of cells creates an environment that is favourable to angiogenesis and collagen deposition. Leucocytes, red cells, and fibrin appear first, followed by macrophages and, after a few days, fibroblasts. Next to the wound space macrophages are found, while fibroblasts replicate just beneath these cells in the 'growth zones'. Behind this layer, regeneration and vessels follow and a dense (1–2 mm) thick hyperaemic layer is found. Between these vessels mature fibroblasts produce collagen fibres at a level of high oxygen tension and a relatively high lactate concentration. This 'module' moves across the ear chamber leaving a relatively acellular, sparsely vascular, fibro-fatty tissue (48, 52).

The oxygen tension in tissues, related to wound healing, is important. No cell division can be found when the oxygen tension is below 20 mmHg (2.7 kPa). In the wound dead space, oxygen tension has been found to range between 0 and 30 mmHg or 4 kPa (53). This energy gradient, spanning across the normal tissue adjacent to the wound into the wound space, seems to stimulate the repair. Our present knowledge is based on combination of gradient of both oxygen tension and lactate in the environment of the wound. While oxygen tension gradients are primarily based on delivery of oxygen through the capillaries, lactate is produced by the cells, especially macrophages, by glycolytic metabolism. In experimental wound environments hypoxia and/or hyperlactated macrophages release substances stimulating angiogenesis (54). Besides the angiogenetic effect on macrophages, lactate has an enhancing effect on collagen synthesis and deposition. Based on this observation, lack of oxygen plus production of lactate in the wound space seems to stimulate angiogenesis and to start collagen synthesis. In this wound environment macrophages continue the healing process by stimulating angiogenesis. The resultant restoration of tissue perfusion may clear lactate in the area and provide oxygen, thus downregulating macrophage activity and thereby suppressing repair when healing is completed and no wound dead space is left.

Tissue perfusion and oxygenation

The supply of nutritive substances is of vital importance for healing. Glycolysis, the pentose-monophosphate shunt, the Krebs cycle, and oxidative phosphorylation all participate in the energy production of reparative tissue. The organism normally has a sufficient store of glucose, protein, and fat. The store of oxygen is small and only lasts a few minutes in the case of an interruption of delivery. For this reason continuous oxygen delivery is pivotal for the normal function of cells. Oxygen delivery depends on the amount of oxygen delivered and exchanged in the lungs, the flow of the blood to and in the tissue, and the capacity of blood to carry oxygen. The second most important factor for tissue oxygenation is the oxygen diffusion capacity in the tissue itself. Finally, the rate of consumption of oxygen in the tissues is related to delivery, to obtain optimal cell function. These variables are influenced by a sensitive control system and external factors. In response to haemorrhage, blood flow to vital organs such as heart and brain is maintained while most other tissues have decreased blood flow (55).

The exchange function of the microcirculation to intestinal fluid occurs by diffusion and filtration across the microvascular walls. Most circulatory exchange function is mediated by capillaries and postcapillary venules, because of their large surface area in relation to flow volume. Respiratory gases (O_2, CO_2) move between the systemic capillary blood and the tissue cells by diffusion, because of higher concentrations of oxygen in the bloodstream in relation to interstitial fluid, while carbon dioxide has the opposite concentration relation and therefore diffuses from cell to blood, but about 20 times faster than oxygen through tissue. For this reason, elimination of carbon dioxide is much less of a problem than oxygen delivery. The differences in partial pressure of oxygen (p_{O_2}) between the surface of the capillary and a point in the tissue can be estimated by the Krogh–Erlangen equation and a three-dimensional model of tissue oxygenation. This model, however, only partly describes the microcirculation but is useful as a simplified calculation for oxygen pressure in the tissue. As oxygen diffuses away from a capillary it is consumed by tissue and the p_{O_2} falls. Therefore, diffusion distance varies directly with the oxygen tension along the length of the capillary. At the venous end of the capillary minor changes in blood p_{O_2} may provide an anoxic region in the intercapillary area. In these cells the partial pressure of oxygen has been measured as low as 1–2 mmHg (133–267 Pa) in cerebral cortex (42). Using this model the effect of hyperbaric treatment at 304 kPa (3 atm) increases the diffusion distance by 2 at the venous, and by 4 at the arterial end of the capillary. This increase of oxygen diffusion distance is important in tissues compromised by infection or local injury. The Krogh model, however, may not be used directly in clinical evaluation because it ignores the kinetics of the oxygen/haemoglobin dissociation curve and the capillaries are more complex than expected from the Krogh model.

The regulation of perfusion through tissue is based on metabolic needs of the tissue ('autoregulation') and the summation of these regional responses determine the overall haemodynamic pattern. The effect of autoregulation is through tissue pressure, myogenic activity of resistant vessels, and the influence of metabolic products in the interstitial fluid surrounding the resistant vessels, which control their state of contraction. During the normal capillary flow range, however, tissue pressure mechanisms are probably not significant, whilst myogenic and metabolic regulation is important. Many vasoactive substances have been suggested as mediators of metabolic control, such as oxygen, carbon dioxide, lactate, and adenosine.

The distribution of blood flow during pathological conditions is altered between different types of organ. Local metabolism will change distribution of blood so organs requiring higher levels of energy receive the greatest flow. Some tissues, like muscle, have the capacity to increase the number of active capillaries. Subcutaneous tissue and the intestinal tract cannot significantly change the number of open capillaries and their perfusion is regulated primarily by automic nerve reflexes. The gastrointestinal tract mucosa is also one of the most sensitive areas in the gut during impaired tissue perfusion in the critically ill. The tissue pH is constant, related to oxygen delivery, until a critical point where oxygen delivery equals oxygen requirement. Below this point the pH in the mucosa falls in parallel, with further decreases in oxygen delivery, and the corresponding fall in oxygen consumption (56). Monitoring systems directed towards measurement in subcutaneous tissue and the mucosa of intestinal tract may give an early warning of tissue hypoperfusion and hypoxia.

Neovascularization is also influenced by perfusion and oxygenation of the tissues. Angiogenesis is enhanced by raised arterial oxygen tension, even though the central space oxygen tension is only minimally changed (57). Both the rate of vessel migration and the number of vessels per unit tissue volume are increased by arterial hyperoxia. Angiogenesis is initiated by macrophages lining the wound space which have been stimulated by increasing lactate concentration and hypoxia, and a direct relation between new vessel formation and arterial oxygen tension has been found (54, 58). Epithelialization consists of replication of epithelial cells and production of basement membrane collagen. The relationship between epithelial healing and tissue perfusion and oxygenation is not fully understood. The mitotic activity of regenerating epidermal cells has been found to be oxygen dependent (59).

The development of infection in injured tissue is also directly related to tissue perfusion and oxygenation. Clinically it is well known, even in the presence of massive contamination, that wounds nearly always heal without infection in patients with normal immune system function. Increased oxygen tension also improves resistance to infection through leucocyte function. Liberated oxygen radicals account for about half of the capacity of granulocytes to kill bacteria (60). The rate of superperoxide production and the bactericidal activity of human leucocytes begins to fall as oxygen tension falls below 30–40 mmHg (4–5 kPa). The clinical relevance of flow and oxygen supply has been shown in experiments in skin flaps in dogs (61–63). In flaps with high tissue oxygen tension, infection does not occur; whereas necrotic infection is seen in the case of an oxygen tension less than 40 mmHg (5 kPa). In problem wounds involving osteomyelitis or irradiated tissue, hyperbaric oxygen treatment increases the rate of resolution (64). The mechanism behind the effect of hyperbaric oxygen has been found to have a reversing effect on the hypocellular-hypovascular-hypoxic tissue bed. The increased oxygen tension induces angiogenesis and fibroplasia. In irradiated tissue, hypoxia develops, compared to normal oxygen tension outside the irradiated field. Hyperbaric treatment increases the tissue oxygen tension both in the centre of such a lesion and in the normal tissue, but the increase is higher in the intact tissue. Therefore, a large oxygen gradient is established between the centre of a wound and normal tissue. This oxygen gradient has been found to be one of the major driving forces of the wound healing process, particularly through improved angiogenesis (57, 58). The gradient has, in this type of patient, been shown to improve angiogenesis healing of post-radiotherapy lesions, both in hard and soft tissue. The success rate of surgical extirpation of avascular, necrotic bone and soft tissue, with ultimate reconstruction, has been significantly improved (65). Hyperbaric oxygen treatment also decreased the amount of bacteria (particularly anaerobes) with prevention of infection.

Important gradients in healing tissue

Gradients of both oxygen tension and lactate have been found important for the stimulation of wound healing as well collagen synthesis and deposition. Hypoxia in the wound edge and hyperoxia in the area of angiogenesis provide an oxygen gradient which becomes the driving force of the wound healing process. During the healing process collagen is synthesized by fibroblasts. This process is also influenced by oxygen tension in the tissue. From ear chamber studies it has been shown that a tissue oxygen tension of 30–40 mmHg (4–5 kPa) is the optimum for replication, while a much higher oxygen tension (probably about 200 mmHg or 2.7 kPa) is the optimum for collagen synthesis (51). Lactate concentrations stimulate fibroblasts to synthesize collagen. Lactate levels in blood rarely rise over about 1 mM, but in wounded tissue they rise to the range of 10–15 mM and sometimes reach as high as 20 mM. Lactate is produced by anaerobic glycolysis as a consequence of hypoxia whereas many wound cells, especially macrophages, are aerobically glycolytic (46). Lactate stimulates collagen synthesis through at least two separate mechanisms (51). First, it is suggested that lactate induces an increase in procollagen mRNA. This effect is through a reduction of the synthesis of poly-ADP-ribose by which collagen gene transcription in fibroblasts is downregulated. Independent of this action on procollagen mRNA levels, lactate also increases the activity of prolyl hydroxylase, a crucial enzyme in collagen biosyntheses (66). Thus, an increased lactate enhances collagen synthesis and deposition as well as angiogenesis (54). Lactate concentration in test wounds is greatest in the central wound space but persists well into the zone of fibrillar collagen synthesis. This means that when angiogenesis in the wound increases oxygen tension, the high lactate concentration continues to stimulate collagen synthesis and deposition. However, when the integrity of the vascular system has reached a point at which lactate can be removed as rapidly as it is produced, the stimulation to angiogenesis and collagen synthesis diminishes. The effect of lactate may even be greater since there seems to be some evidence that lactate also modulates the response of fibroblasts to growth factors (46).

References

1. Schilling, J. A. (1976). Wound healing. *Surg. Clin. N. Am.*, **56**, 859–74.

2. Ehrlich, H. P. and Hembry, R. M. (1984). A comparative study of fibroblasts in healing freeze and burn injuries in rats. *Am. J. Pathol.*, **117**, 218–24.

3. Madden, J. W. and Arem, A. J. (1991). Wound healing: biological and clinical factors. In *Textbook of surgery*, (14th edn), (ed. D. C. Sabiston), pp. 164–77. W. B. Saunders, Philadelphia.

4. Fenton, J. W. 2nd, Ofosu, F. A., Brezniak, D. V., and Hassouna, H. I. (1993). Understanding thrombin and hemostasis. *Hem-Onc. Clin. N. Amer.*, **7**, 1107–19.

5. Morgan, B. P. (1995). Physiology and pathophysiology of complement: progress and trends. *Crit. Rev. Clin. Lab. Sci.*, **32**, 265–98.

6. Mosesson, M. W. (1992). The roles of fibrinogen and fibrin in hemostasis and thrombosis. *Sem. Hem.*, **29**, 177–88.

7. Bennett, J. S. and Kolodziej, M. A. (1992). Disorders of platelet function. *Disease-A-Month*, **38**, 577–631.

8. Clark, R. A. (1993). Regulation of fibroplasia in cutaneous wound repair. *Am. J. Med. Sci.*, **306**, 42–8.

9. Martin, P., Hopkinson-Woolley, J., and McCluskey, J. (1992). Growth factors and cutaneous wound repair. *Progress in Growth Factor Research*, **4**, 25–44.

10. Simpson, D. M. and Ross, R. (1972). The neutrophilic leukocyte in wound repair: a study with antineutrophil serum. *J. Clin. Invest.*, **51**, 2009–23.

11. Coleman, R. M., Lombard, M. F., Sicard, R. E., and Rencricca, N. J. (eds) (1987). *Fundamental immunology*, pp. 234–45. Wm C. Brown, Dubuque, Iowa.

12. Choi, M., Rabb, H., Arnout, M. A., and Ehrlich, H. P. (1995). Preventing the infiltration of leukocytes by monoclonal antibody blocks the development of progressive ischemia in rat burns. *Plast. Reconst. Surg.*, 74.

13. Leibovich, S. J. and Ross, R. (1975). The role of the macrophage in wound repair. *Am. J. Path.*, **78**, 71–91.

14. Morgan, C. J. and Pledger, W. J. (1992). Fibroblast proliferation. In *Wound healing: biochemical and clinical aspects*, (ed. I. K. Cohen, R. F. Diegelmann, and W. J. Lindblad), pp. 63–76. Saunders, Philadelphia.

15. Alexander, S. A. and Donoff, R. B. (1979). The identification and localization of wound hyaluronidase. *J. Surg. Res.*, **27**, 163–7.

16. Skalli, O., Schurch, W., Seemayer, T., Lagace, R., Montandon, D., Pittet, B., and Gabbiani, G. (1989). Myofibroblasts from diverse pathological settings are heterogeneous in their content of actin isoforms and intermediate filament proteins. *Lab. Invest.*, **60**, 275–2.

17. Gabbiani, G. (1992). The biology of the myofibroblasts. *Kidney Int.*, **41**, 530–2.

18. Majno, G., Gabbiani, G., Hirschel, B. J., Ryan, G. B., and Statkov, P. R. (1971). Contraction of granulation tissue *in vitro*: similarity to smooth muscle. *Science*, **173**, 548–50.

19. Hembry, R. M., Bernake, D. H., Hayashi, K., Trelstad, H. P., and Ehrlich, H. P. (1986). Morphological examination of mesenchymal cells in normal and tight skin mice healing wounds. *Am. J. Pathol.*, **125**, 81–9.

20. Ehrlich, H. P. and Rajaratnam, J. B. (1990). Cell locomotion forces versus cell contraction forces for collagen lattice contraction: An *in vitro* model of wound contraction. *Tissue Cell*, **22**, 407–17.

21. Desmouliere, A., Redard, M., Darby, I., and Gabbiani, G. (1995). Apoptosis mediates the decrease in cellularity during the transition between granulation tissue and scar. *Am. J. Pathol.*, **146**, 56–66.

22. van der Rest, M. and Garrone, R. (1991). Collagen family of proteins. *FASEB J.*, **5**, 2814–23.

23. Bailey, A. J., Sims, T. J., LeLouis, M., and Bazin, A. (1975).

Collagen polymorphism in experimental granulation tissue. *Biochem. Biophys. Res. Commun.*, **66**, 1160–5.

24. Birk, D. E., Zycband, E. I., Winkelmann, D. A., and Trelstad, R. L. (1990). Collagen fibrillogenesis *in situ*: discontinuous segmental assembly in extracellular compartments. *Ann. N. Y. Acad. Sci.*, **580**, 176–94.

25. Peacock, E. E., Madden, J. W., and Trier, W. C. (1970). Biological basis for the treatment of keloids and hypertrophic scars. *South. Med. J.*, **63**, 755–9.

26. Clark, E. R. and Clark, E. L. (1939). Microscopic observations on the growth of blood capillaries in the living mammal. *Am. J. Anat.*, **64**, 251–301.

27. Folkman, J. and Klagsburn, M. (1987). Angiogenic factors. [Review.] *Science*, **235**, 442–7.

28. Knighton, D. R., Silver, I. A., and Hunt, T. K. (1981). Regulation of wound healing angiogenesis – effect of oxygen gradients and inspired oxygen concentrations. *Surgery*, **90**, 262–70.

29. Desmouliere, A., Redard, M., Darby, I., and Gabbiani, G. (1995). Apoptosis mediates the decrease in cellularity during the transition between granulation tissue and scar. *Am. J. Pathol.*, **146**, 56–66.

30. Ehrlich, H. P. and Kelley, S. F. (1992). Hypertrophic scar: an interruption in the remodeling of repair – a laser Doppler blood flow study. *Plast. Reconstr. Surg.*, **90**, 993–8.

31. Ehrlich, H. P., Desmouliere, A., Diegelmann, R. F., Cohen, I. K., Compton, C. C., Garner, W. L., *et al.* (1994). Morphological and immunochemical differences between keloids and hypertrophic scar. *Am. J. Pathol.*, **145**, 105–13.

32. Krummel, T. M., Mast, B. A., Haynes, J. H., Diegelmann, R. F., and Cohen, I. K. (1991). Characteristics of fetal repair. In *Clinical and experimental approaches to dermal and epidermal repair.* Wiley-Liss, New York.

33. Somasundaram, K. and Prathap, K. (1970). The effect of exclusion of amniotic fluid on intrauterine healing of skin wounds in rabbit fetuses. *J. Pathol.*, **10**, 81–6.

34. Burrington, J. D. (1971). Wound healing in the fetal lamb. *J. Ped. Surg.*, **6**, 523–8.

35. Rowlatt, U. (1979). Intrauterine wound healing in a 20 week human fetus. *Virchows Arch.*, **381**, 353–61.

36. Hallock, G. G. (1985). *In utero* cleft lip repair in A/J mice. *Plast. Reconstr. Surg.*, **75**, 785–90.

37. Hunt, T. K., Twomey, P., and Zederfeldt, B. (1967). Respiratory gas tensions in healing wounds. *Am. J. Sur.*, **114**, 302–7.

38. Silver, I. A. (1969). The measurement of oxygen tension in healing tissue. In *Progress in respiration research III*, (ed. H. Herzog), pp. 124–35. Karger, Basel.

39. Niinikoski, J., Heughan, C., and Hunt, T. K. (1972). Oxygen tension in human wounds. *J. Surg. Res.*, **12**, 77–82.

40. Gottrup, F., Firmin, R., Hunt, T. K., and Mathes, S. (1984). The dynamic properties of tissue oxygen in healing flaps. *Surgery*, **95**, 527–37.

41. Hunt, T. K. (1988). Physiology in wound healing. In *Trauma, sepsis and shock. The physiological basis of therapy*, (ed. G. H. A. Clowes), pp. 443–71. Marcel Dekker, New York.

42. Grote, J. (1989). Tissue respiration. In *Human physiology*, (ed. R. F. Smidt and G. Thews), pp. 598–612. Springer, Berlin.

43. Myllyla, R., Tuderman, L., and Kivirikko, K. I. (1977). Mechanism of the prolyl hydroxylase reaction. 2. kinetic analyses of the reaction sequence. *Eur. J. Biochem.*, **80**, 349–57.

44. De Jong, L. and Kemp, A. (1984). Stoichiometry and kinetics of the prolyl 4-hydroxylase partial resection. *Biochimica et Biophysica Acta*, **787**, 105–11.

45. Prockop, D. J., Kivirikko, K. I., Tuderman, L., and Guzman, N. A. (1979). The biosynthesis of collagen and its disorders, Part I. *N. Engl. J. Med.*, **301**, 13–23.

46. Niinikoski, J., Gottrup, F., and Hunt, T. K. (1991). The role of oxygen in wound repair. In *Wound healing*, (ed. H. Janssen, R. Rooman, and J. I. S. Robertson), pp. 165–74. Wrightson Biomedical Publishing, Petersfield.

47. Hunt, T. K. and Pai, M. P. (1972). Effect of varying ambient oxygen tensions on wound metabolism and collagen synthesis. *Surgery in Gynaecology and Obstetrics*, **135**, 561–7.

48. Silver, I. A. (1980). The physiology of wound healing. In *Wound healing and wound infection: theory and surgical practice*, (ed. T. K. Hunt), pp. 11–31. Appleton-Century-Crofts, New York.

49. Niinikoski, J. (1980). The effect of blood and oxygen supply on the biochemistry of repair. In *Wound healing and wound infections: Theory and surgical practice*, (ed. T. K. Hunt), pp. 56–71. Appleton-Century-Crofts, New York.

50. Viidik, A. and Gottrup, F. (1986). Mechanics of healing soft tissue wounds. In *Frontiers in biomechanics*, (ed. G. W. Schmid-Schonbein, S. L. Y. Woo, and B. W. Zweifach), pp. 263–79. Springer, New York.

51. Hunt, T. K. and Hussain, Z. (1992). Wound microenvironment. In *Wound healing. Biochemical and clinical aspects*, (ed. I. K. Cohen, R. F. Diegelmann, and W. J. Lindblad), pp. 274–81. Saunders, Philadelphia.

52. Hunt, T. K., Banda, M. J., and Silver, I. A. (1980). *Cell interactions in post traumatic fibrosis*, pp. 11–31. Ciba Symposium 114. Pitman, London.

53. Hunt, T. K. (1988). Physiology of wound healing. In *Trauma, sepsis and shock. The physiological basis of therapy*, (ed. G. H. A. Clowes), pp. 443–71. Marcel Dekker, New York.

54. Jensen, J. A., Hunt, T. K., Scheuenstuhl, H., and Banda, M. J. (1986). Effect of lactate, pyruvate and pH on secretion of angiogenesis and mitogenesis factors by macrophages. *Lab. Invest.*, **54**, 574–8.

55. Gottrup, F. (1992). Measurement and evaluation of tissue perfusion in surgery (to optimise wound healing and resistance to infection). In *International surgical practice*, (ed. D. J. Leaper and F. J. Branicki), pp. 15–39. Oxford University Press, Oxford.

56. Fiddian-Green, R. G. (1989). Studies in splancnic ischaemia and multiple organ failure. In *Splancnic ischaemia and multiple organ failure*, (ed. A. Marston, G. B. Bulkley, R. G. Fiddian-Green, and U. Haglund). Edward Arnold, London.

57. Knighton, D. R., Silver, I. A., and Hunt, T. K. (1981). Regulation of wound healing angiogenesis: effect of oxygen gradients and inspired oxygen concentration. *Surgery*, **90**, 262–70.

58. Knighton, D. R., Hunt, T. K., Scheuenstuhl, H., Halliday, B. J., Werb, Z., and Banda, M. J. (1983). Oxygen tension regulates the expression of angiogenesis factor by macrophages. *Science*, **221**, 1283–5.

59. Winter, G. D. (1972). Epidermal regeneration studied in the domestic pig. In *Epidermal wound healing*, (ed. H. I. Maibach and D. T. Rovee), pp. 71–112. Year Book Medical Publishers, Chicago.

60. Hunt, T. K., Halliday, B. J., Hopf, H. W., and Scheuenstuhl, H. (1991). Measurement and control of tissue oxygen tension in surgical patients. In *Update in intensive care and emergency medicine. Vol. 12: Tissue oxygen utilisation*, (ed. G. Gutierrez and J. L. Vincent), pp. 337–49. Springer, Berlin.

61. Gottrup, F., Firmin, R., Hunt, T. K., and Mathes, S. (1984). The dynamic properties of tissue oxygen in healing flaps. *Surgery*, **95**, 527–37.

62. Gottrup, F., Orredsson, S., Price, D. C., Mathes, S. J., and Hohn, D. C. (1984). A comparative study of skin blood flow in musculocutaneous and random pattern flaps. *J. Surg. Res.*, **37**, 443–7.

63. Jonsson, K., Hunt, T. K., and Mathes, S. J. (1988). Oxygen as an

isolated variable influences resistance to infection. *Annals of Surgery*, **208**, 783–7.

64. Marx, R. E. and Johnson, R. P. (1988). Problem wounds in oral and maxillofacial surgery: the role of hyperbaric oxygen. In *Problem wounds. The role of oxygen*, (ed. J. C. Davis and T. K. Hunt). Elsevier, New York.

65. Heimbach, R. D. (1988). Radiation effects on tissue. In *Problem wounds. The role of oxygen*, (ed. J. C. Davis and T. K. Hunt). Elsevier, New York.

66. Hussain, M. Z., Ghani, Q. P., and Hunt, T. K. (1989). Inhibition of prolyl hydroxylase by poly (ADP-ribose) and phosphoribosyl-AMP. *J. Biol. Chem.*, **264**, 7850–5.

4

Surgical wounds

D. J. LEAPER and F. GOTTRUP

Definitions – types of wounds

A wound may be defined as the loss of continuity of epithelium, with or without loss of underlying connective tissue (including muscle, bone, and nerves for example), following injury. The injury may follow direct violence or be inflicted by a non-mechanical injury-which may also be responsible for delay in healing. Their may be extensive tissue damage (e.g., contusion or haematoma) with minimal tissue loss.

Incised wounds

Incised wounds involve no loss and minimal damage to tissue. See Fig. 4.1. There are two types.

1. Surgical incisions are usually clean, except when made to treat an infective condition such as an abscess or faecal peritonitis. They are usually placed anatomically to avoid major vessels and nerves, but poor surgical technique can cause undue tissue damage and tissue hypoxia. The methods by which a surgeon can incise or dissect tissues using a scalpel or scissors should minimize tissue shear, tension, and compression (1).

2. Penetrating, non-surgical wounds are caused by injuries inflicted by a knife or other sharp instrument. The random nature of such wounds may involve any tissue or organ and be accompanied by extensive haemorrhage. Haemorrhage may be more life threatening after a penetrating wound because contraction of muscular vessels is less likely. Bleeding can be arrested by the use of ligatures on severed vessels or primary wound closure (as in scalp wounds). The use of tourniquets should be avoided where possible as increased venous pressure can add to blood loss. As a first aid procedure, direct digital pressure is preferable to several layers of packing or bandages.

Most incised wounds can be closed within 6–12h provided they are not particularly contaminated (see delayed primary and secondary closure of incised wounds).

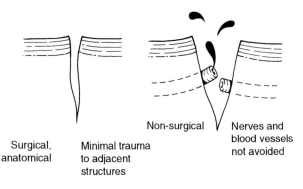

Fig. 4.1 Incised wound.

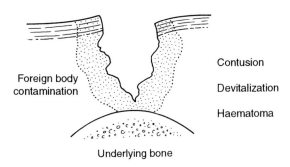

Fig. 4.2 Laceration with contusion.

Lacerated wounds

With this type of wound there may be tissue loss with some tissue damage. See Fig. 4.2. Lacerations are always non-surgical, but their occasional clean appearance should not confused with an incised wound. There is always a traumatic element, usually a blunt compressive force on tissues over an unyielding bony surface beneath. The scalp or face wound following a blow to the head is typical.

The degree of tissue damage may be extensive with a degree of devitalization and bruising or extensive haematoma. The extravasation of blood activates platelets (2) and the coagulation cascade (3), which in turn promotes repair through release of mediators (4).

Lacerated wounds may need exploration to exclude foreign bodies or tissue devitalization. Suspicion of damage to vital or internal organs may arise from careful history taking and the early use of visualization techniques (X-ray, particularly CT scanning, or ultrasound techniques). Many clean uncontaminated lacerations can safely be closed if they are no older than 6–12 h. Interrupted sutures or adhesive strips, particularly in tissues with a good blood supply (such as scalp or face) should be used. Closure, after debridement of devitalized tissue edges with systemic antibiotic cover, may also be feasible. When there is any doubt, delayed primary or secondary suture (or healing by secondary intention) should be undertaken. It is usually not necessary to shave skin, but the skin and damaged tissues should be prepared, cleaned, and irrigated with a dilute aqueous antiseptic such as chlorhexidine or povidone–iodine.

Abrasions

Injury resulting in this type of wound is associated with loss of the superficial layers of epithelium (usually skin). Nerve endings are exposed and the wounds are painful. When extensive, the blood or plasma loss may be substantial and mimic a burn injury. Such wounds need early cleansing with a dilute aqueous antiseptic and, if there is tattooing by dirt particles, brushing of the abrasion with appropriate anaesthesia is necessary. The risk of invasive infection, particularly by *Streptococcus pyogenes*, is high and requires an appropriate systemic antibiotic.

Contusions

These wounds are a more severe form of laceration and follow a much greater energy exchange. The tissue layers are separated and there is often tissue loss leaving an open wound. Closed wounds may obscure the amount of damaged tissue beneath, but this can be estimated from a history and the amount of kinetic energy dissipated in the wound – a function of mass (m) and velocity (v) of the agent ($\frac{1}{2} mv^2$).

When contusions are extensive, devitalized tissue must be debrided and the wound left open for delayed or secondary closure, or be left to heal by secondary intention. Large haematomas need evacuation as they may become infected, but the early stages of resolution and liquefaction may have to be awaited before aspiration is possible using a needle and syringe. Systemic antibiotic cover is advisable and healing may leave extensive scarring. As the haematoma resolves, its colour changes from blue to yellow/green (biliverdin) to brown (haemosiderin). Extensive resolving haematoma may lead to mild jaundice.

Bites, particularly human, may be associated with contusion. Debridement, delayed suture, and systemic broad-spectrum antibiotics are required.

Contamination is usually minimal in operative surgery, but can be severe for example, in operations for faecal peritonitis. Surgical wounds are classified as clean, clean–contaminated, contaminated, and dirty (abscess) and described further in Chapter 7. Contamination can be extreme in military wounds where there is devitalization and tissue loss together with foreign body material in the wound. Debridement, laying open, and later grafting or secondary closure are the mainstay of treatment and this is described later in this chapter and in Chapter 8.

Ulcer

An ulcer (Fig. 4.3) may be defined as a loss of an epithelial surface together with a variable degree of underlying connective tissue. The majority of acute ulcers follow trauma or pyogenic infections and there is usually some loss of connective tissue. The defect is made good by wound contraction and epithelialization (regeneration) and formation of scar tissue

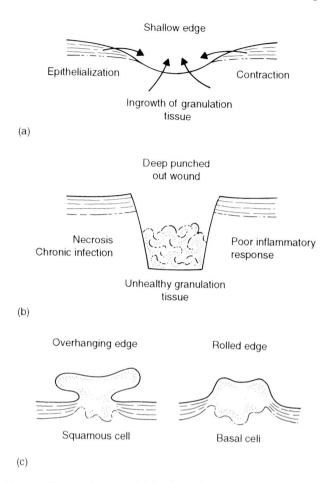

Shallow edge

Epithelialization   Contraction

Ingrowth of granulation
tissue

(a)

Deep punched
out wound

Necrosis   Poor inflammatory
Chronic infection   response

Unhealthy granulation
tissue

(b)

Overhanging edge   Rolled edge

Squamous cell   Basal cell

(c)

Fig. 4.3 Types of ulcers: (a) healing abrasion/venous ulcer; (b) non-healing/chronic infected ulcer; and (c) malignant ulcer.

in the subepithelial layers (repair). The ulcer edge is classically a shelving one (Fig. 4.3(a)), quite different from the punched out chronic ulcer with its indolent edge (Fig. 4.3(b)) or the malignant exophytic ulcer with its rolled edge and umbilication (such as a basal cell tumour of skin) or overhanging edge with central necrosis (such as a squamous cell tumour – Fig. 4.3(c)).

The chronic ulcer is a lesion which fails to heal and its aetiology may be very diverse. The ulcer needs management of the underlying cause (Chapter 10). Objective methods to assess healing are lacking (5), which further contributes to the difficulty of undertaking trials in this field. The only safely determined end point is complete healing.

Healing in surgical wounds

The closure of wounds after surgery or trauma and their healing without complication depends on many factors. One of the most difficult to measure, however, is individual surgeons' technique and expertise, although it is clear that some surgeons enjoy more consistent results than others. The old aphorism still holds true: 'cut well, sew well, get well'.

Surgical procedures should always be undertaken in optimal circumstances with responsibility taken to resuscitate fully when necessary, attend to nutrition and intercurrent diseases with tailored anaesthesia (regional, epidural, general, etc.), and appropriate antibiotic and venous thromboembolic prophylaxis. All this should be combined with informed consent and awareness of resource allocation, avoidance of over-investigation because of medico-legal threats, and compassion to recognize postoperative quality of life.

Most surgery operates on established protocols which can be audited and flexible to change on 'closing the loop' (see Chapter 12). Much surgery, however, is still based on ritual. Lord Moynihan instructed that a surgical wound be made with a clean sweep of the knife (*sic*). The gentle and respectful handling of tissues is much harder to teach, coming with experience. Some ritual is of obvious benefit, such as aseptic technique, rigorously observed, and the swab count at the end of an operation. Surgeons have to practise their craft with as near perfection as possible, quickly and accurately without undue tissue trauma. Haemostasis needs to be obtained but no method, ties and ligation, or diathermy, has clearly been shown to be superior. Natural haemostasis can be relied on to a large extent but patience and pressure may facilitate this. In some vascular fields, topical adrenaline can reduce blood loss; laser surgery is a luxury, and an expensive one.

Wounds should be closed without undue tension and with good opposition. Halsteadian attention to anatomical restoration of wound layers should usually be observed, but in some wounds is not necessary (such as mass closure of the musculoaponeurotic layers of the abdominal wall – Chapter 9, pp. 113–16). Perfect opposition is required in blood vessel anastomoses with permanent strength and immediate haemostasis (Chapter 9, pp. 130–3), whereas in bowel, less perfect tension is required for a leak-proof join and an absorbable suture is appropriate (Chapter 9, pp. 116–20). It is conventional to close, or avoid dead space in wounds, which risks tension, or use drains, but the true value of these techniques has never been proven.

Adequate postoperative care is equally important with further tailored postoperative analgesia, monitoring of progress, and compassion for both patient and relatives. There always needs to be a daily record of the patient's progress until discharge from care.

Delayed primary and secondary closure of incised wounds

Delayed closure of a skin wound to improve resistance to infection has been known for centuries. There are two techniques: delayed primary closure (DPC) and secondary closure (SC).

Delayed primary closure is defined as an anatomically precise closure that is delayed for a few days but undertaken before granulation tissue becomes macroscopically visible (usually within 8 days of wounding). **Secondary closure** refers either to spontaneous closure or to surgical closure after granulation tissue has developed.

For more than a thousand years the timing of wound closure has been debated. To close a wound primarily is a relatively recent concept. Surgeons have recommended the timing of wound closure from half an hour after incision to never closing a wound at all (6). One of the earliest and most clear descriptions of closure after a delay of a few days for the specific purpose of reducing wound infection was written in 1794 by John Hunter (7). In 1854 McKay, a British naval surgeon, practised initial debridement followed by wound closure after 3–7 days. He based his procedure on observations of wound debridement made by earlier naval surgeons (such as John Woodall in 1616 and John Atkins in 1742) (8). Billroth experimentally demonstrated an enhanced resistance to infection in wounds associated with tissue loss. He soaked dressings in liquid faeces and repeatedly applied them to the wound. The wound left open did not develop any sign of infection while those that were closed soon suppurated (9). Friedrich, in his experiments with crush wounds contaminated with street dirt, further emphasized that surgical removal of devitalized tissue and dirt must be undertaken as promptly as possible (10).

French army surgeons in World War I were the first to employ the method of DPC extensively when treating contaminated devitalized wounds (6, 11). Their practice was soon adopted by the British and American forces (12, 13). However, between the World Wars, DPC failed to gain popularity in civilian practice. In World War II increased infection, despite the introduction of sulphonamides, soon re-established DPC, which became the most frequently performed operation, except for debridement (14). Numerous reports during World War II showed the effectiveness of DPC in the prevention of wound infection in nearly all types of tissue damage (15, 16). The Allied victory has even been credited to 'penicillin' and secondary closure of wounds (17). The importance of the delayed closure principle has been re-emphasized during armed conflict in Korea, Vietnam, the Middle East, and more recently (16).

Delayed primary closure has been less frequently used in civilian practice. One reason may be that the risk of infection is lower in civilian circumstances than following military action, and the number of infections prevented by this technique in civilian practice is low compared to the number of DPCs performed. Furthermore, there is a persistent notion that all wounds need to be closed as soon as possible and that delay in closure causes a prolongation of the total healing time. Recently, however, reports of early closure after infection in incisional wounds has been reported (18, 19).

Possible mechanisms of the effect of DPC and secondary closure

Few studies of the detailed effect of delaying wound closure have been published (15). Experimentally, healing rat skin incisions have been studied and mechanical properties, collagen metabolism, blood flow, angiogenesis, and tissue gas tension have been investigated (20). Biomechanical testing shows that wounds closed with delay intervals of 3–6 days were significantly stronger than primarily closed wounds after only 20 days of healing, despite the fact that they had been closed for a shorter time. After 60 days of healing, DPC wounds were almost twice as strong as the primarily closed wound and this persisted 120 days later. Measurement of collagen synthesis demonstrated that there was a more rapid gain in DPC wounds than in primarily closed wounds. Blood flow, angiogenic activity, and tissue oxygen tension in DPC wounds was higher compared to the primarily closed wound. It was concluded that wound strength was enhanced through enhanced metabolism and collagen synthesis. Improved angiogenesis increases blood flow and tissue oxygen tension, which also decreases infection (15). Delayed closure of the wound also quantitatively changes the bacterial population of the wound between the time of operation and the third to fifth postoperative days (21–23). This 'clearing' of some species of bacteria seems to be related both to aerobic and anaerobic bacteria. Stone and colleagues attributed the lack of anaerobic infections to the prolonged exposure to air (24), but it is now clear that increased blood supply and oxygen delivery into the wound are also important factors. It has been supposed that this 'clearing' of some types of bacteria is one of the most important reasons for the efficacy of DPC (25).

Clinical evaluation of the effect of delayed wound closure

No prospective clinical trial comparing DPC and primarily closure has been undertaken. In 1918 Fraser and colleagues found that wound 'failure' (infection or dehiscence) in primarily closed war wounds was 20 per cent after gun shots and 25 per cent after compound fractures. In comparison, failure rates were 4 and 10 per cent, respectively, after DPC. The same results were found in World War II (26). Low infection rates using DPC were found in the Vietnam War. Different types of wounds treated with DPC had an overall infection rate of 2.6 per cent and specific hand injuries had an infection rate of 2.2 per cent (27, 28).

In civilian practice, DPC has failed to gain similar popularity. However, reports of the effect of DPC have been published (16, 26). In patients after appendicectomy the organisms responsible for infection are both anaerobic and aerobic (26). No benefits of DPC were found in patients who had an acutely inflamed appendix, while a decreased infection rate was found in patients who had a perforated appendix (26). One of the difficulties in this type of study is to demonstrate the effect of DPC alone as antibiotics are also used for prophylaxis. In most cases the antibiotic regimen directed against both aerobic and anaerobic organisms will decrease the infection rate in the case of perforated appendix to a level where no beneficial effect can be demonstrated using DPC.

Following gastrointestinal surgery a delay of wound closure results in a decrease in the wound infection rate greater than using antibiotics alone (Table 4.1). The effect is most obvious in contaminated and dirty wounds. If a colostomy is established in the vicinity of the wound the infection rate is as high as 31 per cent compared with 8 per cent when a colostomy is not made (22). Stomas, present at the time of operation, increase the risk of infection in primarily closed wounds to 22 per cent but if the stoma is established during the operation with delayed closure of the wound, the infection rate is 7 per

Table 4.1 Reported wound infections following gastrointestinal surgery (all wounds closed after 1 to 5 days)

Author	Classification	Patient number	Wound infection rate (%)	
			PC	DPC
Bernard and Cole (29)	Clean	22	0	0
	Potential contaminated	69	42	8
Stone and Hester (21)	Colon trauma	126	63	31
	Rectum trauma	9	25	0
Stone and Hester (22)	Clean	695	4	3
	Contaminated	289	49	16
McLachlin and Wall (30)	Clean	134	3	0
	Contaminated	74	0	3
Paul et al. (31)	Contaminated, elective	164	10	4
	Contaminated, emergency	15	38	14
Voyles and Flint (32)	Colon trauma	16	56	0
Verrier et al. (33)	Clean	191	2	20*
	Clean–contaminated	214	4	1
	Contaminated	81	11	5
	Infected	33	33	7

* One out of five patients in DPC group.
PC, primary closure; DPC, delayed primary closure.

cent (the same as the infection rate when a stoma is not raised) (34). The effect of delaying wound closure in gynaecological practice has found that delayed primary closure provided a safe, simple, and effective means of reducing the incidence of wound infection from 23 to 2 per cent. Prophylactic antibiotics in high-risk gynaecological patients has no beneficial effect when delayed closure procedures are used. In open fracture surgery delayed closure decreases the wound infection rate from 44 to 10 per cent (35) and also seems to have a beneficial effect after amputation (36). Recently, the principle of delayed closure has been used for early closure of incisional abscesses in skin (18, 19). It is also possible to make an early closure after incisional abscesses in laparotomy wounds (19). In these studies the delay between drainage of the abscess and closure of the wound was 4–5 days. One study, however, has shown a beneficial effect of early closure after only 2 days of delay (37) although few patients were included. No beneficial effect has been found using conventional secondary closure, after a median time of 12 days, compared to early closure after 4 days (38). An economic evaluation of the advantages of primary suture compared to conventional open treatment has been undertaken for subcutaneous abscesses (39). The abscesses were located on the trunk, limbs, or the perineal/anorectal area. They were incised, septa broken down, and the abscess membrane removed by curettage. The cavity was then either left open using dressings or obliterated by interrupted sutures and antibiotics were given. After primary suture the number of days in hospital decreased by 58 per cent, in the outpatient clinic the decrease was 73 per cent, and visits by the primary health care nurse were decreased by 96 per cent. The healing time was reduced by 66 per cent compared with primary suture.

Recommendation for wound management using delayed closure procedures

In elective surgery for wounds classified as clean or clean–contaminated, delayed procedures are rarely useful. In longer operations (more than 3 h) with wounds which are contaminated or dirty, delayed closure should be considered in addition to antibiotics.

Simple traumatic lacerations caused by sharp instruments like glass or knives are comparable to clean–contaminated elective wounds and may therefore be closed primarily after proper irrigation and debridement within 6 h after injury. In traumatic wounds more than 6 h old, or contaminated by faeces, saliva, purulent exudate, or soil, a delayed closure procedure should be used after debridement. Antibiotics should be added.

Battle wounds and high-velocity missile wounds should be closed after delay, except for wounds of the scalp, face, and neck which require delayed procedures only in the case of heavy crushing or high speed projectile injury.

Wounds near a colostomy or ileostomy can be closed primarily but observed closely for signs of infection. In case of infection and opening of the wound, secondary spontaneous healing is used because closure in such circumstances is followed by a higher risk of development of persistent or recurrent wound infection.

After incisional abscesses following laparotomy a delayed procedure can be used both for subcutaneous wounds and in cases where the abscess goes through the fascia but the peritoneum remains intact. Antibiotics are given when the wounds are reclosed. In most studies the antibiotic is given empirically to cover aerobic and anaerobic organisms.

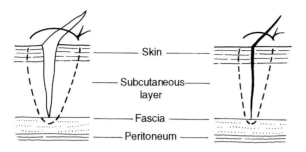

Fig. 4.4 *Left:* the monofilament suture is placed approximately 3 cm from the edge of the wound, but the suture does not run through the wound itself. *Right:* the wound cavity is completely occluded, avoiding collection of blood and tissue fluid. (From Moesgaard *et al.*, ref. 18.)

Technique of wound closure

In delayed closure of a primary wound the most important step is adequate debridement with the removal of all foreign bodies and devitalized tissue. Open-wound management prior to delayed closure involves the use of simple dressings of sterile fine-mesh gauze covered by moist loose absorptive dressings. Antiseptics are not necessary. The optimal time for wound closure has been found to be between 4 and 6 days after wounding, in the case of delayed primary closure. The wound can approximated by sutures, or tape if this is possible. Quantitative microbiology shows a small risk for infection after closure if the bacterial count is less than 10^5 organisms per gram of tissue. If the bacterial count remains higher than this by day 5 the wound should be allowed to heal by either secondary closure or secondary intention.

In early closure after wound infection and abscess the wound management prior to closure is the same. No local antibiotic or antiseptics should be used. After 4–5 days the wound can be closed with appropriate antibiotic cover. Quantitative microbiology is not necessary for management of this type of wound.

Closure procedure

Necrotic tissues must always be excised from the wound margins but extensive curettage of the wound edge should be avoided. The suture technique should secure closure of the wound cavity and avoid accumulation of blood and tissue fluid

in the wound. Foreign material such as sutures increase the risk of infection in contaminated wounds and for this reason a monofilament, non-absorbable suture should be used and sutures in the wound cavity avoided, as shown in Fig. 4.4. In case of an abscess, extending to but not through the peritoneum, sutures closing the defect of fascia are needed. Absorbable sutures may be used successfully (Fig. 4.5). Tension-relaxing incisions may be made to preserve the blood supply. Sutures for delayed closure may be inserted at the first operation and the wound closed later with local anaesthesia. The wound edge can be accurately approximated using skin tapes.

Acquisition of tensile strength in healing wounds

The end point of the wound healing process is to restore continuity between the wound edges and to re-establish the function of the tissue. In adults this process consists of a filling out of the wound cavity with a scar consisting of collagenous connective tissue. In some tissues such as epithelium, endothelium, bone, and to a lesser degree in kidney, liver, and peripheral nervous system, tissue regeneration with re-establishment of original tissue can occur. The principal component of scar tissue is fibrous collagen, which provides mechanical strength, but this can be accompanied by undesirable rigidity as well as constriction.

Wound strength, from a functional point of view, is the most important property for a healing wound and the final functional result. In surgical practice this is critical for the outcome of surgery. The time interval from injury to a healed scar which is strong enough to resist mechanical stress in the tissue, is of great interest. It is essential that an early return to normal life is facilitated with development of significant wound strength. This investigation of acquisition of tensile strength has, for ethical and practical reasons, been based on experimental studies.

In early wounds the tensile strength is low and insufficient to keep the tissue edges together without sutures. Open tissue defects become filled with clotted blood, tissue debris, and fluid early in the inflammatory phase. At this stage the strength of the wound is derived only from fibrin in the clot. Later, in the proliferation (fibroplasia) phase, the strength of a closed wound (such as linear skin wounds sutured after

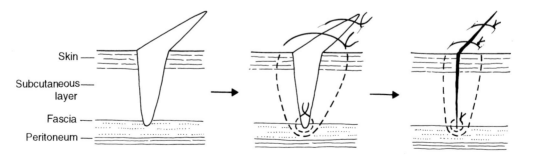

Fig. 4.5 Closure of a wound after an incision abscess extending to the peritoneum. Monofilament sutures are placed 3 cm from the edge of the wound. Defect of fascia is closed by absorbable sutures. (From Gottrup *et al.*, ref. 19.)

incision) increases rapidly as granulation tissue is formed to repair the defect (40–43). Some collagenous elements can be seen already in this phase (after 2–3 days of wounding), but the maximal period of collagen synthesis occurs, for most tissues, around the fifth to seventh day of healing. The collagen fibres are laid down in a random pattern and, in the beginning, possess little mechanical strength. Gradually a more systematic pattern of collagen fibrils develops, leading to stabilization by cross-linking and assembly into fibres. The diameter of the fibrils also increases in some tissues during maturation. Old damaged collagen is broken down enzymatically, as well as some of the new formed elements. There is a 'biochemically active zone' which encompasses tissue up to more than 5 mm from the incisional lines (44–46). After 2–3 weeks the deposition and removal of connective tissue elements reach a steady stage (47). If the wound edges are poorly opposed, the wound healing process may be delayed. In the maturation phase the scar tissue consists of dense connective tissue, which is dominated by collagen fibres. The amount of matrix is less than in granulation tissue and unwounded connective tissue. During this phase the turnover of collagen is still higher than normal and the mechanical strength of tissue continues to increase, but to a less rapid extent than during the phase of proliferation. The further increase in wound strength may be explained by remodelling of the fibre architecture. The change of collagen type III to type I may also contribute. The remodelling process occurs as a response to mechanical (stretching) stimuli and the development of strength is retarded in an immobilized wound (48). Although the collagen fibre pattern becomes more like the pattern in intact connective tissue the regularity of the fibre structure is not regained.

Table 4.2 Tensile strength for healing wounds at day 20 in various tissues (expressed in units of values for intact tissues). Modified from Viidik and Gottrup (42)

Tissue	Tensile strength
Skin	0.12
Tendon	0.10
Fascia	0.55
Muscle	0.74
Colon	0.76
Duodenum	0.86
Corpus ventriculi	1.29

The basic properties of scar tissue probably do not vary significantly from one tissue to another. However, the tissue–scar–tissue complexes may vary considerably, depending on the biomechanical properties of the original tissue. The healing rate, related to the mechanical properties of the original tissue, may show considerable variation from tissue to tissue. The strength of healing tissue has been shown to be related to the content of collagen in the intact tissue. The **relative strength** of a healing wound is defined as the strength of a wounded tissue compared to the strength of the same type of intact tissue. In Fig. 4.6 the relative tensile strengths of different types of tissue are shown (42). In tissues with a low collagen content before injury (e.g. the gastrointestinal tract and intra-abdominal organs) the primarily closed wound has a rapid increase in relative strength. After 10–20 days the intact tissue level is reached. In tissues with a high content of collagen in intact tissue (e.g. tendon, fascia, or skin) the increase in

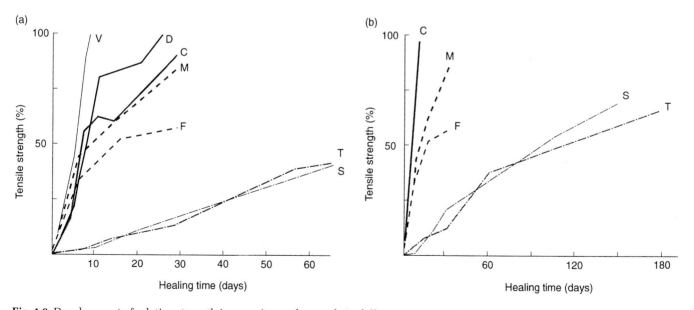

Fig. 4.6 Development of relative strength in experimental wounds in different tissues. (a) Short term healing; (b) long term healing. The tensile strength has been calculated as a percentage of the respective intact tissue. V, ventriculi (corpus; rat); D, duodenum (rat); C, colon (rat); M, lateral abdominal wall muscle (rabbit); F, fascia (*linea alba*, rabbit); S, skin (rat); and T, tendon (*peroneus brevis*, rabbit). (Modified from Viidik and Gottrup 1986.)

relative strength is much lower, and only 20–50 per cent of the intact tissue level is reached after 30 days following wounding. In Table 4.2 the relative tensile strengths for healing wounds at 20 days in various tissues are shown. No data are available for open wounds which have healed by secondary intention.

Tensile strength development in different types of tissue

Tissues with high collagen content

This group of tissues includes tendon, ligaments, fascia, and skin. These tissues are composed of dense and often parallel-fibred connective tissue in which type I collagen dominates. They have a high tensile strength because of the architectural structure of collagen which is the strongest fibrous protein in the body (42, 49, 50). In ligament wounds only 60 per cent of the intact ligament strength is reached 98 days after wounding and, after 280 days, only 70 per cent is reached. As the main role of tendons is to transmit forces and that of ligament to resist them, the influence of stress and immobilization on the development of mechanical strength has been studied. The tissue elements become successfully more organized after the initial phase of healing following partial tenotomy. By controlled passive motion, the normal tensile strength increase can be enhanced from 21 to 35 per cent of intact tendon values after 84 days of healing compared with complete immobilization (51).

Taking into account the three-dimensional meshwork of collagen fibres and the higher degree of vascularization in dermis, compared to tendon, it may be hypothesized that the rate of wound strength increase would be considerably higher. However, this is not the case (Fig. 4.6). The key point is how newly formed collagen fibres connect with those at the wound edges, but this question has not yet been answered. Looking at stress–strain curves it has been found that the curve for scar tissue is always lower and to the right of that of intact skin (i.e. the extensibility is higher and the ultimate strength is lower (52)). Scar tissue in dermis becomes stiffer than in intact tissue but it must be remembered that skin becomes stiffer with maturation and ageing (42). Leaving a skin wound open, under a surgical dressing for 3–6 days, before suturing has been shown to increase the wound strength more than 50 per cent compared to controls after 6 days and this difference is still significant 120 days after wounding (53, 54). Rupture occurs in the wound during early skin healing when mechanically stressed, while later on rupture occurs in the border zone between the scar and the adjacent tissue. This zone has been shown to be active biochemically even after 60 days of healing (45).

Nilsson (55) has investigated various techniques of incision types and suture materials in fascia and abdominal wall. Wounds tend to gain relative strength more rapidly when the incision is placed in muscular areas of the abdominal wall than in fascia (e.g. in *linea alba*). Elastic suture materials (synthetic polymers) that permit a more yielding wound closure than stainless steel sutures seem to stimulate the gain of mechanical strength, while both excessive tension and relaxation seem to impair wound healing from a mechanical point of view (55, 56). It was also suggested that the biochemically active zone around these types of wounds is more pronounced compared to other types of healing wounds (57, 58).

Tissues with low collagen content

In tissues with low collagen content before injury, primary closed wounds have a rapid increase in relative tensile strength. Wounds in the gastrointestinal tract and muscle have been investigated (43, 59). The healing response to injury in the gastrointestinal tract is similar to the general sequence. In the gut, however, the wall is constructed of several layers of tissue and healing has to relate to each of these. Mucosa regenerates with a complete return to normal morphology and without scar formation. Injury penetrating into the submucosa and muscle layer elicits a fibrotic repair and scar formation (60). In relation to the development of tensile strength the submucosa is of most interest. In the alimentary tract the submucosa consists of a loose network, predominantly of collagen with some elastin and numerous vessels. The majority of the collagen in the intestinal wall is in the submucosa and this layer provides most of the strength of an intact intestinal wall (61). Investigations of tensile strength development have principally used the 'blow-out' technique which only yields information of the bursting pressure of what is a geometrically complicated structure. Measurements of true tensile strength in this type of tissue are made with difficulty but have been refined and valuable information have been obtained (59).

The weakest point related to a healing wound in the gastrointestinal tract has been shown to move rapidly from the wound line itself into the biochemically active zone around it and then into intact tissue. The biochemically active zone has been found to be 3–4 mm lateral to the incisional line (62). Healing, measured as gain of relative mechanical strength, is rapid in this type of tissue (Fig. 4.6). More than 50 per cent of the ruptures occur outside the wound area after 10 days of healing (62).

In studies of anastomotic healing of different parts of the gut, the suture holding capacity of the intestinal wall has been used. This concept is defined as the amount and structure of collagen supporting the sutures in the wound margin (63, 64). The tensile strength of a sutured anastomosis is dependent on this concept, together with suture strength and the number of sutures and direction of pull upon them. However, defective modern suture material or tying the knot insecurely would be a rare cause of dehiscence of intestinal anastomosis. In sutured bowel the initial breaking strength of the anastomosis can be almost as strong as that of intact tissue (65, 66). In sutured anastomoses the most critical time for anastomotic integrity is during the first postoperative days, when the suture holding capacity is markedly reduced (65–68). Several explanations have been suggested for these reductions, including collagen degradation, increased collagenolytic activity, and relation to the biochemically active zone. However, early loss of mechanical integrity does not correlate with the amount of collagen, or with the changes in collagen solubility, but the collagen fibres may undergo some structural changes which may not be revealed (61). The early decrease in suture

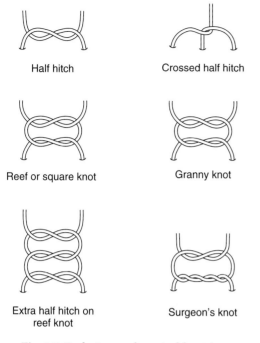

Half hitch   Crossed half hitch

Reef or square knot   Granny knot

Extra half hitch on   Surgeon's knot
reef knot

Fig. 4.7 Techniques of surgical knotting.

holding capacity found 1–3 days after wounding is probably a major factor for the development of anastomotic complications. This early decrease in tissue strength has been related to several factors including infection, trauma, and accumulation of neutrophils in the wound margin (69). Collagen degradation is partly mediated by oxygen free radicals or by the release of proteinases. After 3–4 days collagen synthesis predominates in and around the anastomosis and a rapid net gain in strength follows due to increasing amounts of wound tissue in the incision and increased suture holding capacity of the adjacent intestinal wall. Anastomotic strength with and without sutures has been found the same after one week in colon (70) and after 14 days in ileum (65).

Suture techniques

The development of wound management techniques leading to the manufacture of modern sutures has been described in Chapter 2. By 1920 Lord Moynihan had laid down what he considered to be the criteria for an 'ideal' suture (71):

(1) achieve its purpose (be sufficient to hold parts together)
(2) disappear as soon as its work is accomplished
(3) be free from infection
(4) be non-irritant.

He felt that probably the oldest suture based on animal proteins, catgut, fulfilled these requirements. The chromicization of catgut to prolong integrity by Lord Lister (72) (some 40 years before) added to this conviction. It is not unjust, in

the light of modern knowledge, to say that catgut does not fit with the role of an ideal suture (because it is absorbed too rapidly) and we shall probably see it replaced by synthetic absorbables (which have predictable absorption rates with little tissue reaction) and synthetic non-absorbables (which do not need to disappear because they are non-irritant and do not favour infection). However, many surgeons are not widely aware of the continuing advances of the past 20 years.

It is clear that all sutures must be free from infection. Autoclaving or steeping sutures in antiseptic solutions, which is in itself damaging, has been replaced by large scale sterilization by the manufacturers using irradiation or ethylene oxide which does not weaken the synthetic absorbables. Such large scale sterilization allows presentation of sutures in individual packets.

The security of a suture or ligature also depends on its handling characteristics. Natural materials such as catgut and silk allow easy, secure knots to be tied but they are not as inert in tissue as are the synthetic non-absorbable monofilament sutures, nor do they pass as easily through the tissues. Multifilament or braided sutures allow better handling and knotting, but are rougher in their passage through tissue (unless coated) and are more prone to infection. Natural fibres (catgut and silk) cause the most intense tissue reaction and hydrolysis, measured biochemically and histologically, which can be directly imaged using the ear chamber model (73). The capillarity of a braided suture encourages bacterial migration (74) and enhances the risk of a foreign body in tissues (which in itself logarithmically decreases the number of organisms necessary to establish a wound infection (75)). Knot sinuses caused by persistent infection around suture material left in tissues are more commonly associated with braided material or when an excessive number of knots are used, thereby leaving more suture material in place. Suture abscesses related to the site of entry of a suture in skin closure are also related to capillarity, tissue foreign body reaction, and promotion of infection and leave cosmetically unacceptable scars. A lithogenic effect in the biliary tree or bladder may also follow the use of non-absorbable reactive materials. There is no evidence of increased knot security by throwing more knots than a double, single, double surgeon's square reef knot (76). Handling characteristics of monofilament synthetic materials are also affected by the coefficient of friction (low in polyamide sutures) and memory and elasticity (high in polypropylene sutures). All need to be taken account of when choosing a suture for a particular purpose. Techniques of knotting are shown in Fig. 4.7 and described further in textbooks of operative surgery (76, 77).

Despite advances in technology no single ideal suture has yet been made and the range of materials available remains wide. Wound closure fails because tissues tear (an inadequate bite of tissue is taken by the suture in closing a defect), knots slip, or suture material breaks. In a choice of suture the surgeon must decide which suture best suits the purpose of its use.

1. It must be strong enough to hold tissues together, until healing is complete (in skin a monofilament synthetic non-absorbable removed late is ideal but a synthetic absorbable

Table 4.3(a) Suture materials in common use in surgery – absorbable

Suture	Types	Raw material	Tensile strength retention *in vivo*	Absorption rate	Tissue reaction	Contraindications	Frequent uses	How supplied
Catgut	Plain	Collagen derived from healthy mammals	Lost within 7–10 days. Marked patient variability	Phagocytosis and enzymatic degradation within 70 days	High	Not for use in tissues which heal slowly and require prolonged support	Ligate superficial vessels, suture subcutaneous tissues, stomas, and other tissues that heal rapidly; ophthalmic surgery	6/0–1 with needles; 4/0–3 without needles
Catgut	Chromic	Collagen derived from healthy mammals; tanned with chromium salts to improve handling and to resist degradation in tissue	Lost within 21–28 days. Marked patient variability	Phagocytosis and enzymatic degradation within 90 days	Moderate	As for plain catgut	As for plain catgut	6/0–3 with needles; 5/0–3 without needles
Polyglactin 910 (Coated Vicryl®ᵃ)	Braided multifilament	Copolymer of lactide and glycolide in a ratio of 90:10, coated with polyglactin 370 and calcium stearate	Approx. 60% remains at 2 weeks; approx. 30% remains at 3 weeks	Hydrolysis. Minimal until 5–6 weeks; complete absorption 60–90 days	Mild	Not advised for use in tissues which require prolonged approximation under stress	General surgical use where absorbable sutures required, e.g. gut anastomoses, vascular ligatures. Has become the 'workhorse' suture for many applications in most general surgical practices, including undyed for subcuticular wound closures. Ophthalmic surgery	8/0–2 with needles; 5/0–2 without needles
Poly-glyconate (Maxon®ᵇ)	Monofilament; dyed or undyed	Copolymer of glycolic acid and trimethylene carbonate	Approx. 70% remains at 2 weeks; approx. 55% remains at 3 weeks	Hydrolysis. Minimal until 8–9 weeks; complete absorption by 180 days	Mild	Not advised for use in tissues which require prolonged approximation under stress	Popular in some centres as an alternative to Vicryl and PDS	7/0–2 with needles
Polyglycolic acid (Dexon®ᵇ)	Braided multifilament; dyed or undyed; coated or uncoated	Homopolymer; polyglycolic acid. Available with coating of inert, absorbable surfactant poloxamer 188 to enhance surface smoothness. 97% excreted in urine within 3 days	Approx. 40% remains at 1 week; approx 20% remains at 3 weeks	Hydrolysis. Minimal at 2 weeks, significant at 4 weeks; complete absorption 60–90 days	Minimal	Not advised for use in tissues which require prolonged approximation under stress	Uses as for other absorbable sutures	9/0–2 with needles; 9/0–2 without needles
Polydioxanone (PDS®ᵃ)	Monofilament; dyed or undyed	Polyester polymer	Approx. 70% remains at 2 weeks; approx. 50% remains at 4 weeks; approx. 14% remains at 8 weeks	Hydrolysis. Minimal at 90 days; complete absorption at 180 days	Mild	Not for use in association with heart valves or synthetic grafts, or in situations in which prolonged tissue approximation under stress is required	Uses as for other absorbable sutures, in particular where slightly longer wound support is required	PDS®: 10/0–8/0 with needles; PDS II®: 7/0–2 with needles

ᵃEthicon trademark.
ᵇDavis and Geck trademark.

Table 4.3(b) Suture materials in common use in surgery – non-absorbable

Suture	Types	Raw material	Tensile strength retention *in vivo*	Absorption rate	Tissue reaction	Contraindications	Frequent uses	How supplied
Silk	Braided or twisted multifilament; dyed or undyed; coated or uncoated (with wax or silicone)	Natural protein; raw silk from silkworm	Loses 20% when wet; 80–100% lost by 6 months	Fibrous encapsulation in body at 2–3 weeks; absorbed slowly over 1–2 years	Moderate to high	Not for use with vascular prostheses or in tissues requiring prolonged approximation under stress. Risk of infection and tissue reaction make silk unsuitable for routine skin closure	Ligation and suturing where long term tissue support is unnecessary	10/0–2 with needles; 4/0–1 without needles
Linen	Twisted	Long staple flax fibres	Stronger when wet. Loses 50% at 6 months; 30% remains at 2 years	Non-absorbable; remains encapsulated in body tissues	Moderate	Not advised for use with vascular prostheses	Ligation and suturing in gastrointestinal surgery. No longer in common use in most centres	3/0–1 with needles. 3/0–1 without needles
Surgical steel	Monofilament; multifilament	An alloy of iron, nickel, and chromium	Indefinite	Non-absorbable; remains encapsulated in body tissues	Minimal	Should not be used in conjunction with prosthesis of different metal	Closure of sternotomy wounds. Previously found favour for tendon and hernia repairs	Monofilament: 5/0–5 with needles; multifilament: 5/0–3/0 with needles
Nylon (Ethilon[a] Dermalon[b] Nurolon[a])	Monofilament; braided multifilament; dyed or undyed	Polyamide polymer	Loses 15–20% per year	Degrades at approx. 15–20% per year	Low	None	General surgical use; e.g. skin closure, abdominal wall mass closure, hernia repair. Plastic surgery, neurosurgery, microsurgery, ophthalmic surgery	Monofilament: 11/0–2 with needles (including loops in some sizes); 4/0–2 without needles. Multifilament: 6/0–2 with needles; 3/0–1 without needles
Polyester (Ethibond[a] Tecron[b] Mersilene[a] Dacron[b])	Monofilament; braided multifilament; dyed or undyed; coated (polybutylate or silicone) or uncoated	Polyester polyethylene terephthalate	Indefinite	Non-absorbable; remains encapsulated in body tissues	Low	None	Cardiovascular, ophthalmic, plastic, and general surgery	Monofilament: (ophthalmic) 11/10; 10/0 with needles. Multifilament: 5/0–1 with needles. Ethibond[a]: 7/0–5 with needles
Polybutester (Novafil[b])	Monofilament; dyed or undyed	Polybutylene terephthalate and polytetramethylene ether glycol	Indefinite	Non-absorbable; remains encapsulated in body tissues	Low	None	Exhibits a degree of elasticity. Particularly favoured for use in plastic surgery	7/0–1 with needles
Polypropylene (Prolene[a])	Monofilament; dyed or undyed	Polymer of propylene	Indefinite	Non-absorbable; remains encapsulated in body tissues	Low	None	Cardiovascular surgery, plastic surgery, ophthalmic surgery, general surgical subcuticular skin closure	10/0–1 with needles

[a] Ethicon trademark.
[b] Davis and Geck trademark.

may function as well) or indefinitely (in vascular surgery the monofilament synthetic polymer polypropylene is ideal). The decision may not be clear cut; in abdominal wall, fascial healing strength does not exceed 75 per cent of unwounded strength (78) so that it is not certain whether a suture should be absorbable or non-absorbable.

2. Handling and knotting. The superior qualities of silk and catgut must be weighed against their excessive tissue reaction or unpredictable tensile strength when implanted in tissue. These tissue reactions may predispose to infection, delayed healing, or excessive scarring (hypertrophic or keloid scar).

3. Freedom from infection is a prerequisite for modern sutures. Animal-derived sutures must be derived from uninfected sources, including bovine spongiform encephalitis (BSE). Braids and knots, as well as tissue reaction, predispose to infection.

4. Minimal tissue damage is achieved by the use of eyeless needles and the minimum diameter of suture for optimal strength. Monofilament synthetic materials glide through tissue but braids do not, although this is improved by coating. For the best cosmetic results in skin it is not clearly established whether a removable, non-absorbable monofilament is superior to an embedded absorbable braid.

Classification of sutures

Sutures can be widely defined as natural or synthetic, absorbable or non-absorbable (Table 4.3).

Natural materials
Absorbable

Catgut falls into this category and still has worldwide popularity for anastomosing bowel, in subcutaneous closure, and as a ligature. It is manufactured from the submucosa of sheep and beef intestine twisted into a smooth multifilament suture, which appears and handles as a monofilament. Plain catgut is absorbed within 50–60 days and retains some integrity for up to a third of that time. Chromic catgut is treated with chromic acid salts in a tanning process and this prolongs its absorption up to 70–100 days because hydrolysis and lysosomal enzymatic degradation is delayed. Both forms of catgut are treated with aldehyde which cross-links and strengthens the collagen. When wet this 'stiffness' is lost and catgut handles well and knots are very secure.

The main disadvantage of catgut is its unpredictability in tissues. There is some evidence that the acute inflammatory process involved in its degradation also promotes infection; certainly infection promotes its absorption (79). For this reason it should not be used when suture integrity must be maintained during healing. It is entirely unacceptable for use in the musculo-aponeurotic layers of the abdominal wall, for example (80–83).

Extruded collagen is manufactured from bovine Achilles tendon. It is stiffer than conventional catgut but less reactive, making it suitable for ophthalmic surgery, for example.

Non-absorbable

Silk, linen, and cotton are in this group but only the former remains in widespread use. Silk is presented as a braid with a silicone coating. It handles very well and allows very secure knots. It is biodegradable and leads to a significant tissue reaction and promotion of infection. The capillarity of the braid may allow bacteria to migrate from an epithelial surface into the tissues (84, 85). The promotion of suture abscesses in skin, and the resultant cosmetically unacceptable 'herringbone' scars which result, virtually preclude its use for skin closure.

Synthetic materials
Absorbable

Synthetic sutures can almost be made to order. There are several absorbable alternatives, all of which promote a tissue reaction related to their reabsorption but are much more predictable than catgut with a longer tissue integrity. There is some evidence that they may promote infection (86).

Polyglycolic acid (Dexon®) was the first widely available material in this group. Infection promotes its absorption, much like catgut (87) but it persists in tissues for 60–90 days retaining its tensile strength reliably (unlike catgut) for 20 days. It is a glycolic acid polymer presented as a braid either stained with a non-toxic dye (to be seen easily for general use) or unstained (for use in subcuticular closure to prevent 'tattooing'). As a subcuticular suture it avoids the need for removal but tends to cause some weeping from the wound edge. It has been used for musculo-aponeurotic closure of the abdominal wall (82, 83) with no added significant risk of wound failure compared to non-absorbables, but with the hypothetically reduced risk of persistent knot sinuses.

Polyglactin (Vicryl®) has all the properties of polyglycolic acid with a similar, slightly quicker (88), resorption pattern and tissue integrity (20 days). It is also braided and presented stained or unstained. Polyglactin is a coated copolymer of lactide and glycolide and is widely used for bowel anastomosis and ligatures because it handles well and knots are secure.

Polydioxanone (PDS®) is a monofilament polymer which handles rather like polyamide or polyester (see below) but has a much slower absorption rate (160–180 days) and a tissue integrity of approximately one third of this time. It has promise for abdominal wall closure and for closure of tissues in the presence of infection or persistent inflammation.

Polyglyconate (Maxon®) is another monofilament polymer similar to polydioxanone but without its tissue integrity.

Non-absorbable

There are many materials in this group. All have the advantage of being safe in the presence of infection as they incite no tissue reaction but bulky knots can promote chronic sinuses or painful knots in tissues. Most of the group are monofilaments which glide easily through tissues but handling and knots are relatively poor. Braids improve handling and knots, and if coated (with silicone or polytetrafluoroethylene) to reduce capillarity, can slide through tissues atraumatically. All the materials have high tensile strength which remains indefinitely (although polyamide is very slowly biodegradable in tissue (89)). The low coefficient of friction associated with the monofilament sutures allows easy removal when used to close skin, by the subcuticular method, for example.

Polyamide (Nylon) is the most rigid and maintains a 'memory' of its packed shape. Handling and knots are difficult for the inexperienced although facilitated in braided form.

The polyolefine, polypropylene (Prolene®), is completely inert in tissue and is much more elastic than polyamide, which allows more 'give' in tissues when stressed. It is ideal for abdominal wall closure and vascular anastomosis.

The polyester Dacron® is braided but coated to reduce capillarity and friction. Other sutures in this group include polybutester (Novafil®) and polytetrafluoroethylene (Dacron® and Gore-Tex®).

Stainless steel wire (SSW) needs to be considered in a category of its own. It is unusual to use it now for soft tissue closure as the non-absorbable polymers serve as well, but it is used for closing bony structures such as the sternum after open heart surgery. It is difficult to handle and snaps if loops are allowed to twist, and knots are difficult to tie when main-taining tension. The ends of cut SSW have to be turned in on themselves to prevent painful knot ends.

Suture sizes

The system most widely used for suture sizes is based on the British and North American Pharmacopoeia (BP, USP). It is an empirical measurement varying from 10/0 (the finest) to 2 or 3 (the thickest). It is logical to use the smallest volume of suture required to securely oppose incised tissues until heal-ing is complete, i.e. pull-out strength should match breaking strength (85). Inexperienced surgeons tend to use a suture which is too thick, which presents more foreign body, whereas too fine a suture has a 'cheese-wire' effect and may cut out from tissues if tied too tightly.

Suture needles

Needles (Fig. 4.8) are all now disposable and made with stain-less steel with the suture swaged at one end instead of an eye. This prevents any 'shouldering' between needle and suture to allow smooth passage through tissues. Hand needles are being replaced by instrument needles to minimize needle-stick in-jury and the attendant risk of hepatitis and HIV infection. Needles can be curved or straight, although the latter are really exclusively for hand use to close skin (when the risk of infection transmission by needle-stick injury is minimal anyway).

Needle tips can be round bodied, for atraumatic use on soft structures such as bowel anastomosis; or triangular (with a cutting edge) in cross-section for rigid tissues such as skin, fascia, cartilage, or even bone.

Laboratory and experimental evaluation of sutures

The Instron tensiometer can be used reproducibly to test the tensile strength of sutures (and knots) with a constant rate of shear and stress. Tensile strength is usually expressed in kg/cm^2. Modification after immersion in body fluids (90) or re-lated to the presence of infection (91) can be measured similarly.

Evaluation of sutures has been undertaken widely in ex-perimental wounds (87, 88). Sutures may be implanted into tissues (a seton) and breaking strength assessed after a meas-ured time by pulling out the sutures. The histology of the tissue reaction around an implanted suture can be studied simultaneously. Tissue reaction around sutures can be visual-ized directly in the rabbit ear chamber model (73).

Indications for suture types: clinical applications and recommendations

1. Skin can be closed with most types of suture but catgut does not have a long enough integrity (although it is appropri-ate for closing the subcutaneous layer) and silk causes a cos-metically unacceptable tissue reaction. The scars related to silk involve formation of suture abscesses related to foreign body potentiation of infection (suture abscesses often caused

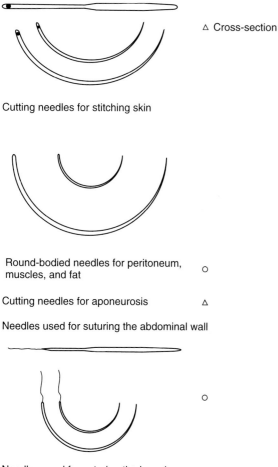

△ Cross-section

Cutting needles for stitching skin

Round-bodied needles for peritoneum, muscles, and fat   o

Cutting needles for aponeurosis   △

Needles used for suturing the abdominal wall

Needles used for suturing the bowel   o
The threads are swaged into the needles

Fig. 4.8 Needles used in surgical practice.

by opportunistic, otherwise innocuous organisms such as *Staphylococcus epidermidis*) and cross-hatched 'herring-bone' scars. Monofilament non-absorbable synthetic polymers (such as Nylon or Prolene®) are ideal, used with an interrupted, simple or mattress, or continuous technique. Subcuticular closure gives the best results, but non-absorbable sutures need removal when healing is complete, whereas closure with a synthetic absorbable suture does not need removal of the suture.

An alternative to sutures for skin closure is the use of stainless steel clips which have been popular for closing neck collar incisions and Pfannenstiel gynaecological abdominal incisions. Clips are certainly preferable to sutures when there is an HIV risk. When supplied on a rail with a forceps applicator (Michel clips) they are cheap but disposable multifire staple units, which allow long skin wounds to be closed quickly, are expensive. Clips give fine supple and cosmetically acceptable scars with a reduction in infection (92) but the choice between them and sutures is not clear (93). The use of stainless steel staples is covered in Chapter 12. They have found wide popularity in gastrointestinal surgery.

Adhesive tapes give equally acceptable scars as clips (94), but are difficult to apply to skin if it is wet. Skin can be dried and application made easier by using tincture of benzoin or a proprietary wipe. Sutures may be replaced by adhesive tapes at 4–5 days when they are easily applied to the dry edge of the wound, but tapes are not very efficient over joints. Modern skin tapes are strong and stretchable (thereby preventing blisters) with good non-allergenic adhesives (95). The use of incise drapes to close wounds (as a giant adhesive tape) is acceptable and in widespread use. They afford a moist wound environment and easy inspection. If such polyurethane film dressings are pulled tight they may cause some skin blistering. Tapes should be applied to Langer's lines and are particularly useful in closing wounds in fractious children or obese skin. There is also the benefit that removal is easy. Excellent cosmetic results can be expected following their use on lacerations as well as incised wounds, possibly related to the low associated infection and rapid acquisition of tensile strength.

2. Bowel and bladder is conventionally anastomosed or repaired using an absorbable suture such as natural catgut or preferably a more predictable synthetic suture such as Vicryl® or Dexon®. Non-absorbable sutures can be used in bowel (the sutures are probably passed in faeces later anyway when healing is complete) but are unacceptable in the biliary or urinary tract because they are lithogenic.

3. Arterial closure or anastomosis needs a suture of adequate strength which can last indefinitely and not cause thrombosis. Separation at a suture line can lead to false aneurysm formation. The monofilament Prolene® is ideal for this purpose.

4. Connective tissues. Bone cannot be sutured unless it is relatively thin. Stainless steel wire or monofilament polymers can be used. The same materials can be used to repair tendon. It is critical not to use catgut and other sutures which incite a tissue reaction to repair nerve because axons may be prevented from entering or redirected from nerve sheaths. Most

of the connective tissues can be closed with absorbables and it is convenient not to have to remove sutures, but in musculo-aponeurotic structures such as the abdominal wall which are exposed to high tension, non-absorbable polymers are safer. Prolene® and Nylon® are the most favoured, but closure with the absorbable polymers PDS® or Dexon® acid show promise without an increased risk of wound failure (burst abdomen or incisional hernia).

5. Sutures can be used for ties or ligatures. Absorbable materials are best as there is little risk of a nidus of infection or irritation in the tissues causing pain. Ties should embrace the least amount of tissue possible to prevent slippage of the knot or to leave too much devitalized tissue beyond the tie. Slipped ligatures from tied vessels may lead to haemorrhage after an operation, which may not be apparent until the patient becomes shocked following excessive blood loss. Bleeding may also be revealed as a haematoma or as continued loss in a drain. When tying a blood vessel cooperation is required between assistant and surgeon, as a haemostatic forceps is removed as the ligature is tied. When the tissue to be tied is bulky a transfixion suture reduces the risk of slipping – a suture on a needle is passed through the tissue to be tied and knotted on both sides.

Techniques of tissue closure using sutures

See also Chapter 9. It is logical to close incisions with an anatomical approach, free from any tension or strangulation of tissue embraced by the suture, when incisions are made in natural crease lines (Langer's lines), or between planes of cleavage. In skin this is perfectly acceptable and a variety of techniques (simple or mattress, interrupted or continuous, or subcuticular) exist (Fig. 4.9). However, this does not apply to connective tissue under tension, as in the abdominal wall, where a wide bite of tissue is required to avoid wound failure. It is recommended that a ratio of 4:1 suture length:wound length be used (96). Sutures are therefore placed outside the biochemically active zone at the wound interface. This is approximately 0.5 cm on each side of the wound, should be wider in the presence of infection, and sutures placed in it are at danger of cutting out, particularly when under tension (97).

It is important to avoid strangulation of tissue as inflammation is increased and in the presence of ischaemia there is a higher risk of wound infection. This is particularly important in skin flaps or grafts for skin loss; and in bowel anastomosis in oesophagus and colon where blood supply may be anatomically tenuous. Excessive use of too many sutures which are too thick for their purpose should also be avoided because of the foreign body complications. Subcuticular skin closure allows less puncture holes to be made in the skin. If a non-absorbable suture is used, this also facilitates removal – only one suture is involved. The technique is safe in contamination (98). The use of an absorbable suture that does not require removal is less certain but this does risk hypertrophic scarring (99), but not if a slow resorption suture is used such as PDS® (100).

Continuous sutures are quicker to insert but are mandatory in arterial anastomosis to achieve the best haemostatic suture

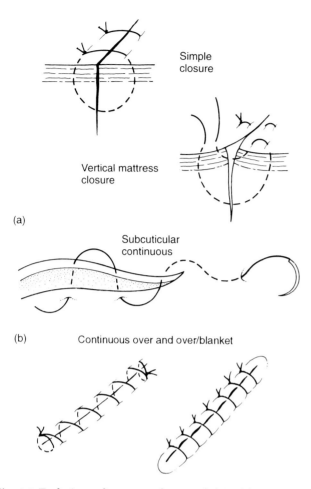

Simple closure

Vertical mattress closure

(a)

Subcuticular continuous

(b)

Continuous over and over/blanket

Fig. 4.9 Techniques for suture closure of skin: (a) various continuous and interrupted techniques; (b) subcuticular closure.

line. Interrupted sutures take longer to place but the mattress technique ensures eversion of skin edges – inversion can give less acceptable and more slowly healing scars. Arterial suture lines should always evert to prevent thrombosis around intimal flaps or atherosclerotic flaps, whereas bowel suture lines heal more acceptably when the mucosa is inverted into the lumen.

Knots are most secure when a double surgeon's knot is followed by a square single knot and a second double knot (2:1:2) (Fig. 4.7).

Techniques of tissue closure using adhesives

Fibrin has been used, not only to close skin (101) but also to reduce bleeding from damaged tissue (102). Fibrin adhesive systems depend on the use of pooled plasma which always causes some concern because of the risk of viral transmission. Any system which can avoid biological systems to polymerize fibrin will be an advance.

Cyanomethacrylate glues have been available for many years and were soon used for bleeding surfaces such as the liver (103). The use of a sterile tube of glue for each operation is a relatively expensive method to close skin. Rapid skin closure is easy provided haemostasis is adequate but fears of a risk of increased infection, and the glue polymer being a barrier to healing, have precluded widespread use.

Technique of incisions

It is obvious that all surgeons should have a gentle respect for tissue but to measure their ability in achieving this is difficult. Surgeons should be aware of the geometry of each shape of scalpel blade (104). To make an incision demands the least energy exchange and tissue disruption. Excessive force damages tissue and invites infection. Very sharp blades or scissors need little energy to divide tissue. Modern disposable scalpel blades soon become dull in tough tissue but blades do not need to be replaced once skin is breached (105). Scissors become blunt through inexpert or forceful use. Lacerating tissue rather than incising it reflects poor technique.

To make a large incision a 10 blade or similar is needed. The skin is stretched between the non-dominant finger and thumb and a sweep of the scalpel, using the belly of the blade, makes the incision. Blade shape and sizes should be chosen for the best results – small incisions require a 15 blade and the scalpel to be held like a pencil.

The making of an incision using diathermy or the more expensive laser has its proponents. Both give localized thermal energy which can divide tissue. The high frequency electrical current used in diathermy can be a monopolar blade or forceps for accurate use, or bipolar for larger areas of tissue haemostasis. Incisions using either technique reduce bleeding in connective tissue and in muscle-cutting operations much less blood is lost overall. Lasers are dangerous when shiny instruments are used (so avoid them) because reflections can damage patients' and operating team's tissues. There is an attendant delay in skin healing using diathermy or laser with a theoretical rather than proven risk of wound infection (106).

Karl Langer of Vienna described the natural tension lines in skin along which the collagen of subcutaneous connective tissue is disposed. Incisions heal best when made in the same direction as these lines. S or Z shaped incisions should be made over the flexor aspects of joints when Langer's lines cannot be followed, and incisions should be avoided over subcutaneous bony surfaces (other than skull) as healing can be delayed (particularly over the tibia). Incisions through musculo-aponeurotic tissues follow similar principles – transverse abdominal incisions heal better than vertical ones, possibly because they also retain a better nerve and blood supply.

Haemostatic measures

Diathermy and lasers can be used to stop bleeding through local heating of tissue. When a significant (>2 mm diameter) vessel, particularly an artery, is bleeding then a ligature is preferable. Of course, traumatic or accidental damage of major vessels should be repaired if feasible. Some surgeons favour widespread use of diathermy for access and haemostasis and report no increased risk of infection, probably related to good anaesthetic and surgical technique and appropriate antibiotic prophylaxis. Simply suturing an incision or laceration can achieve haemostasis; the scalp is a good example. Some tissues pose difficulties in haemostasis – bleeding from a ruptured liver may only be controlled by packing. Never forget natural haemostatic mechanisms – platelets, thrombi, and fibrin and vessel contraction. Most bleeding in an incision is arrested by these means; patience and gentle pressure help achieve them.

In some areas of the body a preliminary injection of adrenaline can be used to reduce haemorrhage and to extend the effective duration of action of local anaesthetics. In vascular areas this is safe (for example the scalp) but is very dangerous (and litigational) when used on digits or areas of poor blood supply. When in any doubt it should not be used.

When a tissue surface continues to ooze with capillary bleeding despite waiting for clot to form with pressure, there are other agents which can be used. Microfibrillar collagen is very effective, expensive, and difficult to manage once wet. Cellulose-derived glucuronic acid, presented as a foam (Oxycel) or gauze (Surgicel) or gelatin sponges soaked in thrombin (Gelfoam®) can also arrest such haemorrhage. Alginate dressings containing calcium are also effective and like some of the foams and gauzes can be used to pack bleeding cavities. Bone wax is used to seal bleeding bone (sternotomy for example) but can delay healing.

Surgeons have traditionally feared leaving dead spaces in tissue. However, it is now realized that serous or wound fluids contain factors which may be beneficial to healing. It is logical to leave a drain when haemostasis is not perfect. These are usually disposable, valved (to avoid infection), suction drains made of inert material but they are rarely effective for more than a few hours. In the presence of infection or body fluid leak, their use may seem more appropriate, but proof of their effectiveness is lacking. Drains are foreign bodies and, although sterile, do promote inflammation and infection.

References

1. Edlich, R. F., Rodeheaver, G., Thacker, J. G., and Edgerton, M. T. (1979). Technical factors in wound management. In *Fundamentals of wound management*, (ed. T. K. Hunt and J. E. Dunphy). Appleton-Century-Crofts, New York.
2. Terkeltaub, R. A. and Ginsberg, H. H. (1988). Platelets and response to injury. In *Molecular and cellular biology of wound repair*, (ed. R. A. F. Clark and P. M. Henson). Plenum, New York.
3. Furie, B. and Furie, B. C. (1988). The molecular basis of blood coagulation. *Cell*, **53**, 505–18.
4. Clark, R. A. F. (1991). Cutaneous wound repair: a review with emphasis on integrin receptor expression. In *Wound healing*, (ed. H. Jansen, R. Rooman, and J. I. S. Robertson). Janssen Biomedical. Science Series Wrightson Biomedical, UK.
5. Walsh, M. S. and Goode, A. W. (1992). A scientific approach to wound measurement: the role of stereo photogrammetry. In *Wound healing*, (ed. H. Janssen, R. Rooman, and J. I. S. Robertson). Janssen Biomedical Wrightson Biomedical, UK.
6. Hepburn, H. H. (1919). Delayed primary suture of wounds. *Br. Med. J.*, **1**, 181–3.
7. Hunter, J. (1794). *Treatise on blood, inflammation and gunshot wounds*, pp. 216–20. Nicol, London.
8. Watt, J. (1976). Delayed wound closure. *J. Roy. Navy Med. Serv.*, **62**, 140–7.
9. Billroth, T. (1865). Beobactungs-Studien über Wundfieber un accidentelle Wundkrankheiten. *Langenbeck Archives Chirurgie*, **VI**, 443–4.
10. Friedrich, P. L. (1898). Die aseptische Versorgung frisher Wunden unter Mittheilung von Thier-Versuchen über die Auseimungzeit von Infectionserregern in frischen Wunden. *Archive Klinishe Chirurgie*, **57**, 288–310.
11. Fraser, F., Dew, J. W., and Tayler, D. C. (1918). Primary and delayed suture of gunshot wounds. A report of research work at CCS. Vol. 6, pp. 92–124.
12. Pool, E. H. (1919). War wounds. Primary and secondary suture. *J. Am. Med. Assoc.*, **73**, 383–7.
13. Coller, F. A. and Valk, W. L. (1940). The delayed closure of contaminated wounds. A preliminary report. *Annals of Surg.*, **112**, 256–62.
14. Rosenfeld, L. (1947). Delayed suture of war wounds. *Surgery*, **21**, 200–7.
15. Gottrup, F., Fogdestam, I., and Hunt, T. K. (1982). Delayed primary closure: an experimental and clinical review. *J. Clin. Surg.*, **1**, 113–24.
16. Gottrup, F. (1985). Delayed primary closure of wounds. *Infections in Surgery*, **4**, 171–7.
17. Foisie, P. S. (1946). The results of secondary closure. *New Eng. J. Med.*, **234**, 320–2.
18. Moesgaard, F., Larsen, P. N., Nielsen, M. L., and Hjortrup, A. (1983). New approach to treatment of severe incisional abscesses following laparotomy. *Diseases of the Colon and Rectum*, **26**, 701–2.
19. Gottrup, F., Gjøde, P., Lundhus, E., Holm, C. N., and Terpling, S. (1989). Management of severe incisional abscesses following laparotomy. *Arch. Surg.*, **124**, 702–4.
20. Fogdestam, I. (1980). Delayed primary closure. Thesis, University of Göteborg, Sweden.
21. Stone, H. H. and Hester, T. R. (1972). Topical antibiotic and delayed primary closure in the management of contaminated surgical incisions. *J. Surg. Res.*, **12**, 70–6.
22. Stone, H. H. and Hester, T. R. (1973). Incisional and peritoneal infection after emergency celiotomy. *Ann. Surg.*, **177**, 669–78.
23. Pettigrew, R. A. (1979). Delayed primary wound closure in gangrenous and perforated appendicitis. *Br. J. Surg.*, **68**, 635–8.
24. Stone, H. H., Kolb, L. D., and Geheber, C. E. (1975). Incidence and significance of intraperitoneal anaerobic bacteria. *Ann. Surg.*, **181**, 705–14.
25. Robson, M. C. and Heggers, J. P. (1970). Delayed wound closures based on bacterial counts. *J. Surg. Oncology*, **2**, 379–83.
26. Gottrup, F. and Hunt, T. K. (1982). Antimicrobial prophylaxis in appendectomy patients. *World J. Surg.*, **6**, 306–11.
27. Heaton, L. D., Hughes, C. W., Rosegay, H., Fisher, G. W., and Feighny, R. E. (1966). Military surgical practices of the United States army in Viet Nam. 1–59.
28. Burkhalter, W., Butler, B., Metz, W., and Omer, G. (1968). Experiences with delayed primary closure of war wounds of the hand in Viet Nam. *J. Bone and Joint Surg.*, **50A**, 945–54.
29. Bernard, H. R. and Cole, W. R. (1963). Wound infections following potentially contaminated operations. Effect of delayed primary closure of skin and subcutaneous tissue. *J. Am. Med. Assoc.*, **814**, 118–20.
30. McLachlin, A. D. and Wall, W. J. (1976). Delayed primary closure of the skin and subcutaneous tissue in abdominal surgery. *Can. J. Surg.*, **19**, 37–40.

31. Paul, M. E., Wall, W. J., and Duff, J. H. (1976). Delayed primary closure in colon operations. *Can. J. Surg.*, **19**, 33–6.

32. Voyles, C. R. and Flint, L. M. Jr. (1977). Wound management after trauma to the colon. *South. Med. J.*, **70**, 1067–9.

33. Verrier, E. D., Bossart, K. J., and Heer, F. W. (1979). Reduction of infection rates in abdominal incisions by delayed wound closure technique. *Am. J. Surg.*, **138**, 22–7.

34. DeGennaro, V. A., Corman, H. L., Coller, J. A., Pribek, M. C., and Veidenheimer, M. C. (1978). Wound infections after colectomy. *Dis. Col. Rec.*, **21**, 567–72.

35. Gustilo, R. B. and Andersonj, T. (1976). Prevention of infection in the treatment of 1025 open fractures of long bones. *J. Bone and Joint Surg.*, **58A**, 453–8.

36. Hudspeth, A. S. (1973). Elimination of surgical wound infections by delayed primary closure. *South. Med. J.*, **66**, 934–6.

37. Hermann, G., Bagi, P., and Christoffersen, I. O. (1988). Early secondary suture versus healing by secondary intention of incisional abscesses. *Surg. Gynec. Obstet.*, **167**, 16–18.

38. Lykkegaard-Nielsen, M., Moesgaaard, F., Larsen, P. N., and Hjorttrup, A. (1984). Early reclosure versus conventional secondary suture of severe wound abscesses following laparotomy. *Scand. J. Infect. Dis.*, (Suppl.), **43**, 67–70.

39. Moesgaard, F., Larsen, P. N., Nielsen, R., Christoffersen, S., and Larsen, T. (1988). Economic advantages of treatment of subcutaneous abscesses by incision and primary suture v. conventional open treatment. *Clinical Trials J.*, **25**, 419–23.

40. Fogdestam, J. and Gottrup, F. (1980). Biomechanical methods in wound healing research, with special reference to skin and gastrointestinal tract. In *Biology of collagen*, (ed. S. Viidik and J. Vuust), pp. 363–71. Academic Press, London.

41. Gottrup, F. (1984). Healing of incisional wounds in stomach and duodenum. An experimental study. (Thesis, University of Aarhus.) *Danish Med. Bull.*, **31**, 32–48.

42. Viidik, A. and Gottrup, F. (1986). Mechanics of healing soft tissue wounds. In *Frontiers in Biomechanics*, (ed. G. W. Schmid-Schonbein, S. L. Y. Woo, and B. W. Zweifach), pp. 263–79. Springer, New York.

43. Gottrup, F. (1993). Models for studying physiology and pathophysiology of wound healing and granulation tissue formation in surgical research. In *Animal modelling in surgical research*, (ed. B. Jeppsson). Harwood Academic, Philadelphia.

44. Adamson, R. A., Musco, F., and Engquist, I. F. (1966). The chemical dimension of healing incisions. *Surg. Gynec. Obstet.*, **123**, 515–21.

45. Danielsen, C. C. and Fogdestam, I. (1981). Delayed primary closure. Collagen synthesis and content in healing rat skin incisions. *J. Surg. Res.*, **31**, 210–17.

46. Gottrup, F. (1981). Healing of incisional wounds in stomach and duodenum. Collagen distribution and relation to mechanical strength. *Am. J. Surg.*, **141**, 222–7.

47. Danielsen, C. C. and Gottrup, F. (1981). Healing of incisional wounds in stomach and duodenum. Collagen synthesis. *Eur. Surg. Res.*, **13**, 194–201.

48. Hunt, T. K. and Van Winkle, W. (1979). Normal repair. In *Fundamentals of wound management*, (ed. T. K. Hunt and J. E. Dunphy), pp. 2–67. Appleton-Century-Crofts, New York.

49. Frank, C., Woo, S. L. Y., Amiel, D., Harwood, F., Gomes, M., and Akeson, W. H. (1983). *Am. J. S. Med.*, **11**, 379–89.

50. Hutton, P. and Ferris, B. (1984). Tendons. In *Wound healing for surgeons*, (ed. T. E. Bucknall and H. Ellis), pp. 286–96. accents Tindall, London.

51. Woo, S. L. Y., Gelbermann, R. H., Cobb, N. G., Amiel, D., Lothringer, K., and Akeson, W. H. (1981). *Acta Orthopedica Scandinavica*, **52**, 615–22.

52. Viidik, A. (1975). The 'dynamic' connective tissue. In *Annals of Estonia medical association*, (ed. J. Kauda), pp. 155–69. Förlags A B Eesti Post, Malmö.

53. Fogdestam, I. (1980). Delayed primary closure. An experimental study on the healing of skin incisions. Thesis, University of Göteborg, Sweden.

54. Fogdestam, I. (1981). Biomechanics of healing rat skin incisions. *Surg. Gynec. Obstet.*, **153**, 191–9.

55. Nilsson, T. (1983). Abdominal wound repair. An experimental study of the wound healing mechanism in the rabbit. (Thesis.) *Danish Medical Bulletin*, **30**, 394–407.

56. Thorngate, S. and Ferguson, D. J. (1958). Effect of tension on healing of aponeurotic wounds. *Surg.*, **44**, 619–24.

57. Nilsson, T. (1982). The relative rate of wound healing in longitudinal and transverse laparotomy incisions. *Surg. Gynec. Obstet.*, **148**, 251–6.

58. Leaper, D. J. (1984). Blood vessels. In *Wound healing for surgeons*, (ed. T. E. Bucknall and H. Ellis), pp. 221–40. Bailliere Tindall, London.

59. Gottrup, F. (1993). Experimental tissue trauma and healing in the GI-tract with especial reference to surgery. Harwood Academic, Chur, Switzerland.

60. Morson, B. C. and Dawson, I. M. P. (1979). *Gastrointestinal pathology*, (2nd edn), pp. 125–9. Blackwell Scientific Publications, Oxford.

61. Graham, M. F., Blomquist, P., and Zederfeldt, B. (1992). The alimentary canal. In *Wound healing. Biochemical and clinical aspects*, (ed. I. K. Cohen, R. F. Diegelmann, and W. J. Lindblad), pp. 432–49. Saunders, Philadelphia.

62. Gottrup, F. (1981). Healing of incisional wounds in stomach and duodenum. Functional interaction between normal and wounded tissue. *Am. J. Surg.*, **141**, 706–11.

63. Howes, E. L. and Harvey, S. C. (1929). The strength of the healing wound in relation to the holding strength of the catgut suture. *New Engl. J. Med.*, **200**, 2185–90.

64. Howes, E. L. (1940). The immediate strength of the sutured wound. *Surg.*, **7**, 24–31.

65. Jönsson, K., Jiborn, H., and Zederfeldt, B. (1983). Breaking strength of small intestinal anastomoses. *Am. J. Surg.*, **145**, 800–3.

66. Högstöm, H. and Haglund, U. (1985). Postoperative decrease in suture holding capacity in laparotomy wounds and anastomoses. *Acta Chirurgica Scandinavica*, **151**, 533–5.

67. Wise, L., McAlister, W., Stein, T., and Schuck, P. (1975). Studies on healing of anastomoses of small and large intestines. *Surg. Gynec. Obst.*, **141**, 190–4.

68. Hesp, F. L. E. M., Hendriks, T., Lubbers, E. J. C., and de Boer, H. H. M. (1984). Wound healing in the intestinal wall. A comparison between experimental ilial and colonic anastomoses. *Dis. Col. Rect.*, **27**, 99–104.

69. Murphy, P. (1976). *The neutrophil*. Plenum, New York.

70. Blomquist, P., Jiborn, H., and Zederfeldt, B. (1985). Effect of diverting colostomy on breaking strength of anastomoses after resection of the left side of the colon. *Am. J. Surg.*, **149**, 712–15.

71. Moynihan, B. G. A. (1920). The ritual of a surgical operation. *Br. J. Surg.*, **8**, 27–35.

72. Lister, J. (1881). Presidents Address. *Trans. Clin. Soc. Lond.*, **14**, XLiii–LXiii.

73. Leaper, D. J., Foster, M. E., Brennan, S. S., and Silver, I. A. (1986). The rabbit ear chamber: a study of cell interaction. In *Interaction of cells with natural and foreign substances*, (ed. N. Crawford and D. E. M. Taylor), pp. 221–9. Plenum, New York.

74. Bucknall, T. E., Teare, L., and Ellis, H. (1983). The choice of suture to close abdominal fascia. *Eur. Surg., Res.*, **15**, 59–66.

75. Elek, S. D. and Conen, P. E. (1957). The virulence of *Staphylococcus pyogenes* for man: a study of the problems of wound infection. *Br. J. Exp. Pathol.*, **38**, 573–86.

76. Leaper, D. J. (1994). Instruments and materials. In *General surgical operations*, (ed. R. M. Kirk and R. C. N. Williamson). Churchill Livingstone, Edinburgh.

77. Taylor, F. W. (1938). Surgical knots. *Ann. Surg.*, **107**, 458–68.

78. Douglas, D. M. (1952). The healing of aponeurotic incisions. *Br. J. Surg.*, **40**, 79–84.

79. Lawrie, P., Angus, G. E., and Rees, A. J. M. (1959). The absorption of surgical catgut. *Br. J. Surg.*, **46**, 638–42.

80. Tagart, R. E. B. (1967). The suturing of abdominal incisions. A comparison of monofilament nylon and catgut. *Br. J. Surg.*, **54**, 952–7.

81. Goligher, J. C., Irvin, T.T., Johnston, D., *et al.* (1975). A controlled clinical trial of three methods of closure of laparotomy wounds. *Br. J. Surg.*, **62**, 823–9.

82. Leaper, D. J., Rosenberg, I. L., Evans, M., and Pollock, A. V. (1976). The influence of suture materials on abdominal wall wound healing assessed by controlled clinical trials. *Eur. Surg. Res.*, **8**, 75–6.

83. Leaper, D. J., Pollock, A. V., and Evans, M. E. (1977). Abdominal wound closure: a trial of nylon, polyglycolic acid and steel sutures. *Br. J. Surg.*, **64**, 603–6.

84. Bucknall, T. E. (1981). Abdominal wound closure: choice of suture. *J. Roy. Soc. Med.*, **74**, 580–5.

85. Capperauld, I. and Bucknall, T. E. (1984). Sutures and dressings. In *Wound healing for surgeons*, (ed. T. E. Bucknall and H. Ellis), pp. 78–80. Bailliere Tindall, Eastbourne.

86. Foster, G. E., Hardy, E. G., and Hardcastle, J. D. (1977). Subcuticular suturing after appendicectomy. *Lancet*, **i**, 1128–30.

87. Hermann, J. B., Kelly, R. J., and Higgins, G. A. (1970). Polyglycolic acid sutures: laboratory and clinical evaluation of a new absorbable suture material. *Arch. Surg.*, **100**, 486–90.

88. Craig, P. H., Williams, J. A., Davis, K. W., *et al.* (1975). A biologic comparison of polyglactin and polyglycolic acid synthetic absorbable sutures. *Surg. Gynecol. Obstet.*, **141**, 1–10.

89. Crawford, N. and Taylor, D. E. M. (1986). *Interaction of cells with natural and foreign substances*. Pleneum, New York.

90. Holbrook, M. C. (1982). The resistance of polyglycolic acid sutures to attack by infected human urine. *Br. J. Urol.*, **54**, 313–15.

91. Durdey, P. and Bucknall, T. E. (1984). Assessment of suture materials for use in colonic surgery. *J. Roy. Soc. Med.*, **77**, 472–7.

92. Johnson, A., Rodeheaver, G. T., Durand, L. S., *et al.* (1981). Automatic disposable stapling devices for wound closure. *Ann. Emerg. Med.*, **10**, 631–3.

93. Harrison, I. D., Williams, D. F., and Cuschieri, A. (1975). The effect of metal clips on the tensile property of healing skin wounds. *Br. J. Surg.*, **62**, 945–9.

94. Forrester, J. C., Zederfeldt, B. H., Hayes, T. L., and Hunt, T. K. (1970). Tape-closed and sutured wounds: a comparison by tensiometry and scanning electron microscopy. *Br. J. Surg.*, **57**, 729–36.

95. Rodeheaver, G. T., Halversen, J. H., and Edlich, R. F. (1983). Mechanical performance of wound closure tapes. *Ann. Emerg. Med.*, **12**, 203–6.

96. Jenkins, T. P. N. (1976). The burst abdominal wound: a mechanical approach. *Br. J. Surg.*, **63**, 873–6.

97. Adamsons, R. J., Musco, F., and Enquist, I. F. (1966). The chemical dimensions of a healing incision. *Surg. Gynecol. Obstet.*, **123**, 515–21.

98. Hopkinson, G. B. and Bullen, B. R. (1982). Removable subcuticulo skin suture in acute appendicitis. *Br. Med. J.*, **284**, 869.

99. Simpson, J. E. P., Ornstein, M., Spicer, C. C., and Cox, A. G. (1979). Hypertrophic scarring: Dexon suture in a randomised trial. *Br. J. Surg.*, **66**, 281–2.

100. Leaper, D. J. and Benson, C. E. (1985). A controlled trial of polypropylene or polydioxanone sutures for subcuticular skin suture after inguinal surgery. *J. Roy. Coll. Surg. Ed.*, **30**, 234–6.

101. Jorgensen, P. H., Jensen, K. H., and Andreassen, T. T. (1987). Mechanical strength in rat skin incisional wounds treated with a fibrin sealant. *J. Surg. Res.*, **42**, 237–41.

102. Spotnitz, W. D., Dalton, M. S., Baker, J. W., *et al.* (1987). Reduction of perioperative haemorrhage by anterior mediastinal spray application of fibrin glue during cardiac operations. *Ann. Thor. Surg.*, **44**, 529–33.

103. Marable, S. A. and Wagner, D. E. (1962). The use of rapidly polymerising adhesives in massive liver resections. *Surg. Forum.*, **13**, 264–70.

104. Edlich, R.F., Rodeheaver, G., Thacker, J. G., and Edgerton, M. T. (1979). Technical factors in wound management. In *Fundamentals of wound management*, (ed. T. K. Hunt and J. E. Dunphy). Appleton-Century-Crofts, New York.

105. Hasselgren, P. O., Hagberg, E., Malmer, H., *et al.* (1984). One instead of two knives for surgical incision. Does it increase the risk of postoperative wound infection? *Arch. Surg.*, **119**, 917–21.

106. Cruse, P. J. E. and Foord, R. (1973). A five-year prospective study of 23 649 surgical wounds. *Arch. Surg.*, **107**, 206–10.

5

Experimental models in wound healing

H. P. EHRLICH and F. GOTTRUP

Introduction

Tissue injury resulting in irreversible cell death and connective tissue disruption initiates the repair process. The number of causes that produce tissue injury and tissue loss outnumber the responses the host has to repair the defect. In a superficial injury, where only the epidermal surface is damaged and destroyed (such as a sun burn), the repair process is limited to cellular replacement. Through a process of epidermal cell migration and duplication, the defect is resurfaced in a regenerative manner in the absence of scarring. In contrast, with deeper tissue loss where the connective tissue matrix is destroyed, healing occurs by scarring with the introduction of new cell populations residing in a newly constructed connective tissue matrix and having a new blood supply. The chemical components of a scar are similar to those which make up the normal dermis surrounding the defect, but the organization of the scar connective tissue components differs from that of normal dermis. The inability to reassemble the connective tissue components identically to normal dermis designates that scar tissue has been formed.

One of the initial reactions in the repair process is the re-establishment of homeostasis by the process of coagulation. The acute inflammatory response follows, which protects the host from microbial infection, clears the wound site of debris, and signals the next phase of the repair process. The proliferative phase of repair, with the infiltration of fibroblasts into the wound site, is characterized by an accumulation of a high density of fibroblasts, the ingrowth of new blood vessels, and the deposition of a new connective tissue matrix. These components make up granulation tissue which is the transitional matrix that matures into scar tissue. During the remodelling phase of repair the density of fibroblasts diminishes, the number of blood vessels declines, and the connective tissue matrix undergoes a reorganization whereby the fine collagen fibrils condense into thicker, more dense fibres. The completion of the repair process, a scar, is represented as a newly organized connective tissue matrix composed of collagen fibres arranged in lines parallel to the skin surface, a modest cell number, and sparse density of blood vessels. The epidermal surface of the scar lacks the ingrowth of rete pegs into the underlying connective tissue matrix. There is no regeneration of lost subepidermal appendages, such as hair follicles, in scar.

Biochemical considerations of the repair process

The major biochemical components of the repair process include DNA from cell proliferation, RNA for the coding of new messenger RNA, and amino acid incorporation into newly synthesized proteins. Since the deposition of a new connective tissue matrix is the major component of a scar, changes in its protein composition is a means to follow the progress of the repair process. Collagen is the major protein unit that makes up the fibres of the new connective tissue matrix of the scar. The collagen molecule is composed of three polypeptide chains each having a 95 000 Da molecular weight and a glycine residue at every third amino acid. These three chains are wrapped together in a triple helical configuration. This arrangement of the polypeptide chains gives great rigidity to the basic molecule unit. These rigid rods self-assemble into collagen fibrils which are also quite rigid and have great tensile strength. There are numerous different types of collagen based upon the amino acid composition of their polypeptide chains. Currently more than 16 types of collagens based upon unique gene products have been reported (1). In granulation and scar tissue matrices, types I and III collagens make up about 95 per cent of the collagen. The proportions of types I and III collagens vary. In normal dermis type III collagen makes up 20 per cent of the matrix, in granulation tissue 30 per cent is type III collagen, and in mature scar tissue it is reduced to 10 per cent (2, 3). Besides these differences in the proportion of collagen types between dermis, granulation tissue, and scar, the organization of collagen fibres also differs. With dermis, the collagen fibres are arranged in a basket weave pattern; in granulation tissue, collagen is in fine filaments arranged in random arrays; and in scar, collagen fibres are organized parallel to the skin surface. Though collagen molecules can self-assemble under physiological conditions into collagen fibrils, the further organization of these fibrils into fibres requires cellular interventions. The cellular organization of collagen fibres is important for the integrity of a scar in terms of volume, stability, and strength. Changes in the collagen content of a healing wound can be monitored by the concentration changes of the imino acid, hydroxyproline (hyp). Hyp is a post-translational modification of peptide-bound proline within collagen polypeptide chains. As the number of hyp residues increases in the polypeptide chains, the tighter and more rigid the triple helical configuration of the molecule becomes. With types I and III collagens, about 10 per cent of the amino acid residues are hyp. The quantity of connective tissue deposited at a healing wound site can be monitored by its hyp content. To measure tissue hyp, the tissue is hydrolysed in 6 N hydrochloric acid in a sealed tube with a nitrogen-enriched atmosphere at 108°C for 18 h. The hydrolysate is assayed for hyp using either a colorimetric method (4) or a column chromatographic method (5).

To quantify the collagen types in wound healing, the best technique is cyanogen bromide (CnBr) digestion and peptide analysis. Other methods of solubilizing collagen and analysing the denatured polypeptide chains are restricted because of the variability of the solubility of collagen as granulation tissue matures. With CnBr digestion, consistently greater than 95 per cent of the tissue will be solubilized. Fresh tissue is placed in a sealable tube containing a five-fold greater volume of degassed 70 per cent formic acid. A volume of solid CnBr equivalent to the tissue is added, the tube sealed under vacuum, and incubated at 42°C for 4 h. The CnBr digest is diluted in 20 volumes of distilled water, frozen, and lyophilized to dryness. The dried residue is redissolved in water, frozen, and relyophilized. The dried material is weighed, dissolved in water at 10 mg/ml, and stored as a solution. The analysis of the CnBr peptides can be done by column chromatography separation (6) or by polyacrylamide gel electrophoresis (PAGE) (3).

Histological considerations of the repair process

The histology of a healing wound changes rapidly over the initial three weeks post-trauma. Initially, the wound site is filled with fibrin filaments and wound debris. At the wound edges, populations of inflammatory cells accumulate, particularly neutrophils initially, followed by macrophages later. Macrophages and fibroblasts enter the wound site and, utilizing the fibrin filaments as highways, repopulate the necrotic wound site. In time, the density of fibroblasts increases within the repair site from about day 4 until about day 14. After day 14 the density of fibroblasts in the repair site diminishes. Granulation tissue is generated from synthesis of a new connective tissue matrix by the fibroblasts. This transitional tissue, early granulation tissue, has a great density of fibroblasts and an extensive build up of a new blood vessel network. As time goes on there is an increase in the accumulation of collagen fibres in the granulation tissue, as determined by stains such as Sirius red stain, and a decline in cell numbers and blood vessel density.

Standard haemotoxylin and eosin staining will demonstrate the changes in the cell populations in granulation tissue in the initial stages of healing and later as there is maturation into scar. Using immunohistological staining techniques changes in the presence, location, or density of specific cell types such as macrophages, endothelial cells, myofibroblasts, lymphocytes, and mast cells can be followed during the early development and later maturation of granulation tissue. The connective tissue matrix of granulation tissue is undergoing change as that tissue matures, and the progress of collagen fibres at the wound edges can be followed as the volume of scar needed to repair the defect, which is minimal in wounds healing by the first intention.

Sutured closed wounds in experimental animals show that wound breaking strength is about 3 per cent of its final obtainable strength at one week, a time when sutures are commonly removed. The final breaking strength of an incisional wound is about 80 per cent of that of intact skin. The inability of a scar to obtain the equivalent strength of skin may be based on the suboptimal organization of the collagen fibres in the newly formed scar and a weakness in the splice between the new scar tissue collagen fibres and the old dermal collagen fibres. The re-weaving of the collagen fibres at the interface between the old and new tissues is incomplete and breaking strength testing of such wounds causes them to separate at that junction.

The breaking strength of an anastomosis in rabbit intestine is manifested as a rupture in the intestinal wall adjacent to the suture line (7). The weakest area in the intestinal repair is not at the suture line but in the intestinal wall distant from it. A weakness in the intestinal wall develops because collagen is lost in that weakened area due to an increased local collagenolytic activity. The speculation is that a portion of the released collagen is recruited to the suture line and re-utilized in the developing scar. The concept of intact collagen re-utilization has been proposed and studies have been reported (8). Radioisotope studies demonstrate that intact collagen is recruited to the wound site and that collagen is incorporated into the developing scar tissue. Wound breaking strength can be studied in skin incision wounds (9) or in modified sponge implants where the sponge implant is cut in half and the halves re-approximated prior to implantation (10).

Implant models

The examination of granulation tissue and wound fluid is facilitated by implanting a chamber or sponge in a subcutaneous pocket. A wound chamber is a hollow tube implant which operates as a dead space, where granulation tissue develops at the periphery of the chamber and the central reservoir is filled with wound fluid. These chambers are commonly made of stainless steel mesh and can be implanted in rabbits (11). Repeated wound fluid samples can be taken from such implanted chambers. Reliable samples can be obtained from wound chambers after seven days and continued sampling can be carried out for more than four weeks. In this experimental study a single rabbit was maintained in the vivarium with implanted wound chambers for seven months. These chambers were harvested and found to retain a central cavity surrounded by a thick capsule. A single large vein occupied the centre of the chamber cavity with some branches incorporated into the capsule tissue at the chamber edges.

These wound chambers have been used in a variety of experiments to determine the metabolic state as the repair process proceeds (12), the release of factors in response to burn or freeze trauma (13), and obtain activated macrophages for *in vitro* studies (14). These wound chambers offer the advantage of frequent sampling of wound fluid and the harvesting of large quantities of granulation tissue. The disadvantage is their size and the time required to obtain harvestable granulation tissue.

The sponge implant is a popular technique for the study of granulation tissue deposition and how it is related to wound healing. The polyvinyl alcohol (PVA) sponge implant is the most commonly used material. The PVA sponge implant is very useful for histological evaluations as well as biochemical analysis of granulation tissue. It can be used for wound breaking strength experiments as well (10, 15).

The organization of collagen into thick fibres and their further stabilization with covalent cross-links is critical for the continued gain in wound breaking strength and the increasing integrity of the scar. The organization of collagen fibres in scars differs from collagen fibre organization in dermis (Fig. 5.1). The collagen fibres of scar tissue are thinner in diameter and tend to be organized parallel to the skin surface. Dermal collagen fibres are organized in a 'basket weave' pattern with fibres running parallel as well as perpendicular to the skin surface. Scar collagen fibres never develop a basket weave pattern identical to that seen in intact dermis.

The collagen fibre organization of hypertrophic scar and keloid differ from that seen in normal scar (16). Hypertrophic scars have nodular structures; keloids do not have these structures. The collagen on the surface of the hypertrophic scar nodule is arranged in parallel sheets like that of an onion skin. The collagen within the centre of the nodule is composed of fine, disorganized fibrils which appear similar to collagen in

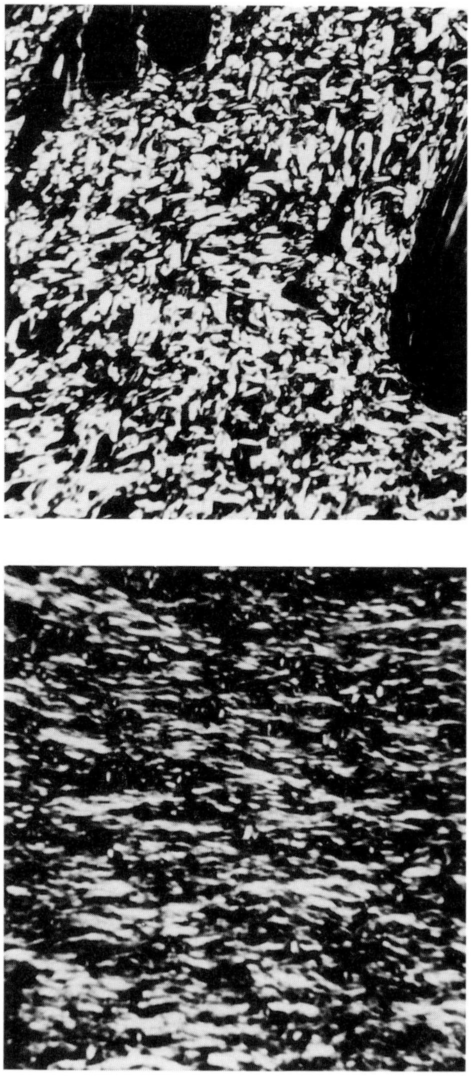

(a)

(b)

Fig. 5.1 Rat skin and scar biopsies were excised, fixed, and processed for polarized light microscopy (for details see ref. 16): (a) shows the birefringence pattern of normal adult rat dermis, having thick collagen bundles arranged in a basket weave pattern; (b) shows a healed wound scar of an adult rat harvested seven weeks after injury. The collagen fibres are arranged in moderately thick bundles that run parallel to the skin surface. Magnification ×120.

early granulation tissue. Keloids, which lack nodules, have their collagen fibres arranged in thick bands composed of numerous fine collagen fibrils running parallel to one another (16).

Tensiometry

Wound bursting strength is the measure of progress in the repair of sutured wounds healing by first intention. The gain in wound breaking strength is the force required to disrupt or pull apart the edges of the wound. During the initial two weeks of repair the gain in wound breaking strength parallels the quantity of collagen deposited within the wound site. After two weeks the collagen content of the wound does not increase but wound breaking strength continues to rise. That increase is due to an increase in the proportion of insoluble collagen as a consequence of the synthesis of intra- and intermolecular chemical, covalent, collagen cross-links (17). Besides the insolubility of collagen and the formation of chemical covalent cross-links, the increasing thickening of the newly deposited collagen fibres is also important for the continued gain in wound breaking strength (18). The animal model which is closest to the human for studying the modulations and alterations in wound breaking strength is the rat where experimental wound breaking strength measurements are similar to those in man (19).

Intact skin tensile strength has been shown to correlate to its insoluble collagen content. The daily injection of cortisol to male rats will reduce the soluble collagen content of intact skin but increase the insoluble collagen content as well as tensile strength in intact skin (20). In contrast, with wound repair, the systemic introduction of cortisol will inhibit collagen deposition and the gain in wound breaking strength (9). Likewise blocking the formation of covalent collagen cross-links will inhibit the gain in wound breaking strength (21). Thyroid hormone, oestrogen, vitamin E, and ascorbate are other agents that also inhibit this gain in strength (22).

It has been reported that the addition of soluble collagen or cartilage powder to wounds will increase wound breaking strength (15, 23). Peptide growth factors such as transforming growth factor (TGF) and platelet derived growth factor (PDGF) have been shown to stimulate wound healing and enhance the gain in wound breaking strength during the initial two weeks of repair (24, 25). The stimulating effects of most factors is lost after two weeks and the levels of wound breaking strength of treated and controls are equivalent. This implies that the initial stimulation of wound breaking strength is due to a rise in collagen deposition, but the continued organization of that collagen and increasing fibre integrity are responsible for final wound breaking strength.

Healing open wounds (culture systems)

A deep open defect which occupies an area too large to approximate the wound edges heals by secondary intention. Healing such a defect requires a large volume of new connective tissue, epithelialization for resurfacing and closing of the defect, and wound contraction to reduce the volume of scar tissue required to fill the defect. During the proliferative phase of repair, granulation tissue fills up the defect which has a high density of fibroblasts, an immature connective tissue matrix, and no epidermal surface. A large volume of granulation tissue fills a healing wound. This well vascularized, densely cell populated, collagen-rich transitional tissue is a barrier to microbial invasion and supports the migration of epidermal cells. The appearance of red coloured granulation tissue filling an open defect indicates the healing process is progressing through the proliferative phase of repair. The over-abundance of granulation tissue contributes to the formation of hypertrophic scars.

The remodelling phase of open wound repair involves wound contraction where intact surrounding skin is pulled into and over the defect by cellular forces generated within the granulation tissue. Wound contraction is more evident in certain areas of the body, examples being the back of the neck and buttocks (26). The closure of open wounds by wound contraction is desirable, since the volume of scar is reduced and skin fills a major portion of the defect. In contrast to wound contraction, the process of scar contracture, with the compaction of scar tissue, occurs late in the remodelling phase of repair and when wounds are completely closed by epithelialization. Wound contraction occurs early in the repair process, when open wounds are not closed by epithelialization.

Many proposals have been presented to explain the mechanism of wound contraction (27). The concept of cell-generated forces being responsible for wound contraction was introduced by Abercrombie and colleagues (28). The cellular forces are generated by the sliding of cytoplasmic actin-myocin filaments are part of microfilaments in response to myosin ATPase activity. The rearrangement of collagen fibrils by these cellular forces produces the pulling that moves the surrounding skin into the defect. If the surrounding skin is tightly locked in place and the granulation tissue-generated forces are not great enough to move that skin, then no wound contraction occurs. If, on the other hand, the skin is loosely attached to the underlying tissue, then the granulation tissue's cellular forces will translocate the skin. In loose-skinned laboratory animals, such as the rat, an excisional wound on the back closes by 50 per cent in 7 days, and by 21 days the wound is completely closed with a small residual scar.

There have been discussions concerning the cellular mechanism of wound contraction and whether a specialized cell, the myofibroblast, is responsible for contraction. Majno and Gabbiani were the first to describe the presence of the myofibroblast in contracting, 7 day old, excisional rat wounds (29). The myofibroblast is a differentiated fibroblast with a high density of thick cytoplasmic stress fibres composed of aggregates of microfilaments. These stress fibres contain alpha smooth muscle actin, an isoform of actin present in contractile cells such as arterial smooth muscle cells, but absent in dermal fibroblasts (30). It is proposed that myofibroblasts, which are present as sheets of cells in high density within maturing granulation tissue, have numerous cell-to-cell contacts and that a synchronized, multicellular contraction occurs which translocates the surrounding collagen fibrils. The proposed myofibroblast mechanism for wound contraction is based upon a multicellular contraction unit which reorganizes collagen fibres. Another proposal is that cell-generated 'locomotion' forces translocate the organized collagen fibrils (31). The myofibroblast is assumed to be a differentiated fibroblast which is no longer actively involved in generating the contractile forces for ongoing wound contraction. The less differentiated fibroblast is proposed as the cell responsible for generating the force required for wound contraction.

The experimental evidence for cells' locomotion forces organizing collagen is based upon *in vitro* and *in vivo* studies.

Myofibroblasts are not identified in rat wounds until day 7 post-wounding, a time at which 50 per cent of the wound area has been reduced by wound contraction (32). During the initial 7 days of wound contraction, some cell other than a myofibroblast generates the forces of wound contraction. The contraction of excisional wounds in the tight skin (Tsk) mouse showed a three week delay in the initiation of wound contraction (33). Histologically the granulation tissue of the non-contracted wound was rich in myofibroblasts. The Tsk mouse wounds begin to contract after 21 days and contract at a rate equal to normal mouse wound contraction. Hence the inhibition of wound contraction in the Tsk mouse is a delay in the initiation of the process. During the first week of re-established wound contraction in the Tsk mouse, myofibro-

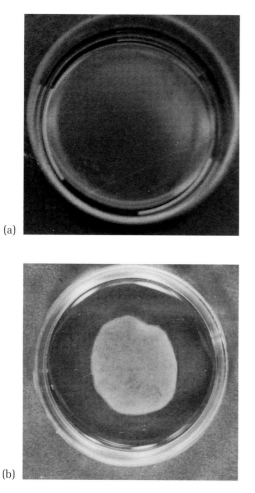

(a)

(b)

Fig. 5.2 A fibroblast populated collagen lattice (FPCL) was manufactured with 40 000 human dermal fibroblasts and 1.25 mg of rat tail tendon, acid extracted, salt purified collagen per millilitre of DMEM supplemented with 10% fetal bovine serum. A total volume of 2.0 ml of the mixture was pipetted into a 35 mm Petri dish which was transferred to a 37°C incubator, where the collagen polymerized, entrapping the cells in a collagen matrix. (a) shows a newly cast polymerized FPCL (time 0) which fills the entire 35 mm Petri dish. (b) shows that same FPCL 2 h later when the FPCL has decreased in size – referred to as lattice contraction.

blasts are not present in the granulation tissue. Fibroblasts are the major cell population present during the delayed initiation of wound contraction. At 5 weeks, when wound contraction is more than 50 per cent completed, the myofibroblasts reappear. It is proposed that myofibroblasts dedifferentiate back into fibroblasts in order to organize collagen fibres and produce the contractile forces needed for wound contraction.

In vitro studies have used the fibroblast-populated collagen lattice (FPCL) model, introduced by Bell and his co-workers, to study the cellular organization of collagen (34). To manufacture an FPCL, a suspension of cultured fibroblasts is placed in a Petri dish in medium containing serum and soluble collagen, at 37°C. The collagen polymerizes, trapping the cells in the rapidly forming matrix. Within 24 h of manufacture the FPCL is reduced in size, which is referred to as lattice contraction (Fig. 5.2). Experimentation has demonstrated that individual cells located in the more central regions of the lattice produce the forces of lattice contraction through cell locomotion rather than cell contraction (31).

Polarized light optics demonstrate that fibroblast organization of collagen in FPCL produces birefringent collagen fibres. The mechanism for lattice contraction is fibroblast translocation of collagen fibrils and their organization into thicker fibres. The collagen make-up of the FPCL influences the rate and degree of lattice contraction. The greater the concentration of collagen the less contraction; the greater the number of cells the more contraction (34). FPCLs made with type III collagen contract faster, and to a greater degree, than lattices made with type I collagen (35). It should be noted that granulation tissue, which generates the forces of wound contraction, is enriched in type III collagen (2).

The functioning of the fibroblast's cytoskeletal machinery is required for translocation of collagen fibrils. Agents which disrupt the functioning of microfilaments, actin polymerization, or depolymerisation, or myosin ATPase activity, inhibit lattice contraction. Cytochalasins and phalloidin disrupt actin polymerization and both of these agents inhibit lattice contraction (34). Myosin ATPase is required for the generation of contractile forces in actin–myosin filaments and its activity is regulated by the phosphorylation of its associated myosin light chains (36). Elevating the level of intracellular cAMP prevents the phosphorylation of myosin light chains and inhibits lattice contraction (37). Disruption of microtubule polymerization by colchicine also inhibits lattice contraction (34). The attachment of collagen fibrils to the fibroblast cell surface involves the $\alpha_2\beta_1$ integrin (38). Application of antibodies to this integrin blocks collagen attachment to the cell and inhibits lattice contraction.

Measurement of tissue perfusion and tissue oxygenation

Peripheral tissue perfusion and tissue oxygenation is vital for the metabolic processes of cells because 95 per cent of body energy is generated by aerobic pathways. Whilst the stores of energy resources are normally adequate for long term starving, the entire oxygen store of the body would only support resting needs for a maximum of 5 minutes (39). Continuous delivery of an adequate volume of oxygen and a sufficient partial pressure for cell metabolism therefore is critical for normal tissue function. The consequences of inadequate oxygen delivery are that cellular metabolism is disturbed leading to hypoxia and aerobic conditions, followed by a decreased resistance to infection and impaired wound healing (40). Monitoring of tissue perfusion and maintaining oxygen supply therefore is of importance in all types of patients.

Routine clinical evaluation of peripheral perfusion has been based on blood pressure, cardiac output, urine output, skin temperature, and capillary return. Routine measurements of haemodynamic variables such as systemic blood pressure (MAP), heart rate, pulmonary artery pressure (PAP), cardiac output (CO), and mixed venous blood oxygenation are performed in critically ill patients in order to evaluate peripheral tissue perfusion. These measurements, however, are indirect indices of perfusion and little is known to what extent the peripheral tissue oxygenation is fulfilling the demand for oxygen in peripheral tissues. Tissue oxygenation is a result of two main factors: oxygen delivery (D_{O_2}) and oxygen consumption (V_{O_2}), and the supply/demand ratio (D_{O_2}/V_{O_2}) becomes, from a physiological point of view, of great interest. Measuring oxygen delivery and oxygen consumption are cumbersome, time consuming, of questionable accuracy, and difficult to apply in routine clinical situations. Clinical evaluation of systemic blood pressure, pulse rate, and urine output has been found to be a poor assessment of tissue perfusion (41). A system is required which permits monitoring of the cardio-respiratory status and adequacy of tissue oxygenation in all tissues of the body. In clinical practice few, if any, methods achieve this goal. A reason may be that tissue perfusion and tissue oxygenation are poorly established concepts. Most clinicians equate tissue perfusion with blood flow or oxygen delivery, while others have a combined concept of blood flow and nutritional supply, including oxygen. The concept of tissue oxygen perfusion (TOP) has been suggested for this reason (40). This parameter permits monitoring of both tissue perfusion and oxygenation, and is a measure of the ability of the central cardiovascular system to deliver an adequate volume of oxygen to the periphery to meet the metabolic demands of the tissues.

Many monitoring systems have been claimed to evaluate peripheral perfusion and tissue oxygenation. Few have been employed in clinical practice and are of unproven use in relation to wound healing. The following techniques are presently available:

(1) laser Doppler flowmetry
(2) pulse oximetry
(3) tissue oxygen tension measurements.

Laser Doppler flowmetry (LDV)

This technique was introduced 20 years ago (42) to measure skin blood flow and is based on the principle that light scattered by moving particles, mainly erythrocytes, undergoes a shift in frequency compared with light reflected by non-moving structures (43). This frequency shift may be used to evaluate the quantity of blood moving in tissue. The method has been refined with better signal-to-noise ratio and has become clinically useful (44, 45).

Laser Doppler flowmetry has been applied to measurement of perfusion in different types of tissue, such as skin; gastric blood flow; and graft viability in plastic surgery (40). LDV provides information only about relative changes in perfusion rather than absolute values of blood flow. In skin it has also been difficult to determine which part of the microcirculation produces the signal, and probably only a small fraction of the recorded signal is due to blood flow in skin capillaries. In patients with peripheral vascular disorders marked discrepancies between total circulation, measured by laser Doppler techniques, and vital capillary microscopy have been recorded (46).

The advantage of LDV is that this method is non-invasive and continuous and can be used on any body surface. The major disadvantage is that it does not measure tissue oxygenation and therefore does not fulfil TOP. Other disadvantages are that depth resolution has not been clarified, that blood flow may be altered due to tissue compression or mechanical stimulation, and that absolute figures or values of blood flow cannot be provided.

Pulse oximetry

This method is based on a combination of an optical method for measuring oxygen and photoplethysmography which enables the assessment of oxygen saturation in pulsating arterial blood. Several techniques have been developed for pulse oximetry measurement (47).

The primary use of pulse oximetry has been in intensive care units and during anaesthesia. The method is an important tool for evaluating the function of the lung related to transport of oxygen from the respiratory tract to arterial blood. Evaluation of blood saturation is easily performed using probes placed non-invasively on fingertips, ear lobes, or other peripheral sites. The measurement and interpretation is easy, and constant results with high accuracy are obtained.

Pulse oximetry has also been suggested for measurement of tissue perfusion with interpretation of the plethysmographic pulse curve and therapy and thereby to be another non-invasive method for assessing circulatory function (47). Evaluation of tissue perfusion using this method has not proved to be of value in routine clinical use. The methods cannot indicate the quality of oxygen transport and tissue oxygenation, and during hypoperfusion pulse oximetry reveals only the quality of oxygen uptake, providing a value of 93 per cent saturation when tissue oxygen tension is decreased to less than 20 per cent of baseline values (48). It is not possible to distinguish an oxygen saturation of 100 or 500 mmHg (13 or 67 kPa) or more in the presence of 98–100 per cent saturation. At low oxygen saturation there are other limitations (49, 50).

This method has advantages in being a continuous, non-invasive procedure with high accuracy. The disadvantages are that it provides only information on arterial oxygen saturation, reflecting only the quality of oxygen uptake of the

Table 5.1 Methods for evaluation of peripheral perfusion

Laser Doppler velocimetry
Post-capillary venous pressure measurements
Skin temperature measurements
Vital capillary microscopy
Pulse oximetry
Intramural pH measurements in stomach and bowel
Tissue oxygen tension measurements
Other methods
    Nuclear magnetic resonance spectroscopy
    Infrared techniques for cytochrome a_3

lungs. No information regarding oxygen transport, tissue oxygenation, and the oxygen supply and demand relationship is obtained.

Tissue oxygen tension measurements

The most important criterion on which to judge oxygen supply to organ tissues is the cellular oxygen partial pressure (51). The cell wall has no barrier to oxygen and the interstitial fluid close to the cell has the same partial pressure as the inside of the cell. Measurement of tissue oxygen tension, therefore, can be used to evaluate TOP. This measurement has not become routine because of methodological problems, but recent developments allow clinical measurements to be made, both invasively and non-invasively. In patients where information on general tissue perfusion oxygenation is desired, measurements can be performed in subcutaneous tissue. Subcutaneous tissues are the first type of tissue to suffer during hypovolaemia and appear to be the best for measurement of peripheral perfusion and oxygenation (52). The theory that subcutaneous tissue is representative of perfusion states of other peripheral tissues has been tested by means of microsphere technology (53). When tissue oxygen tension is normal and responding to changes in external oxygen tension, it can be assumed that perfusion and oxygenation of all other tissues and organs is also normal. After haemorrhage, tissue oxygen tension returns to normal only after blood has been reinfused (48, 54). If a low oxygen tension has returned to normal it can be assumed that perfusion and oxygenation of the tissue may be adequate. Recent work has shown that tissue oxygen measurement in the subcutaneous tissue is an important parameter for observation of tissue perfusion and oxygenation experimentally, as well as in clinical practice (41, 54–57). Tissue oxygen tension in subcutaneous tissue has been shown to be dependent on both cardiac output and tissue perfusion, normovolaemia, and hypovolaemia; a close relationship to oxygen delivery/oxygen consumption ratios has also been found (58).

Tissue oxygen tension measurement in subcutaneous tissue is a measure of TOP in experimental and clinical practice. The advantages of this method are that it is continuous, simple, rapid, and relatively cheap. Measuring the net result of oxygen supply and demand of the tissues, it fulfils the criteria of TOP and may also be a predictor of postoperative complications. The disadvantages of the method are that to obtain direct measurements of tissue perfusion and oxygenation in some tissues it is invasive.

Basic principles of measuring tissue oxygen tension

A variety of techniques are available to measure wound oxygen tension, each having special properties and limitations (Table 5.1).

The best proved method for measuring tissue oxygen tension is polarographic. This principle is based on an electrode system having a noble metal (gold or platinum) as a cathode and reference electrode of silver/silver chloride. The resulting current flow in the system is proportional to the number of oxygen molecules reduced and to the partial pressure of oxygen of the solution (59). This system has been available for more than 50 years, but was not useful until 1956 when Clark (60) placed a cathode adjacent to the anode in an electrolyte solution behind an oxygen-permeable polyethylene membrane, thus solving the problem of 'protein poisoning'. The advantages of this technique are that it has been used for many years, it is relatively easy to handle, and the sensor and monitor are relatively small and cheap. The disadvantages are 'drift' during use (with need for frequent calibration, temperature dependence, sensitivity to movement, and sensitivity to anaesthetic agents, notably halothane).

The basic principle of mass spectrometry is gas diffusion through a permeable membrane located at the end of a probe placed in a tissue. In the mass spectrometer the gas mixture is separated and measured quantitatively according to molecular weight. The advantage of this method is that it can measure several tissue gases and the recording is stable. The disadvantages are that the response time is long and the method consumes oxygen from the tissues during the measuring procedure. Furthermore, the system is large and expensive.

The third major system for measuring tissue oxygen in tissue is optical fluorescence. This principle is based on the sensitivity of certain fluorescent dyes to quenching by oxygen. The optical sensors in this system are called optodes. Recently a fibre optic sensor containing an optical fibre with a dye incorporated has been developed for measuring oxygen in blood (61). This type of optode has been used for measuring oxygen directly, particularly in subcutaneous tissue. The advantages of the optical fluorescent system are that no oxygen is consumed during the measurements; that it is probably not influenced by protein in the tissue; it is not sensitive to movement; and it requires less frequent calibration. Although

Table 5.2 Basic principles of measuring tissue oxygen tension

Polarographic
Mass spectrometry
Optical fluorescence
Others
    Gas chromatography
    Radioactive oxygen
    Magnetic resonance imaging
    Radioisotope imaging

Table 5.3 Methods of measuring tissue oxygen tension

Direct, in tissue	Wire mesh cylinders
	Microelectrodes
	Tonometer
Indirect, on surfaces	Transcutaneous
	Conjunctival
	Trans-serosal

optodes are temperature-sensitive instruments, they can be compensated internally. The main disadvantage is that the system is still being developed and has not been used in clinical practice. Other methods for measuring tissue oxygen tension are under further development (Table 5.2).

The goal of measuring tissue oxygen tension is to obtain a true value of oxygen tension during all physiological and pathological conditions. To achieve this in different tissues and organs two fundamental methods are available: direct measurement in tissue itself and indirect measurement on tissue surfaces (Table 5.3).

Direct measurement of tissue oxygen tension

Tissue oxygen tension can be measured directly in different ways. Microelectrodes with a 1–5 µm diameter have been used by Silver (62) to measure oxygen tension in the rabbit ear chamber. This microelectrode can provide a profile of tissue oxygen but multiple measurements have to be made if a mean value of tissue oxygen is wanted. In order to measure a reproducible oxygen tension measurement with a sensor, a certain area of tissue, including several capillaries, must be investigated. The sensor must either be placed directly in the tissue (coated, in order not to be contaminated by protein) (Fig. 5.3), or placed inside a Silastic tissue tonometer (1 mm outer

diameter, 0.8 mm inner diameter) implanted in the tissue (63). The values of tissue tonometry measurements are based on a single integrated mean of tissue oxygen tension (64). Perfusion of anoxic saline through the tonometer with measurement of the equilibrated saline in a Clark gas monitor system or in a chamber with a membrane-covered transcutaneous oxygen electrode has been used to investigate different types of tissue (55, 65, 66). As single electrodes, both the polarographic electrode and the optode based on optical fluorescence are available. For implantation of the tonometer an 18-gauge spinal needle is used while only a 21-gauge needle is needed for placing the sensor or optode directly into the tissue, which is even less traumatic than inserting an intravenous cannula. After insertion of such a needle only 2–3 h are needed before normalization of the microcirculation following insertion (67).

Indirect measurement of tissue oxygen tension

These methods are non-invasive and measure oxygen tension through a tissue surface. Three types of measurement have been used both experimental and clinically: transcutaneous, conjunctival, and trans-serosal.

Transcutaneous oxygen tension is based on a Clark polarographic electrode containing a heating element and a thermistor. The electrode must be heated to 43–44°C in order to produce measurable oxygen tension values and this value will, in most situations, closely approximate the blood values of the dilated underlying capillaries. This technique has been used for evaluating arterial oxygen tension and as an indicator of amputation levels in patients with vascular diseases and of healing in chronic leg ulcers (68–70).

Conjunctival oxygen tension and trans-serosal oxygen tension are based on measurements taken where the barrier to oxygen diffusion is only a few cell layers thick and there is

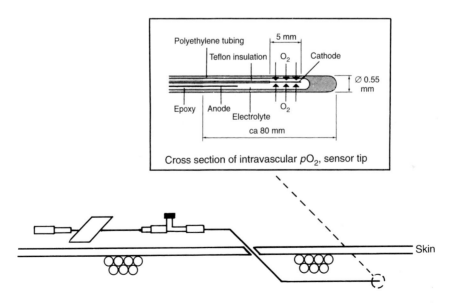

Fig. 5.3 A schematic drawing of a coated polarographic oxygen sensor placed in the subcutaneous tissue. The catheter is only 0.55 mm in diameter.

local temperature control, therefore no heating is needed. Both types of sensors normally consist of a membrane-covered polarographic electrode and a thermistor. The conjunctival sensor is placed on a specially designed ophthalmic conformer of a material used in the manufacture of hard contact lenses (Fig. 5.4). This method has been used to evaluate arterial oxygen tension, the oxygen delivery to the brain, and during unstable haemodynamic conditions, as an indicator of TOP (48, 71). Different types of trans-serosal oxygen tension measuring techniques have been developed. Typically the system consists of a membrane-covered Clark electrode and a thermistor. This system is constructed as a small electrode directly applied by hand on the surface of an organ during abdominal surgery (Fig. 5.5). This method has been used for predicting failure of colonic anastomotic healing (72–75). Recently a vacuum-fixed electrode has been tested for oxygen tension measurements in the gastrointestinal tract (76).

Conclusions

Survival of an organism depends upon its ability to recover function following trauma. In lower animals the recovery of function is based upon regenerative repair. A lost limb will be replaced with a new one. At the other end of the animal kingdom, regenerative repair does not occur to any significant degree. Here scar tissue patches the defect and, in most cases, a high degree of normal function is restored. However, in some cases the scar may limit function. With too little scarring and the dehiscence of a wound, a catastrophic end point occurs. With the over-production and deposition of unstable scar, a different catastrophic end point occurs. Besides the volume of scar tissue deposited, the organization of that tissue is important for determining the integrity and stability of that scar.

The deposition and maturation of scar tissue is dependent upon a cooperation between the resident cell populations, composition and quantity of the deposited connective tissue matrix, and the interactions between the contractile forces within the defect and adjacent structures. Here, the focus has been limited to the regulation of wound healing in regard to collagen fibre reorganization. As our understanding of that process increases in terms of cell–cell association, cell–connective tissue interactions, and the effects of released soluble factors, the better the wound care that can be offered to the patient. The goal is to heal a defect in such a way that it resembles regeneration, where collagen fibres are organized more like dermal fibres. New therapies need to be developed which will eliminate weak scars, excessive scarring, and fibrotic tissue contractures. It may take many years before regenerative repair is achievable, but a scar tissue which shares characteristics similar to that which was lost may not be too far off in the future.

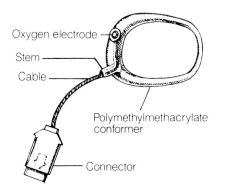

Fig. 5.4 Conjunctival eyelid sensor for indirect measurement of oxygen tension. When the conformer is placed in the eye, tissue oxygen tension can be measured on the palpebral conjunctiva.

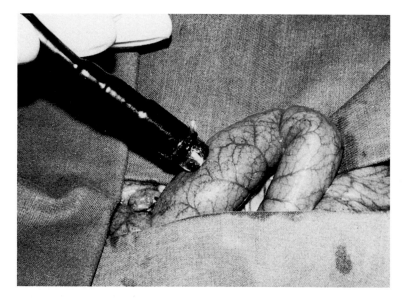

Fig. 5.5 Trans-serosal sensor for indirect measurement of oxygen tension. The sensor is placed on the surface of a bowel.

References

1. Van Der Rest, M. and Garrone, R. (1991). Collagen family of proteins. *FASEB J.*, **5**, 2814–23.
2. Bailey, A. J., Sims, T. J., LeLouis, M., and Bazin, A. (1975). Collagen polymorphism in experimental granulation tissue. *Biochem. Biophys. Res. Commun.*, **66**, 1160–5.
3. Scott, P. G., Telser, A. G., and Veis, A. (1976). Semiquantitative determination of cyanogen bromide peptides of collagen SDS-Polyacrylamide gels. *Anal. Biochem.*, **70**, 251–7.
4. Blumenkrantz, N. and Ashoe-Hansen, G. (1973). A quick and specific assay for hydroxyproline. *Anal. Biochem.*, **55**, 288–91.
5. Cheung, D. T., Benya, P. D., Perelman, N., Dicesage, P. E., and Nimni, M. E. (1990). A highly specific and quantitative method for determining TYPE III/I collagen ratios in tissues. *Matrix*, **10**, 164–71.
6. Deshmukh, K. and Nimni, E. (1973). Isolation and characterisation of cyanogen bromide peptides from the collagen of bovine articular cartilage. *Biochem. J.*, **133**, 615–22.
7. Hawley, P. R., Faulk, W. P., Hunt, T. K., and Dunphy, J. R. (1970). Collagenase activity in the gastrointestinal tract. *Br. J. Surg.*, **57**, 896–900.
8. Klein, L. and Rudolph, R. (1972). H³-collagen turnover in skin grafts. *Surg. Gynecol. Obstset.*, **135**, 49–57.
9. Sandberg, N. (1964). Time relationship between administration of cortisone and wound healing rates. *Acta Chir. Scand.*, **217**, 446–52.
10. Hatz, H. A., Kelly, S. F., and Ehrlich, H. P. (1989). The tetrachlorodecaoxygen complex reverses the effect of cortisone on wound healing. *Plast. Reconst. Surg.*, **84**, 953–9.
11. Hunt, T. K., Twomey, P., Zederfeldt, B., and Dunphy, J. E. (1967). Respiration gas tension and pH in healing wounds. *Am. J. Surg.*, **114**, 302–7.
12. Greenberg, G. B. and Hunt, T. K. (1978). The proliferative response *in vitro* of vascular endothelial and smooth muscle cells exposed to wound fluids and macrophages. *J. Cell Physiol.*, **97**, 353–60.
13. Ehrlich, H. P., MacGarvey, U., McGrane, W. L., and White, M. E. (1987). Ibuprofen as an antagonist of inhibitors of fibrinolysis in wound fluid. *Thromb. Res.*, **45**, 17–28.
14. Hunt, T. K., Andrews, W., Haliday, B., Greenburg, G., Knighton, D., Clark, R., and Thakral, K. (1981). Coagulation and macrophage stimulation of angiogenesis and wound healing. In *Surgical wound*, (ed. P. Dineen and G. Holdrick-Smith), pp. 1–18. Lea and Febiger, Philadelphia.
15. Vijanto, J. and Kulonen, E. (1962). Correlation of tensile strength and chemical composition in experimental granuloma. *Acta Path. Microbiol. Scand.*, **56**, 120–6.
16. Ehrlich, H. P., Desmouliere, A., Diegelmann, R. F., Cohen, I. K., Compton, C. C., Garner, W. L., *et al.* (1994). Morphological and immunochemical differences between keloid and hypertrophic scar. *Am. J. Path.*, **145**, 105–13.
17. Nimni, M. (1980). The molecular organisation of collagen and its role in determining the biophysical properties of connective tissues. *Biorheology*, **17**, 51–83.
18. Doillon, C. J., Dunn, M. G., Bender, E., and Silver, F. H. (1985). Collagen fibre formation in repair tissue: development of strength and toughness. *Coll. Rel. Res.*, **5**, 481–92.
19. Lindstedt, E. and Sandblom, P. (1975). Wound healing in man: tensile strength of healing wounds in some patient groups. *Ann. Surg.*, **181**, 842–6.
20. Vogel, H. G. (1974). Correlation between tensile strength and collagen content in rat skin. Effect of age and cortisol treatment. *Conn. Tiss. Res.*, **2**, 177–82.
21. Hoffman, D. L., Owen, J. A., and Chvapil, M. (1983). Healing of skin incision wounds treated with topically applied BAPN free vbase in the rat. *Exp. Molec. Path.*, **39**, 154–62.
22. DiPasqual, G., Tripp, L., and Steinetz, B. G. (1968). Effects of lysosomal labilizers and pro-inflammatory substances on connective tissue repair as measured by tensile strength. *Proc. Soc. Exp. Biol. Med.*, **127**, 529–32.
23. Heimburger, S., Wolf, M., Cherry, G., and Myers, M. B. (1967). An evaluation of cartilage powder on wound healing. *Arch. Surg.*, **94**, 218–23.
24. Mustoe, T. A., Pierce, G. F., Thomason, A., Gramates, P., Sporn, M. B., and Deuel, T. F. (1987). Accelerated healing in incisional wounds in rats induced by TGF. *Science*, **237**, 1333–6.
25. Pierce, G. F., Brown, D., and Mustoe, T. A. (1991). Quantitative analysis of inflammatory cell influx, procollagen type I synthesis, and collagen cross-linking in incisional wounds: influence of PDGF-BB and TGF 1 therapy. *J. Lab. Clin. Med.*, **117**, 373–82.
26. Edwards, L. C. and Dunphy, J. E. (1958). Wound healing: injury and abnormal repair. *N. Engl. J. Med.*, **259**, 275–80.
27. Van Winkle, W. Jr (1967). Wound contraction. *Surg. Gynecol. Obstet.*, **125**, 131–42.
28. Abercrombie, M., Flint, M. H., and James, D. W. (1956). Wound contraction in relation to collagen formation in scorbutic guinea pigs. *J. Embryo. Exp. Morphol.*, **4**, 167–75.
29. Majno, G., Gabbiani, G., Hirschel, B. J., and Ryan, G. B. (1971). Contraction of granulation tissue *in vitro*: similarity to smooth muscle. *Science*, **173**, 548–50.
30. Gabbiani, G. (1992). The biology of the myofibroblast. *Kidney Int.*, **41**, 530–2.
31. Ehrlich, H. P. and Rajarartnam, J. B. M. (1990). Cell locomotion forces versus cell contraction forces for collagen lattice contraction: an *in vitro* model of wound contraction. *Tiss. Cell*, **22**, 407–17.
32. Majno, G., Gabbiani, G., Hirschel, B. J., and Ryan, G. B. (1971). Contraction of granulation tissue *in vitro*: similarity to smooth muscle. *Science*, **173**, 548–50.
33. Hembry, R. M., Bernanke, D. R., Hayahashi, K., and Trelstad, R. L. (1986). Morphologic examination of mesenchymal cells in healing wound of normal and tight skin mice. *Am. J. Path.*, **125**, 81–9.
34. Bell, E., Ivarsson, B., and Merrill, C. (1979). Production of a tissue-like structure of contraction of collagen lattice by human fibroblasts of different proliferative potential *in vitro*. *Proc. Natl. Acad. Sci. USA*, **76**, 1274–8.
35. Ehrlich, H. P. (1988). The modulation of contraction of fibroblast populated collagen lattices by type I, II and III collagen. *Tiss. Cell*, **20**, 47–50.
36. Ehrlich, H. P., Rockwell, W. B., Cornwell, T. L., and Rajaratnam, J. R. M. (1990). Demonstration of a direct role for myosin light chain kinase in fibroblast-populated collagen lattice contraction. *J. Cell. Physiol.*, **147**, 1–7.
37. Ehrlich, H. P. and Griswold, T. R. (1974). Epidermolysis bullosa dystrophica recessive fibroblasts produce increased concentrations of cAMP within a collagen matrix. *J. Invest. Dermatol.*, **83**, 230–3.
38. Klein, C. E., Dressel, D., Steinmayer, T., Mauch, C., Eckes, B., Krieg, T., *et al.* (1991). Integrin α2 is unregulated in fibroblasts and highly aggressive melanoma cells in three-dimensional collagen lattices and mediates the re-organisation of collagen I fibrils. *J. Cell Biol.*, **115**, 1427–36.
39. Kreuzer, F. and Cain, S. M. (1985). Regulation of the peripheral vasculature and tissue oxygenation in health disease. *Critical Care Clinic*, **1**, 453–70.
40. Gottrup, F. (1992). Measurement and evaluation of tissue perfusion in surgery (to optimize wound healing and resistance

to infection). In *International surgical practice*, (ed. D. J. Leaper and F. J. Branicki), pp. 15–39. Oxford University Press, Oxford.

41. Jonsson, K., Jensen, J. A., Goodson, W. H., West, J. M., and Hunt, T. K. (1987). Assessment of perfusion in post-operative patients using tissue oxygen measurements. *Br. J. Surg.*, **74**, 263–7.

42. Tanaka, T., Riva, C., and Ben-Sira, I. (1974). Blood velocity measurements in human retinal vessels. *Science*, **186**, 830–1.

43. Stern, M. D. (1975). *In vivo* evaluation of micro-circulation by coherent light scattering. *Nature*, **254**, 56–8.

44. Holloway, G. A. and Watkins, D. W. (1977). Laser Doppler measurements of cutaneous blood flow. *J. Invest. Derm.*, **69**, 306–9.

45. Nilsson, G. E., Tenland, T., and Oberg, P. A. (1980). A new instrument for continuous measurement of tissue blood flow by light beating spectroscopy. *IEEE Transactions: Biomedical*, **27**, 12–19.

46. Fagrell, B. (1986). The use of capillaroscopy in evaluation of skin viability. *Progress in Applied Microcirculation*, **11**, 40–6.

47. Striebel, H. W. and Kretz, F. J. (1989). Advantages and limitations of pulse oximetry. In *Clinical aspects of O_2 transport and tissue oxygenation*, (ed. K. Reinhart and K. Eyrich), pp. 212–29. Springer, Berlin.

48. Gottrup, F., Gellett, S., Kirkegaard, L., Hansen, E. S., and Johansen, G. (1989). Effect of haemorrhage and resuscitation on subcutaneous, conjunctival, and transcutaneous oxygen tension in relation to haemodynamic variables. *Crit. Care Med.*, **17**, 904–7.

49. Sendak, M. J., Harris, A. P., and Donham, R. T. (1988). Accuracy of pulse oximetry during arterial oxy-haemoglobin desaturation in dogs. *Anaesthesiology*, **68**, 111–14.

50. Severinghaus, J. W. and Naifeh, K. H. (1987). Accuracy of response of six pulse oximeters to profound hypoxia. *Anaesthesiology*, **67**, 551–8.

51. Grote, J. (1989). Tissue respiration. In *Human physiology*, (ed. R. F. Smidt and G. Thews), pp. 598–612. Springer, Berlin.

52. Gottrup, F., Niinikoski, J., and Hunt, T. K. (1991). Measurement of tissue oxygen tension in wound repair. In *Wound healing*, (ed. H. Janssen, R. Rooman, and J. I. S. Robertson), pp. 155–64. Wrightson Biomedical, Petersfield, England and Blackwell, Oxford.

53. Hunt, T. K., Halliday, B. J., Hopf, H. W., Scheuenstuhl, H., and West, J. M. (1991). Measurement and control of tissue oxygen tension in surgical patients. In *Update in intensive care and emergency medicine Vol. 12: tissue oxygen utilization*, (ed. G. Gutierrez and J. L. Vincent), p. 336. Springer, Berlin.

54. Gottrup, F., Firmin, F., Rabkin, J., Halliday, B. J., and Hunt, T. K. (1987). Directly measured tissue oxygen tension and arterial tension assess tissue perfusion. *Crit. Care Med.*, **15**, 1030–6.

55. Chang, N., Goodson, W. H., Gottrup, F., and Hunt, T. K. (1983). Direct measurement of wound and tissue oxygen tension in post-operative patients. *Ann. Surg.*, **197**, 470–8.

56. Kuttila, K. (1989). Tissue perfusion and oxygenation in cardiac surgery. *Scan. J. Thor. Cardiovasc. Surg.* (Suppl.), **38**.

57. Hjortdal, V. E., Awwad, A., Gottrup, F., Kirkegaard, L., and Gellett, S. (1997). Tissue oxygen tension measurement for monitoring musculocutaneous and cutaneous flaps. *Scan. J. Plas. Recon. Surg.* (In Press).

58. Gottrup, F. (1991). Tissue oxygen tension monitoring: relation to haemodynamic and oxygen transport variables. In *Update in intensive care and emergency medicine Vol. 12: tissue oxygen utilization*, (ed. G. Gutierrez and J. L. Vincent), pp. 322–36. Springer, Berlin.

59. Fatt, I. (1976). Polarographic oxygen sensors. Its theory of operation and its application in biology. In *Medicine and technology*. CRC Press, Cleveland.

60. Clark, L. C. (1956). Monitor and control of blood and tissue oxygen tension. *Transactions of the American Society of Artificial and Internal Organs*, **2**, 41–6.

61. Baker, S. J., Tremper, K. K., Hyatt, J., Heitzmann, H. A., Holman, B. K., Pike, K., *et al.* (1987). Continuous fibre optic arterial oxygen tension measurements in dogs. *J. Clin. Mon.*, **3**, 48–52.

62. Silver, I. A. (1969). The measurement of oxygen tension in healing tissue. In *Progress of respiration research III*, (ed. H. Herzog), pp. 124–35. Karger, Basel.

63. Gottrup, F., Firmin, R., Chang, N., Goodson, W. H., and Hunt, T. K. (1983). Continuous direct tissue oxygen tension measurement by a new method using an implantable silastic tonometer and oxygen polarography. *Am. J. Surg.*, **146**, 399–403.

64. Hunt, T. K. (1964). A new method of determining tissue oxygen tension. *Lancet*, **ii**, 1370–1.

65. Niinikoski, J., Heughan, C., and Hunt, T. K. (1972). Oxygen tension in human wounds. *J. Surg. Res.*, **12**, 77–82.

66. Larsen, P. N., Moesgaard, F., Gottrup, F., and Helledie, N. (1989). Characterization of the silicone tonometer using a membrane-covered transcutaneous electrode. *Scan. J. Clin. Lab. Invest.*, **49**, 523–9.

67. Henriksen, T. B., Hjortdal, V. E., Kjolseth, D., Hansen, E. S., Djuurhus, J. C., and Gottrup, F. (1989). The microcirculatory changes in the surroundings of silastic catheters and the relationship between tissue oxygen tension and microcirculation. An experimental study in pigs. *Eur. Surg. Res.*, **21** (Suppl. 2), 75–6.

68. Katsamouris, A., Brewster, D. C., Megerman, J., Cina, C., Darling, R. C., and Abott, W. M. (1984). Transcutaneous oxygen tension in selection of amputation level. *Am. J. Surg.*, **147**, 510–17.

69. Pecoraro, R. E., Ahroni, J. E., Boyko, E. J., and Stensel, V. L. (1991). Chronology and determinants of tissue repair in diabetic lower-extremity ulcers. *Diabetes*, **40**, 1305–13.

70. Sheffield, P. J. (1988). Tissue oxygen measurements. In *Problem wounds. The role of oxygen*, (ed. J. C. Davis and T. K. Hunt), pp. 17–51. Elsevier, New York.

71. Abraham, E., Oye, R. K., and Smith, M. (1984). Detection of blood volume deficits through conjunctival oxygen tension monitoring. *Crit. Care Med.*, **12**, 931–4.

72. Sheridan, W. G., Lowndes, R. H., and Young, H. L. (1987). Tissue oxygen tension as a predictor of colonic anastomotic healing. *Dis. Colon Rec.*, **30**, 867–71.

73. Sheridan, W. G., Lowndes, R. H., and Young, H. L. (1990). Intraoperative tissue oximetry in the human gastro-intestinal tract. *Am. J. Surg.*, **159**, 314–19.

74. Kallehave, F. and Gottrup, F. (1991). The profile of serosal tissue oxygen tension in patients in surgery. *Eur. Surg. Res.*, **24** (Suppl. 1), 93.

75. Kallehave, F., Hovendal, D. P. H., and Gottrup, F. (1992). Surface tissue oxygen tension in assessment of local perfusion in colonic interposition in infants. *Surgical Research Communications*, **13**, 239–43.

76. Larsen, P. N., Naver, L. P. S., Helledie, N., Gottrup, F., Kirkegaard, P., and Moesgaard, F. (1991). Tissue oxygen tension in the gastrointestinal tract measured by a vacuum fixated transcutaneous oxygen electrode. *Scan. J. Gastro.*, **26**, 409–18.

6

Factors influencing wound healing

G. D. MULDER, B. A. BRAZINSKY, K. G. HARDING, and M. S. AGREN

Relationship of ageing to wound repair

Traditionally, the elderly are classified as those individuals 65 years of age and older. This section addresses the effect of age-associated skin changes, peripheral vascular disease, diabetes, musculoskeletal diseases, infection, drugs, and nutrition on the wound healing process.

Age-associated skin changes

The perceived age of an individual is often based upon skin appearance. Gross inspection of skin in the elderly reveals dryness, wrinkling, thinning, laxity, uneven pigmentation, and decreased hair growth. Although individuals respond differently to ageing, certain characteristics are associated with the ageing process (Table 6.1).

Recent studies indicate that the rate of wound repair declines with age. The inflammatory response, proliferative phase (cell migration, proliferation, and maturation), and remodelling phase (tertiary bonding of collagen), have all been shown to be altered with age (1–3). The phases of repair tend to start later and proceed more slowly. These age-related changes have been determined by measuring decreased epidermal turnover rates, collagen deposition, and regeneration of blister roofs (4).

Microscopic examination of aged skin reveals a thinning epidermis, resulting in less resistance to shear forces, rendering the skin more susceptible to trauma (3). An age-related decrease in the barrier function of the stratum corneum has also been observed, predisposing the body to chronic infections, including tineal and bacterial superinfections (3). A flattening in the dermal–epidermal junction is one of the most significant changes which occurs. This results in fragile tissue with diminished nutrient transfer capacity, decreased melanocytes necessary for ultraviolet protection, and decreased vitamin D production (5).

Elderly patients are predisposed to ecchymosis due to a relative avascularity of the skin. Thinning vascular walls have a 35 per cent decrease in venular cross-sectional area (6, 7). This has a deleterious affect on hair bulbs, eccrine, apocrine, and sebaceous glands, as well as the cutaneous end-organs responsible for perception of pressure and touch (Table 6.2). These changes in vascular response increase chances of skin breakdown and impede normal healing capabilities.

Table 6.1 Ageing, skin changes, and wound healing

Changes in skin with ageing	Effects of ageing on healing
Decreased vascularity	Decreased wound contraction
Decreased tissue barrier function	Decreased biological activity
Decreased epidermal proliferation	Decreased breaking strength
Increased vulnerability to trauma	Delayed cellular migration and proliferation
Diminished pain perception	Decreased wound capillary growth
	Delayed collagen remodelling
	Altered metabolic response
	Increased rate of wound dehiscence

Table 6.2 Skin functions that decrease with age

Barrier function	Sensory perception
Chemical clearance	Sweat production
Epidermal turnover	Thermo regulation
Immune function	Vascular response
Injury response	Vitamin D production
Sebum production	Wound healing

The most important affects of ageing skin result in changes in collagen. Collagen is a major structural protein of the skin and is responsible for most of its strength. The collagen of a younger individual appears random in structure. With age, elastins and the extracellular matrix (of which the dermis is comprised along with collagen), decrease. Collagen fills in the empty spaces creating more dense collagen fibres. The structure of the collagen cross-links changes, increasing tensile strength while decreasing elasticity and stretchability of the skin (3). The amount of collagen decreases by 1 per cent per year and secondary to thickening in the elderly, becomes less soluble, has less ability to swell, decreases the breaking potential, and predisposes the skin to the negative affects of trauma. Therefore, it is not the decreased tensile strength which affects wound healing in ageing. On the contrary, tensile strength increases with age, but the amount of time necessary to form the collagen molecules increases, prolonging wound repair.

Tissue friability is one of the most important considerations when treating the elderly. It is extremely important to avoid damaging the intact skin in an effort to close a wound. Manual debridement, forceful scrubs, and frequent dressing changes may cause even more damage to a wound. Adhesive materials may remove healthy tissue or cause a contact dermatitis. Caustic agents such as povidone–iodine, acetic acid, and hydrogen peroxide may irritate the surrounding skin and initiate inflammation. Wet-to-dry dressings should be used reluctantly to debride necrotic tissue as they may cause further skin trauma.

When dealing with the geriatric patient, extreme care must be taken to prevent further tissue damage which delays wound healing.

Peripheral vascular disease (PVD)

Blood delivers oxygen, nutrients, cells, and other important materials necessary for wound repair. Approximately 20 per cent of the geriatric population experience varying degrees of peripheral vascular disease (8). Many will progress to arterial and venous obstruction which may hinder wound healing, increasing the risk of ulceration and infection (see Chapter 10). A decreased or interrupted vascular supply will result in delayed wound healing and may result in an acute wound becoming a chronic one.

A diminished blood flow also decreases the removal of necrotic, bacterial, or foreign material, all of which slow the healing process, from a wound site. If toxins are introduced into the wound, which act as inhibitors to healing, they are less rapidly cleared. It has been shown that a decrease or cessation of blood flow is a major contributor to development of pressure injury to the skin, resulting in an increased risk of pressure ulcers in the elderly (9).

Ageing has been shown to decrease the transcutaneous partial pressure of oxygen (Tcp_{O_2}) in patients with PVD. This leads to an increase in skin rigidity and greater subcutaneous tissue pressure (9). Geriatric patients may, therefore, be more susceptible to outside environmental factors which put additional stress on the skin.

In the geriatric patient with PVD, exercises, leg elevation, compression stockings, sequential compression devices, and vascular bypass as indicated are all important adjuvant therapies which aid in the rapid closure and healing of a wound.

Diabetes

More than 20 per cent of the geriatric population is affected by diabetes mellitus, a destructive endocrine disease (10). Non-insulin dependent diabetes is more common in the elderly and is related to heredity, obesity, and diet. The effects of diabetes are manifested in the skin, vasculature, nerves, and bones and play a vital role in the wound healing process.

Diabetes mellitus may include both micro- and macrovascular disease. The most frequently involved vessels are those below the knee; the tibial and peroneal arteries, as well as their smaller branches, consequently the manifestation of symptoms in the lower extremity are more common. These vascular changes make the diabetic more susceptible to gangrene. In a study by Bell, it was found that gangrene was 156 times more common in diabetics in the 5th decade, 85 times more common in the 6th, and 53 times more common in the 7th decade, than in the non-diabetic (11). Clotting factors are also deranged by diabetes, leading to atherosclerosis and, in turn, an adverse effect on wound repair (Table 6.3).

The development of neuropathy, primarily the loss of pain and temperature sensation, may lead to painless trauma, resulting in ulceration of the diabetic foot. Infection is also very common with diabetic ulceration, as is the chance of osteomyelitis. Alteration in the autonomic nervous system may lead to anhydrosis which can cause skin fissuring and the increased predisposition of the skin to ulceration and infection. Autonomic neuropathy also leads to decreased skin oxygenation

Table 6.3 Effects of diabetes on platelet function

Increased platelet turnover
Increased platelet adhesiveness
Increased platelet aggregation

Table 6.4 Musculoskeletal diseases associated with the elderly

Rheumatoid arthritis
Osteoarthritis
Gout and pseudo-gout
Osteoporosis
Septic arthritis
Paget's disease of bone
Diffuse idiopathic sclerosing hyperostosis
Polymyalgia rheumatic and giant cell arteritis
Systemic lupus erythematosus
Sjögren's syndrome
Polymyositis

through an inadequacy of capillary flow, tissue oedema, arterio-venous shunting, and atypical microvasculature responses to stimuli, all of which negatively affect wound repair (12, 13). Neuropathy may lead to the diabetic Charcot foot, with disfigurement of the bones of the foot. Muscle atrophy may also occur, resulting in alterations of gait and normal bone alignment. Patients with neuropathy tend to develop extremely high pressures beneath the forefoot (14) which frequently leads to ulceration.

One major factor affecting wound repair in the diabetic is blood sugar control. It has been shown that geriatric patients with poorly controlled diabetes have a delay in wound closure of up to three times that of elderly non-diabetic patients (13). Well controlled sugar levels may help prevent as well as stabilize PVD, although this still remains controversial (15, 16).

Diabetes remains an important factor influencing wound healing potential, and its affects must be strictly controlled. Patient education is important in assuring daily skin evaluation. Help should be sought at initial signs of ulceration to prevent infection and any further skin damage. Treatment should include debridement, pressure relief via non-weight-bearing aids, or appropriate treatment including contact casting, special shoes, and when indicated, surgery.

Musculoskeletal disease

Elderly patients are frequently afflicted with diseases of the musculoskeletal system. Individuals over age 65 frequently have joint and muscle pain as their most common systemic complaint. There are no statistics reporting the various arthritides in the elderly, but it is safe to say that 5–10 per cent of individuals who are over 60 experience some form of arthritis (17). Rheumatoid arthritis, osteoarthritis, and gouty arthritis lead this list, with other forms being less common (Table 6.4).

Common manifestations of musculoskeletal diseases are evident as bony prominences and joint subluxations. These deformities place excessive pressure on soft tissue, increasing the risk of skin breakdown and interfering with wound closure. Common areas susceptible to increased pressure include the metatarsal heads on the plantar side, phalanges of the foot dorsally, and metacarpal–phalangeal joints of the hand. These areas are prone to increased loading and shear forces. In response, inflammation and hyperkeratosis occur, contributing to pre-ulcerative lesion formation. Early recognition is important in order to accommodate and treat pre-ulcerative lesions adequately.

Custom moulded shoes with proper insoles and orthotics are important for treatment and prevention of ulcer reccurrence as well as initial formation. Surgery such as panmetatarsal head resections in the foot, digital fusion in the

hands and feet, as well as digital implants may be appropriate for prevention of ulcer recurrence.

Osteoporosis, a decrease in the amount of normal bone mass per unit volume, is present to varying degrees throughout the geriatric population. By age 80, the incidence is almost 100 per cent (17). These patients are at risk of pathological fractures and decreased bone healing. Geriatric patients should perform 3–4 h of weight bearing exercise per week to help increase their bone mass. Additionally, daily calcium supplements of 1500 mg/day as well as vitamin D supplements should be given to post-menopausal women. Calcitonin injections have more recently been used for treatment of osteoporosis.

Infection

The skin naturally acts as a barrier to infection, both actively and passively. Sebum, the secretion of the sebaceous glands of the skin, not only acts as a lubricant, but actively destroys streptococci. Any trauma to the skin, or inflammation, inactivates sebum through the accumulation of serum. This can lead to an overgrowth of streptococci on the skin. The active signs of infections – rubor, dolor, calor, and tumor – may not be manifested in the elderly patient. This is primarily due to poor white blood cell response, decrease in IgM, and increase in complement levels (18, 19).

In the geriatric patient, the stem cells in bone marrow have been shown to decrease in cell division, with a decrease in B cell formation, thereby affecting their immune capacity. The number of B cells does not change with age, but the size of the B cell subpopulations tends to change. Qualitative changes are also evident with age for B cells. B cells have been shown to have an impaired response to T-cell dependent antigens (19–21).

Natural antibodies which aid in humoral immunity have been shown to decrease with age. The number of circulating T cells decreases to a level which is 15 per cent of the level found in adolescents, thereby making the elderly more susceptible to infection (22). Many intracellular changes have been identified as well which inhibit the immune response. Various studies have shown a decrease in development of delayed hypersensitivity reactions in the elderly. After age 70, approximately 70 per cent of individuals will elicit a contact sensitivity reaction (23). The failure of any part of the immune and inflammatory responses allows infection to occur and impairs wound healing. The rate of wound dehiscence has been shown to increase 2–3 times in patients over 60 (24).

Medications and drugs

The geriatric patient with open chronic wounds is frequently being treated with medications for concomitant illnesses. Treatment is usually focused on wound care, without particular attention to the effects of the individual's medications on the wound healing process. Drugs such as anti-inflammatory drugs, steroids, and immunosuppressives have a deleterious effect on wound repair.

Non-steroidal anti-inflammatory drugs (NSAIDs) are prescribed for treatment of illnesses ranging from chronic pain to arthritis. Colchicine, used frequently for the treatment of gout, has been shown to reduce the tensile strength of connective tissue. It is believed that colchicine may reduce blood supply to a wound through a vasoconstrictive effect, thereby affecting the initial inflammatory phase of healing (25). It has been shown that NSAIDs do not affect re-epithelialization or dermal collagen synthesis, but topical indomethacin has been shown to delay corneal re-epithelialization in domestic pigs (26).

The primary action of oral NSAIDs is to reduce the inflammatory process, thereby reducing pain. Inflammation is an important factor in early wound repair and acute wounds, but its precise role in chronic wound repair has yet to be clarified.

Corticosteroids have a major effect on the healing process. A large percentage of geriatric patients with arthritis use corticosteroids. Therefore, it is important to determine whether a patient is consuming any type of steroid which may inhibit wound repair. Some of the documented effects of corticosteroids include the inhibition of collagen synthesis, as well as slowing of the wound healing process when administered just prior to or just after the occurrence of the injury (27, 28). Tensile strength, as well as healing of open wounds, has been found to be affected by corticosteroids. Steroids may impair wound repair by inhibiting several important factors in the repair process, including fibroblast function, thereby inhibiting collagen synthesis (29–31). The influence of steroids on cellular components would affect the phagocytic and antibacterial components of wound repair. The overall effect is delayed or altered wound healing. Rheumatologists agree that less than 15 mg of prednisone daily has no significant effect on wound healing, but larger doses may impair the inflammatory phase of healing.

Topical steroids may be used to treat various skin abnormalities associated with ageing. For example, patients with severe venous disease may suffer from venous-stasis-dermatitis. Topical corticosteroids have varying affects on the epidermis and dermal synthesis of collagen (32). One such effect may be a delay in wound healing and when applying topical steroids to these patients care should be taken to avoid the ulcer surface.

Immunosuppressive drugs such as cyclosporin have been found to have varying effects on wound repair. When compared to methylprednisolone, no effect on hydroxyproline (an indicator of collagen levels) or macrophages has been found.

There is a suggestion that it may impair wound healing (33, 34). Azathioprine and prednisone therapy have been shown to cause significant reduction in breaking strength of cutaneous wounds (35).

It is important to realize that patients on immunosuppressive drugs will not respond to conventional therapy so extra care must be taken to avoid inflicting trauma to the wound.

Several other drugs have also been found to affect wound repair (Table 6.5). Therefore, it is extremely important to determine a patient's exact medication before initiating and selecting wound therapy.

Nutrition

One of the most important factors essential for adequate wound repair is nutritional status. Unfortunately, due to ill health or poor eating habits, significant numbers of the geriatric population suffer from malnutrition. Fluid, protein, and calorie intake in the elderly are often reduced, yet the requirements for vitamins and minerals does not decrease with age (Table 6.6).

Table 6.5 Drugs which delay wound healing

Non-steroidal anti-inflammatory drugs (NSAIDs)
Immunosuppressive agents
Steroids
Anticoagulants
Anti-neoplastic drugs
Antiprostaglandins

Table 6.6 Nutrient requirements of young compared with older adults

Nutrient	Young adult (<50 years)	Older adult (51+ years)
Calcium	800 mg	800 mg
Iron	10 mg (male)–18 mg (female)	10 mg
Protein	0.8 g/kg body weight	0.8 g/kg body weight
Vitamin A	800–1000 RE*	800–1000 RE*
Vitamin B_1 (thiamine)	1.0–1.4 mg	1.0–1.2 mg
Vitamin B_2 (riboflavin)	1.2–1.6 mg	1.2–1.4 mg
Vitamin B_3 (niacin)	13–16 mg[†]	13–15 mg NE[†]
Vitamin B_{12} (cobalamin)	3.0 µg	3.0 µg
Vitamin C (ascorbic acid)	60 mg	60 mg
Vitamin D (calciferol)	400 IU	400 IU

*RE = retinal equivalence.
[†]NE = niacin equivalence.

The prevalence of protein calorie malnutrition (PCM) of hospitalized patients in the United States alone is approximately 50 per cent. PCM results in malabsorption, decreased visceral protein stores, flaky dermatitis, and altered immune function (36). Additionally, patients with PCM develop oedema secondary to low serum colloid osmotic pressure, which results in accumultation of interstitial fluid. Peri-wound oedema can impair healing by increasing the distance that oxygen and other nutrients must travel to reach the cells and by inhibiting movement of cellular waste products causing build-up around the wound.

The deleterious effects of malnutrition can be seen in various phases of the wound repair process. An altered inflammatory response can be related to the effects of malnutrition on the immune function. Animals fed protein-free diets have been shown to have a decrease in several components of fibronectin and complement, which are important chemotactic factors for fibroblasts and macrophages (37). In children with the kwashiorkor protein deficiency, a decreased *in vitro* activity against fungi and bacteria by polymorphonuclear leucocytes has been demonstrated (38). Later, the wound healing process is affected by disorders in collagen synthesis, fibroblast proliferation, and neovascularization. Vitamin A deficiency results in decreased collagen synthesis and also affects epithelialization (38). Vitamin C deficiency results in decreased collagen synthesis, decreased membrane integrity, and decreases the threshold for pressure injury (38). An adequate level of enzymes to serve as cofactors in certain biochemical reactions is necessary for normal wound repair. Many of the enzymes are derived from trace minerals like copper, iron, and zinc. Therefore, their deficiency will have an adverse affect on wound repair (Table 6.7).

Serum proteins have been used for detecting general protein status. Serum albumin is the only protein which is not affected by increased age (36). An albumin level of less than 35 g/l (depending on local laboratory values) indicates the need for further assessment of nutritional status. Albumin breakdown increases in response to injury in the skin and albumin synthesis decreases with trauma (39). If utilization increases at the wound site and synthesis decreases, then serum albumin falls. An albumin level of less than 30 g/l results in major impairment of wound healing. Several studies have shown that pressure ulcers are associated with hypoalbuminaemia (40).

Although diagnosis of PCM is difficult, a clinician should suspect its presence with a history of recent change in mental status, recent weight loss, and lymphocytopenia. The affects of PCM are similar to normal ageing, so it must actively be considered (36). Table 6.8 describes a quick screening process for patients at risk of poor wound healing.

Nutritional management is important for elderly patients. If dietary intake is insufficient to meet calculated nutritional needs, supplements should be instituted. Table 6.9 provides a formula to estimate protein and calorie needs. The goal is to obtain a calorie intake of approximately 35 kcal/kg based on ideal body weight. Only 10 per cent of the elderly with PCM can consume food voluntarily, therefore supplementation is necessary.

Table 6.7 Necessary nutrients for wound healing in elderly patients

Nutrients	Function	Deficiency effects
Vitamin A	Collagen synthesis Epithelialization	Poor healing
Vitamin C	Membrane integrity	Poor wound healing Capillary fragility Scurvy
Zinc	Enzyme cofactor Cell proliferation	Slow healing Anorexia
Protein	Wound repair Collagen synthesis Fibroblast proliferation White blood cell production and migration Clotting factor production Neovascularization Wound remodelling	Hypoalbuminaemia Lymphopenia Impaired cellular immunity Poor wound healing
Fats	Prostaglandin production Provide essential fatty acids Cellular energy Cell membrane production	Poor wound helaing
Carbohydrates	Spare protein Cellular energy	Muscle and visceral protein stores used for energy

Table 6.8 Protein – calorie malnutrition screen

History	Recent change in mental status Recent weight loss – greater than 10% of normal weight
Physical examination	Weight less than 80% of ideal body weight Oedema Easy hair pluckability
Laboratory analyses	Low serum albumin (less than 30 g/l) Lymphocytopenia (count of less than 1500) $\times 10^6$/l

Table 6.9 Nutritional needs for elderly patients with wounds

Daily protein needs	$1.5 \times$ weight in kg	
Daily calorie needs	$1.2–1.5 \times$ BEE	
Harris Benedict equations for BEE	Men:	BEE $= 66.47 + 13.75\,W + 5.0\,H - 6.76\,A$
	Women:	BEE $= 655.1 + 9.56\,W + 18.5\,H - 4.68\,A$

BEE, base energy expenditure.
W, weight in kg; H, height in cm; A, age in years.

For those patients with normal gastrointestinal tracts, enteral hyperalimentation via a nasogastric tube is the ideal route. Infusion should begin at a continuous rate of 25 ml/h with the rate increasing such that after 48 h the total daily protein and calorie requirements are met (36). Hospitalized patients with severe PCM may require total parenteral nutrition (TPN) to improve the serum albumin level, but TPN is associated with many related complications.

Chronic wounds such as pressure ulcers have been shown to improve following vitamin C supplements (41). This low-cost, low-risk treatment may be advised for all elderly patients with wounds. Elderly patients may also benefit from a multi-vitamin and zinc supplementation. Additional vitamin A has not yet been shown to be essential, and being fat soluble, may be toxic.

Biology of impaired wound healing in relation to systemic diseases

Impaired wound healing may be due to local and systemic factors. Systemic diseases by their nature often produce multiple pathological effects. Clinical impressions might suggest that diabetes, uraemia, and jaundice are associated with wound related complications, but evidence in support of this is lacking, particularly when considering human wounds. This section considers the local effects of these conditions on cellular proliferation, granulation tissue formation, and wound breaking strength.

Uraemia

Evidence suggests that renal failure results in a general inhibition of cell proliferation (42). The use of animal models has shown that wound complications associated with acute renal failure appear to be related to inadequate production of granulation tissue. Experimentally induced acute uraemia in rabbits has been found to be associated with a decrease in both fibroblast activity and collagen deposition in abdominal wounds (43). Decreased granulation tissue formation with an associated reduction in the percentage of actively proliferating fibroblasts and capillary endothelial cells has been found in mice rendered acutely uraemic by intraperitoneal injection of uranyl nitrate (a nephrotoxic heavy metal salt) or by urinary obstruction. Results obtained from the mice treated with uranyl nitrate may be complicated by the intense nephritis and proteinuria it causes which can lead to hypoproteinaemia. The decrease in granulation tissue formation was only demonstrated if uraemia was present during the proliferative phase of wound healing. Inhibition of cellular proliferation of fibroblasts and endothelial cells was most marked when renal failure was severe and rapidly progressive (44). Cell population kinetic studies of skin epithelia in experimental acute renal failure in mice demonstrated a prolongation of the cell cycle with an increase in the duration of the DNA synthetic phase (45).

More recently it has been shown, by quantitative electroimmunoassay, that the plasma fibronectin concentration was significantly reduced, independent of haemodialysis, in patients with chronic renal failure. It has been postulated that poor wound healing may be related to reduced plasma fibronectin, but this deficiency has not been demonstrated in the tissues (46). Studies employing steel-mesh cylinders implanted in the backs of uraemic and control rats have also shown a reduction in the production of granulation tissue, but

the content of collagen in the granulation tissue was normal (47). As a further measure of the wound healing process the strength of linear wounds in rats was studied for eight weeks after wounding. Wound strength appeared to be reduced but after correction for reduced skin thickness, was found to be normal (48). Using rat skin fibroblasts in culture, Colin (49) demonstrated marked inhibition of fibroblast growth when either urea or uraemic rat serum was added to the culture medium. This was confirmed by autoradiographs using tritiated thymidine to label actively dividing cells.

Animal studies certainly suggest that uraemia impairs wound healing by a combination of decreased fibroblast and endothelial cell growth and an overall decrease in granulation tissue formation. Collagen content of granulation tissue, however, is not adversely affected and thus wound breaking strength is not significantly diminished.

Jaundice

Any study to determine the effects of jaundice or established liver failure on wound healing is complicated by the multiple biochemical and clinical features of the conditions. *In vitro* studies can therefore be more useful than those *in vivo*, as the pathologies associated with liver failure such as renal impairment, 'the hepato-renal syndrome', hypoproteinaemia, and sepsis, can be excluded as causal factors in impaired wound healing. The aetiology of the liver pathology also influences the biology of wound healing. Jaundice may be due to benign or malignant disease. Benign causes include infection, which can be acute or chronic, and obstruction, which may be due to stones or stricture. Acute events such as an obstructing gallstone, which can readily be treated endoscopically or surgically, are less likely to cause impaired healing than malignant obstructing disease. In all cases the results of *in vitro* studies should be considered in the light of full clinical and biochemical information so that an appropriate interpretation can be made. Prospective human studies of the effect of jaundice on wound healing have been performed (50–52) but further work is necessary to clarify results of previous work.

Morphological changes and impaired growth of dermal fibroblasts have been shown in tissue culture experiments where bilirubin and jaundiced human sera are added to the culture medium (53). Whether these findings in themselves lead to clinically impaired healing have been cast into doubt by a study of abdominal wound mechanical strength in jaundiced rats (54). It was found that despite a significant delay in the accumulation of collagen in the wounds this did not manifest itself as decreased mechanical strength. A decrease in the mechanical strength of abdominal wounds has been found, however, in similar studies (55, 56). Jaundice, induced by ligation and division of the common bile duct in all of these studies, becomes clinically apparent after two days and the serum bilirubin concentration remains steady at a concentration of 170 mmol/l during the subsequent five weeks (55). In the initial period after the onset of jaundice complications due to alterations in haematocrit, prothrombin time, urea, electrolytes, and total protein levels are not observed.

A feature of hepatic failure is excessive ammonia production, which can lead to a relative deficiency of the amino acids ornithine and arginine. In such a state ornithine becomes the rate-limiting factor for urea cycle function, leading to decreased urea synthesis. Optimal growth in several animal species requires 0.4–1.0 per cent arginine in the diet, and it is recognized that diets deficient in arginine are associated with poor wound healing (56). Further determination of the role of jaundice in wound healing has been provided by studies using cultured fibroblasts (53, 57). In the first study (53) the addition of bilirubin or sera from jaundiced patients to fibroblast culture media led to both morphological changes and impaired growth of the fibroblasts. Interestingly, whilst morphological changes were seen, these only occurred when the cells were grown in a medium containing *un*conjugated bilirubin (57). Conjugated bilirubin (bilirubin diglucuronide), in contrast, produced no such changes. These data suggest that wound failure should be less common in patients with obstructive jaundice than in these with non-obstructive jaundice. These examples serve to illustrate that even though the mechanisms by which healing is impaired may be complex, ultimately they may act via common pathways, such as impaired nutrition (58) or the direct toxic effects of abnormal metabolic products on cells whose activity is essential to healing (57).

The use of oral sodium taurocholate (a bile salt) in jaundiced rats has been demonstrated to cause a significant increase in abdominal wound bursting strength at six days postoperatively compared with rats who were not given oral bile salts (56). In the same study hydroxyproline content was estimated in the excised wounds, with no significant difference found between jaundiced rats, jaundiced rats given bile salts, and control rats. It was postulated from this work that reduced bursting strength was due to reduced *quality* rather than quantity of collagen in the wound, but this is not supported by histological evidence (59). However, this latter study also demonstrated minimal collagen formation in rat peritoneal defects at eight days postoperatively. One possible explanation for the role of bile salts in preserving wound strength is that they absorb endotoxins associated with biliary obstruction. It is believed that if absorbed, these endotoxins impair vascular ingrowth into the healing wound, a possible cause of reduced wound strength (59).

Histologically, it has been shown in gastric and peritoneal wounds in rats that there is a delay in fibroplasia and decreased new vessel formation which lead to delayed healing (55). This delay in angiogenesis has further been shown by micro-angiography of gastric wounds in jaundiced animals. These experiments showed little new vessel formation even by eight days post-wounding (59). In an experiment to determine the effect of jaundice on the migration of reticuloendothelial cells and fibroblasts into experimental foreign body granulomata (60) significant inhibition was found in the first week after the formation of the granuloma. No histological confirmation of the nature of the cells invading the granuloma was made, however, and further studies are required to determine directly the effect of jaundice on the migratory activity of fibroblasts. Other histological findings associated with healing in jaundiced animals include increased acute inflammation at a pancreatico-jejunostomy site in dogs as compared with control dogs (61). As acute inflammation is an essential early process in wound healing it is

difficult to determine whether this finding correlates with the clinical picture of impaired healing.

Using the activity of the enzyme prolyl hydroxylase as an index of collagen synthesis and therefore collagen turnover, several workers have found that its activity in the skin of jaundiced patients was significantly lower than that of normal controls (62). This activity was normalized in patients with benign, obstructive jaundice after curative surgery, indicating that in these patients impaired healing is reversible. In patients with malignant obstruction, however, biliary bypass increased activity but to a level that remained below normal values (50). In the same study dehiscence of the abdominal wound (a catastrophic example of failure of the healing process) was more common in jaundiced than anicteric patients and it has therefore been postulated that this complication appears to be associated with low skin prolyl hydroxylase activity and thus low rates of collagen synthesis.

Despite evidence that points to a direct effect of raised bilirubin on the wound healing process, in the clinical situation it remains difficult to separate the causal factors when wound failure occurs. A multivariate and univariate analysis (51) of factors relating to wound dehiscence and incisional hernia in a group of surgical patients with and without obstructive jaundice found that a raised plasma bilirubin was not of independent significance for either event. From this it was concluded that reduced healing in jaundiced patients is due to the associated features of poor nutrition such as low haematocrit, low albumin, and malignancy and not to raised bilirubin *per se*.

Jaundice clearly has the potential to impair wound healing. Based on the result of studies to date, however, it is equally certain that much remains to be done to elucidate the specific underlying mechanisms.

Diabetes mellitus

Clinically, diabetes mellitus is associated with a generalized defect in connective tissue metabolism, which is characterized by features including decreased growth, poor wound healing, and osteopenia. Vascular insufficiency, peripheral and autonomic neuropathy, and impaired immune response create an environment within the organism that is not generally conducive to optimal wound healing. Abnormalities at tissue and cellular level further frustrate the natural tendency of the body to repair itself. Hyperglycaemia leads to osmotic diuresis and subsequent decreased oxygenation and perfusion. It also limits polymorphonucleocyte functioning and impairs nutrition by increasing circulating levels of the hormones that cause catabolism (63).

The duration of the cell cycle and its component phases measured by ^{3}H-thymidine autoradiography are reduced in diabetic rats (64). The reduced rate of cell proliferation may contribute to the slow rates of healing seen in subjects with diabetes mellitus.

It has been demonstrated that granulation tissue formation in diabetic rats is reduced both in quantity and in its collagen content (65). Malnutrition and renal failure were also found to cause a reduction in granulation tissue formation *without* a decrease in collagen content. From this it has been deduced that low collagen content in the granulation tissue is related specifically to diabetes, as the phenomenon was prevented by insulin treatment. The replicative capacity of fibroblasts in diabetics has been shown to be diminished (66), which may in part account for the findings of reduced collagen content. Further evidence in support of the theory of impaired healing due to collagen abnormalities has been been provided by a study of experimental myocardial infarction in diabetic rats (67). Using ^{3}H-thymidine and ^{3}H-proline it was found that retarded formation of collagen fibres in diabetic animals is caused by a reduced number of tropocollagen-synthesizing fibroblasts and by a diminished synthesizing performance of the individual cells. Histologically, the fibroblast arrangements are also found to be abnormal (68). Excised wounds from diabetic rats have shown that the expected increase in tropocollagen occurs later than in normal controls but subsequent to this the level rises above normal. Even 30 days after wound formation the mature collagen content of the wound had still to reach 80 per cent of its preoperative level (68). Surprisingly, however, measurements of skin prolyl hydroxylase (an index of collagen synthesis) showed no evidence of reduction in diabetic patients (69).

Numerous growth factors are released from platelets on degranulation. Platelet derived growth factor (PDGF), for example, is involved in atherogenesis and in the generation of vascular alterations in diabetes mellitus (70). The mitogenic stimulation of fibroblasts by platelet extract was significantly reduced in diabetics compared to controls. It has thus been postulated that platelet mitogens are released into the circulation with a resulting acquired platelet defect. A trial of topical epidermal growth factor (EGF) in diabetic rats (71) demonstrated promotion of early synthesis of type I collagen and was associated with increased wound protease activity. Whether EGF is deficient, abnormal, or inhibited in diabetic wounds remains to be seen. Understanding of the complex nature of the growth factor interactions that facilitate wound healing in normal subjects remains a challenge; consideration of growth factors in isolation, or without considering their receptors and carrier molecules, may only further complicate the picture.

In order to assess possible circulating factors in diabetes which could be responsible for the abnormalities of collagen and fibroblasts, the effect of diabetic rat serum on cartilage has been investigated (72). In this study, collagen and non-collagen protein production were reduced by addition of the serum. Addition of insulin did not reverse defective collagen production and, moreover, addition of glucose or ketones to normal rat serum did not induce changes in collagen production. The inhibitory activity of the diabetic serum was found to be in a high molecular weight fraction, but its identity has yet to be determined. A similar study, however, whilst confirming the reduced production of collagen, did not show any change in non-collagen protein production (73). The effect on collagen could be demonstrated only two weeks after the induction of diabetes. Clearly, a deficiency of collagen in the granulation tissue of diabetics contributes to the clinical problem of impaired healing.

Non-enzymatic glycosylated haemoglobin is a familiar biochemical parameter used to monitor control in diabetic subjects. This phenomenon can also be shown to affect serum proteins. The extent of non-enzymatic glycosylation of granulation tissue soluble proteins in diabetic rats is significantly greater than in normal controls (74). There is also a significant decrease in the free amino acid groups in soluble proteins from diabetic tissues with greater activities of cathepsins B and D. It is possible therefore that increased non-enzymatic glycosylation of soluble proteins and increased proteolysis could have a role in impaired wound healing in diabetic subjects.

Integrity of the wound healing process is not only dependent on the quantity and quality of collagen present. Fibronectin plays a fundamental role in wound healing and acts as an opsonin for phagocytosis of foreign antigens (75). However, there is no evidence to suggest that diabetic patients on insulin exhibit any alteration in plasma fibronectin function, despite raised circulating glucose. Fibrin, another component of the extracellular matrix, does have its form and function modulated by the diabetic state. Fibrin nets accumulate poorly within the wound and are coarse and fragile in nature (68). The increase in plasma fibrinogen consequent on wounding occurs more slowly than normal, further evidence that the mechanisms of healing are globally retarded by diabetes.

As mentioned previously, the inflammatory response in diabetics is impaired. It has been shown, however, that alkaline phosphatase activity, a marker for polymorphonuclear leucocytes, is raised in granulation tissue (76), which may be a reflection of a prolonged, or more accurately, a delayed inflammatory phase. Histologically, in the wound environment the inflammatory response is minimal and occurs later than in non-diabetic subjects (68). Examination of wound fluid from diabetic rats has shown that altered leucocyte infiltration occurs principally during the late inflammatory phase of wound healing (77) and that this is associated with diminished levels of interleukin 6 (IL-6) at the same time. Both these factors indicate that in diabetes, the normal immunological response to injury, which is an essential prerequisite to tissue repair, is not achieved.

Epithelial healing problems and abnormalities of the basement membrane have been observed in the corneas of patients with diabetes. Epithelial healing problems may be related to damage to the basement membrane, with resulting poor adhesion of regenerating epithelial cells (78). Unlike type I and type III collagen, type IV collagen synthesis is increased in diabetes mellitus (79); this then accumulates in thickened basement membranes. This situation is further exacerbated by the fact that type IV collagenase, secreted by endothelial cells cultured in high glucose concentrations, appears to show diminished activity (79). Aldose-reductase inhibitors such as Sorbinil have been shown to prevent basement membrane thickening and overproduction of type IV collagen but did not demonstrate an increase in mechanical strength of wounds in diabetic rats. The role of basement membrane thickening in diabetic retinopathy and nephropathy has benefited from intense scientific interest, but further work now needs to be done on the relevance of basement membrane thickening to impaired wound healing.

Measurements of wound mechanical strength are a useful

method of assessing the adequacy of the healing mechanism. Despite wound strength being reduced in diabetic animals, this can be improved with treatment with insulin, especially if diabetic control is rigorously maintained (80). Even, after correction for diminished skin thickness, mechanical strength remains subnormal. Temporal examination of the changes in wound strength (66) reveal that for up to 14 days after wounding there may be no increase in wound strength. Any increase occurs slowly and, unlike normal controls, the pre-wound level may never be achieved.

It is clear that the factors responsible for impaired wound healing in diabetes act at multiple cellular and tissue loci, and a single responsible circulating factor is unlikely to be found.

Effect of vitamins A and C and zinc on wound healing

General malnutrition impairs wound healing. Scurvy is the classical example of the vital importance of a single nutrient (vitamin C) to wound healing. Fat-soluble vitamin A was found in 1916 to be essential for growth and its role in night blindness was elucidated two decades later. Zinc is also necessary for growth. Although other vitamins (vitamin E, pyridoxine, riboflavin, thiamin, and vitamin K) and trace elements (Fe, Cu, Mn, Mg, Se) are required for normal function of the body and may theoretically play a role during wound healing, the three aforementioned nutritional factors appear to be linked most closely with wound healing. Therefore emphasis in this section will be placed on vitamin A, vitamin C, and zinc.

Vitamin A

In this section not only will the parent molecule, retinol (vitamin A) and its derivatives be reviewed, but also other retinoids, i.e. retinaldehyde (vitamin A aldehyde) and derivatives and retinoic acid (vitamin A acid) and derivatives. By definition, retinoids are naturally occurring compounds with vitamin A activity and synthetic analogues with or without biological activity.

More than 90 per cent of the vitamin A stores are in the liver. Recommended daily intake has been estimated at 750 RE (retinol equivalents) for an adult (81). Hypovitaminosis A is still prevalent, especially in young children and in developing countries. Although easily obtained, plasma or serum levels (normal 30 µg/dl) do not accurately reflect the body's status when the liver is not critically depleted or excessively saturated with vitamin A. Liver biopsy for diagnosis is out of the question, and instead one has to rely on dietary assessment and the clinical picture.

Retinoids have profound effects on epithelial differentiation. In the classical experiment performed by Fell and Mellanby (82), addition of retinol or retinyl acetate inhibited the keratinization process and induced the skin to produce mucus (mucous metaplasia). These original observations have been confirmed and extended by other investigators and it is now well established that retinoid deficiency increases differentiation of most epithelia, whereas excess of retinoids inhib-

its differentiation. Apart from these morphological changes, fewer high-molecular weight keratins and an altered response to Ca^{2+} concentration shifts were seen in retinoid treated cells.

The effect of retinoids on keratinocyte proliferation depends on the culture system used and the origin of the keratinocytes. Retinoids (preferably retinoic acid) increase DNA synthesis in normal keratinocytes (at $<10^{-5}M$) when added at the time of plating but not afterwards. Conversely, retinoids are antiproliferative to neoplastic cells. The demonstration of multiple retinoic acid nuclear receptors provides the basis for the mechanism of action (83). Retinoids are also capable of increasing the production by keratinocytes of transforming growth factor β2 and interleukin-1, and possibly also of other cytokines (84, 85).

Another effect of retinoids relevant to wound healing is decreased collagenase production by keratinocytes as well as by fibroblasts exposed to retinoic acid (86). Vitamin A is also an important micronutrient in host resistance but information on the effect of vitamin A on phagocytic cell functions is limited.

Wound healing

Vitamin A deficiency was shown in early research to retard wound repair and increase the incidence of wound infection (87). More recent studies have shown that even marginal vitamin A deficiency impairs wound healing, as evidenced by decreased tensile strength on postoperative day 5 but not on day 14. These findings indicate a physiological role of vitamin A during the inflammatory phase. The impaired healing ability was restored in animals fed the recommended dietary allowance by retinyl acetate and β carotene (88).

The situation is different when there is no true deficiency. Most studies on the effect of systemic megadose vitamin A administration suggest that systemic vitamin A has no or only a marginal effect on wound healing in well-nourished animals (89, 90). On the other hand, an increased tensile strength was found on day 5 but not on day 14 when rats were fed five times the recommended daily intake of retinyl acetate and retinoic acid (88).

When applied topically, vitamin A (retinoic acid) promotes granulation tissue formation (90–92). Increased infiltration of macrophages has been proposed as one mechanism of action (89). It is also known that retinoids can increase proliferation of cultured fibroblasts, one important component in the formation of granulation tissue (93). In one study, retinoic acid increased fibroblast proliferation (at $>10^{-6}M$) whereas retinol had no effect (93). This may be one explanation why some early investigators failed to find any effects of vitamin A on wound healing in normal animals.

Topical application of vitamin A to skin wounds does not enhance epithelialization, another mechanism in the closure of wounds, but may on the contrary retard it. However, two studies attest to the positive effect on epithelialization of pre-treating the skin of the prospective wound sites with retinoic acid (Fig. 6.1). These findings may be explained by the mitogenic effect of retinoic acid when applied to normal skin (94). Epithelial defects in the cornea, on the other hand, healed faster with retinoic acid (0.1 per cent) applied 2–5

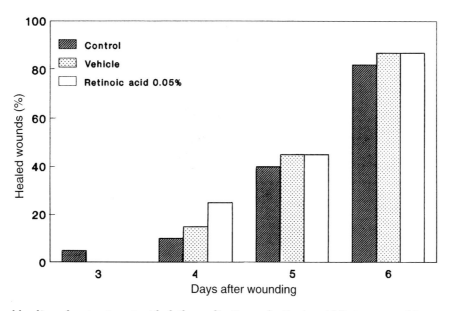

Fig. 6.1 Effect on wound healing of pretreatment with daily applications of retinoic acid (0.05 per cent) in a cream vehicle to pig skin for 10 days prior to making partial thickness wounds (figure based on data in Table 1 in Hung *et al.*, ref. 89.)

times daily (95, 96). Retinyl palmitate, retinyl acetate, and 13-cis-retinoic acid were ineffective (96).

Retinoid treatment seems to be beneficial for impaired healing caused by corticosteroids, uncontrolled diabetes, irradiation, or malignancies (97–100). Ehrlich and Hunt were the first to report the antagonistic effect of retinoids (palmitate) on cortisone-retarded healing (97). Vitamin A must be given for at least seven days postoperatively to be effective. These novel findings on the healing of skin wounds have also been found during healing of intestinal anastomoses (100). One theory is that the stabilizing property of steroids on lysosomes is reversed by the labilizing influence of retinoids. Rats fed high doses of vitamin A developed lymphocytosis, monocytosis, and a relative neutropenia (101). Although the results are impressive, supplemental vitamin A has not gained widespread clinical popularity, possibly due to the relatively high, albeit subtoxic, doses of vitamin A that are required for these indications (91). For example, the plasma vitamin A level was increased five-fold when therapeutic doses of vitamin A (300 RE) were given to rats intramuscularly. Suppressed weight gain was seen even at doses as low as 30 RE (102).

Vitamin C

Scurvy was described in 1500 BC, but it was not until 1753 that James Lind prevented it by giving citrus fruits. In 1932, the antiscorbutic substance vitamin C was identified. Carefully monitored experiments in humans have shown that vitamin C deprivation leads to fatigue, hyperkeratoses around hair follicles, haemorrhages, loose teeth, and after about 180 days of ascorbic acid withdrawal, poor wound healing follows (103). Concentrations of >200 mg/l of leucocyte ascorbic acid are normal, while levels <40 mg/l are found after about 80 days on an ascorbic-acid-free diet. By then total body stores of ascor-

bic acid have decreased from about 1500 mg to 300 mg. A daily intake of about 40 mg of ascorbic acid is required to prevent depletion.

One important biochemical function of ascorbic acid is its action as a cofactor for the dioxygenases prolyl and lysyl hydroxylase. The hydroxylases also require α-ketoglutarate and oxygen as co-substrates. Ascorbic acid acts primarily as a reductant for Fe^{3+} and does not seem to take part directly in the hydroxylation reaction (104). Without these enzymes being active, collagen molecules will not be hydroxylated and thus cross-linking and stabilization of the triple helix is delayed or may cease. Ascorbic acid influences the rate of collagen synthesis at several levels, from gene transcription, mRNA stabilization, and translation to secretion (105). Ascorbic acid is also necessary for the formation of intercellular proteoglycans. Further, supplements of ascorbic acid to neutrophils and macrophages in culture can increase their motility and phagocytotic capability (106, 107).

Defective collagen is produced in the absence of vitamin C which leads to blood vessel disruption (haemorrhage) and dehiscence of wounds (108). Vitamin C deficiency decreases collagen deposition in wounds, resulting in reduced wound strength. Despite the decreased collagen formation, wound contraction is not affected in scorbutic guinea-pigs (109). Treatment of scorbutic animals and humans with ascorbic acid rapidly restores the healing capabilities (110).

Megadose therapy using vitamin C was introduced in the 1970s. The rationale was that humans should receive amounts of vitamin C equivalent to those of lower animals who are able to make ascorbic acid themselves (e.g. mice, rats, rabbits, who have L-gulono-γ-lactone oxidase). Direct beneficial effects of extra ascorbic acid in *in vitro* experiments on important wound healing parameters such as increased phagocytosis, fibroblast proliferation (10 mg/l), and collagen synthesis have been demonstrated (111, 112). During wound healing ascorbic acid seems to accumulate preferentially in repair tissue (113, 114). More of the oxidized form of ascorbic acid, dehydroascorbic acid, is also seen in repair tissue than in adjacent uninjured skin (115). Thus, early investigators claimed that there is an increased demand for ascorbic acid after extensive skin injuries such as burns and major surgery. A 40 per cent reduction in the leucocyte ascorbic acid concentration has been reported after extensive surgical trauma on the first postoperative day although this reduction may be explained by the postoperative increase in the number of polymorphonuclear leucocytes (116). A supplement of 1–2 g of ascorbic acid to prevent wound complications in these patients has been recommended.

A placebo-controlled trial in 1977 gave direct support for this concept in wound healing (117). In a total of 20 elderly patients with pressure sores, 10 received 1 g/day of oral ascorbic acid and the other 10 a placebo. The healing rate was twofold in the vitamin C group after four weeks of treatment. Despite the normal leucocyte ascorbic acid levels the authors speculated that their patients may have been vitamin C deficient. Although the results of this small-size trial are promising they need to be reproduced in larger scale clinical trials. However, vitamin C supplementaion had no effect on the healing of wounds in non-deficient cornea and gingiva (118, 119). Vitamin C might, however, be useful in the prevention of skin ulcers because a low leucocyte ascorbic acid level was found to be a predisposing factor for developing pressure sores (120).

Zinc

The need of living organisms for zinc was first reported for microorganisms in 1869, for plants in 1926, for rats in 1934, for pigs in 1955, and for man in 1961. Zinc is required for the activity of several metalloenzymes, i.e. enzymes in which zinc is tightly bound to the active site and takes part in the catalytic process. There are at least 200 known zinc-dependent metalloenzymes involved in different biological processes, such as protein and nucleic acid synthesis or degradation, and carbohydrate and lipid metabolism. Although the biological action of zinc is commonly attributed to its role in these enzymes, zinc is also important for the structure and function of biomembranes. Intensive research during the past decade has identified zinc-containing proteins which seem to regulate gene expression (121).

Theoretically, zinc may interact with the wound healing process in many ways. Since zinc is important for chromatin and DNA polymerases, it plays a role in cell division and proliferation. Cell growth is retarded in zinc-depleted media. Protein synthesis is also adversely affected by zinc deficiency. Recently, Hicks and Wallwork showed that the primary defect in protein synthesis in zinc deficiency occurred at the translational rather than at the transcriptional level (122). Zinc can also modulate the activity of inflammatory cells by interacting with their membranes and intracellular reactions.

Skin zinc stores are not depleted unless both zinc and proteins are severely restricted. However, zinc appears to accumulate in wounded skin, indicating a specific demand for this trace element in wound healing (123). Patients with delayed healing have lower zinc levels in granulation tissue than patients with adequate healing. Although surgical trauma is associated with a transient fall in serum zinc the effect of zinc deficiency on primary healing in humans is not known. It is known, however, that surgical patients on total parenteral nutrition (TPN) without trace element supplements, develop typical signs of zinc deficiency, which are relieved by zinc administration. In dogs it was found that animals on zinc-free TPN accumulated only half the amount of hydroxyproline (as a measure of collagen accumulation) in intestinal wounds compared with control animals given adequate zinc (124). More than 10 controlled clinical trials with zinc have been performed in patients with leg ulcers (for a review see Ågren, ref. 125). These studies have shown that zinc sulphate given orally (usually as capsules or tablets 220 mg three times a day in combination with meals) is effective only in patients with subnormal serum zinc levels. One has to be aware that serum zinc measurements do not always reflect the zinc status. Rats fed a zinc-deficient diet have poor healing of skin incisions and gastric ulcers (126–128).

Topical application of different zinc-containing preparations has been practised for many years. The use of topical zinc seems to be based on empirical rather than scientific grounds since wound healing experiments in normal, non-deficient rats and guinea-pigs have not been able to attest to any beneficial effects. We have investigated the effects of zinc oxide applied topically to both chronic and acute wounds in controlled experiments. In a double-blind trial, zinc oxide promoted the healing of leg ulcers (128). Since the patients had subnormal serum zinc levels it could not be concluded that topical zinc oxide was effective in patients with normal zinc status. In subsequent experiments zinc was tried in the form of zinc oxide and also in the form of the water-soluble zinc sulphate in nutritionally balanced domestic pigs. Zinc oxide enhanced re-epithelialization by 30 per cent above control, whereas topical zinc sulphate had no beneficial effect on the healing rate at any of the three concentrations (Fig. 6.2). In another study, topical application of zinc oxide increased the mitotic index by 30 per cent in uninjured and incised mouse skin (129). In more recent studies we have also shown that topical zinc oxide significantly increases the wound closure rate of full-thickness cutaneous wounds (Fig. 6.3).

These results indicate that when zinc is added as zinc oxide to wounds it may exert a pharmacological action on wound healing apart from being an essential nutrient. The pig was chosen as an experimental animal in these experiments because of the similarity of its skin to human skin. This may be one explanation why other investigators, using rodents as experimental animals, found no beneficial effects of topical zinc oxide. The choice of vehicle is also important. For example, zinc oxide was found to be ineffective when incorporated in a hydrocolloid dressing (123).

In pharmacokinetic studies it was further shown that local treatment with zinc oxide resulted in constant zinc concentrations in wound fluid and wounded tissue, whereas in local treatment, with zinc sulphate, the zinc concentrations declined as a function of time (131, 132). Therefore the mode of delivery of zinc is critical to achieve a beneficial effect. We hypothesized that zinc oxide provides a depot of zinc which

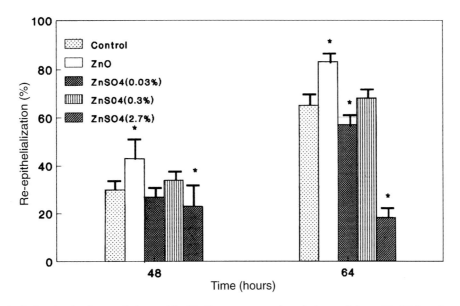

Fig. 6.2 Effect of topical zinc in the form of zinc oxide (ZnO, 1.4 per cent) and zinc sulphate ($ZnSO_4$) at three concentrations on re-epithelialization (mean ± SEM) of partial thickness wounds in pigs (reconstructed from Table 1 in Ågren *et al.*, ref. 130.) Statistical significance ($p < 0.05$) relative to control values is indicated by an asterisk above the relevant bar.

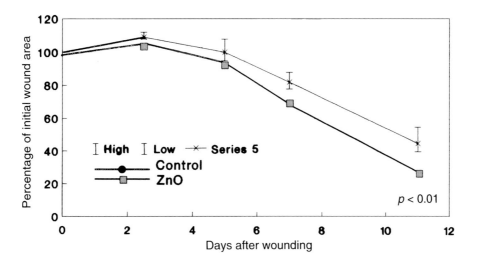

Fig. 6.3 Effect of zinc oxide (ZnO, 1.4 per cent) on the closure time (mean ± SEM, $n = 8$) of full-thickness wounds (2.2 cm × 4.4 cm) in two domestic pigs. Control wounds ($n = 8$) were treated with the vehicle for zinc oxide alone. (From Tarnow *et al.*, ref. 131.)

releases zinc ions at a proper rate to stimulate healing over an extended period.

The reasons for the beneficial effects of topical zinc oxide are unknown. Because neither cell proliferation nor protein or collagen synthesis are stimulated by zinc *in vitro*, zinc most likely acts by some indirect mechanisms *in vivo*. An antibacterial effect of topical zinc oxide has been found *in vivo* (133). The antibacterial activity of zinc oxide in wounds is not only a direct one but zinc oxide appears to augment the phagocytic function of polymorphonuclear leucocytes (134). We have also shown recently that zinc can increase the gene expression of one growth factor – insulin-like growth factor-1 – in full-thickness wounds in pigs (131).

Oxygen and perfusion in wound healing

Tissue repair in living organisms is a complex process which is affected by a host of endogenous and exogenous factors. However, it has long been recognized that clinically adequate wound healing and scar formation can still occur in the face of less than perfect conditions. The extent to which each individual factor influences the outcome of the healing mechanism has been the subject of intense investigation for many years. One of the most exciting scientific and clinical debates that has arisen is over the role of oxygen in tissue repair (see also Chapters 3 and 5).

It has been clear to surgeons, from clinical observations,

that the presence of ischaemia leads to an increased incidence of wound failure and breakdown, anastomotic dehiscence, and wound infection, all of which represent a major cause of patient morbidity and mortality. Based on this evidence, much of modern surgical management is aimed at optimizing blood and oxygen delivery to the wound during the healing phase (135). Locally, blood supply is maintained by a knowledge of the arterial anatomy, careful planning of incisions, anastomoses, and flaps and by minimizing local dissection of vulnerable structures such as the ureter or the oesophagus. Some surgical texts still advocate the aggressive correction of postoperative anaemia, maintaining the level of haemoglobin at or above 10 g/dl (136), to facilitate oxygen delivery to the wound. Scientific justification for this recommendation is lacking. Local tissue ischaemia is thought to be the underlying cause of skin breakdown and persistent non-healing of decubitus ulcers, though reperfusion injury following the period of ischaemia may be important. Respiratory hypoxia, hypovolaemia, and all forms of circulatory collapse have been implicated in poor wound healing, though the underlying mechanism is unclear.

It has only been within the past 30 years that scientific techniques which allow detailed investigation of the microenvironment of the wound have been developed, leading to a better understanding of the role of oxygen delivery and consumption at a microscopic level in both the normal and the abnormal wound (see Chapter 3). Initial experimental evidence of the hypoxic nature of wounds and the effect of oxygen on healing came from Niinikoski (137). At the same time the use of microelectrodes to measure tissue oxygen tensions, within the rabbit ear chamber model of an acute wound, revealed that a diffusion gradient, with a tissue p_{O_2} as low as 3 mm/Hg (400 Pa) in areas furthest away from capillary loops, existed in the granulation tissue (138). The discovery that a certain degree of hypoxia was a normal feature of healing wounds generated two further questions. Would any increase in the tissue oxygen tension augment either the rate of healing or the strength of the wound and to what extent would further reductions in the tissue oxygen level retard the repair process?

Normal wounds extract and consume very little of the oxygen that is supplied to them (139), yet both animal and human studies have shown a direct relationship between local oxygen tension and both the rate of collagen deposition by fibroblasts and, consequently, the tensile strength of the wound (140–142). Despite this, there is little clinical evidence to support the view that merely increasing the fraction of inspired oxygen (FiO_2) leads to enhanced tissue repair in normal subjects, though some patients with marginally hypoxic wounds may benefit from such simple measures (143). The modest improvement in tissue oxygenation provided in this way may, however, exert a beneficial effect on successful wound healing through the enhancement of the bactericidal activity of neutrophils and macrophages (144). Animal models of tissue infection with *Escherichia coli* have demonstrated that supplemental oxygen therapy can produce an antibacterial effect equivalent to that of antibiotic prophylaxis (145).

The nature of the oxygen saturation curve for haemoglobin allows almost complete saturation under normal physiological conditions and increases in the fraction of inspired oxygen (FiO_2) up to 100 per cent, in the absence of respiratory disease, will make very little difference to the oxygen delivered to the tissues. The oxygen saturation of the plasma, whilst being only a very minor component under normal conditions, has enormous carrying capacity for oxygen delivered at pressures greater than atmospheric. The use of hyperbaric oxygen can increase the arterial oxygen pressure (p_{aO_2}) from 100 mmHg (13 kPa), when breathing 100 per cent O_2 at 1 ATA, to 2000 mmHg (270 kPa) at 3 ATA. At 4 ATA enough oxygen is carried by the plasma to allow the survival of pigs despite the absence of haemoglobin following the removal of all erythrocytes from their circulating blood volume (146). The higher arterial p_{O_2} leads to a greater diffusion radius and therefore increases the levels of tissue oxygen at greater distances from the capillaries (147). If the oxygen diffusion radii increase to such an extent that they overlap, the hypoxic areas commonly seen in wound granulation tissue will be abolished. It can be seen from this reasoning that it is the arterial oxygen tension rather than the arterial oxygen content that will lead to increased tissue perfusion and hence wound healing (140, 148, 149). Some clinical evidence does exist to support the use of measures to increase the local oxygen concentration. The rate of re-epithelialization of a wound is increased in the presence of increased local p_{O_2} (150) and clinical trials of hyperbaric oxygen therapy in the healing of chronic wounds and pedicled skin flaps have shown a limited degree of success (151–153).

There is good evidence to support the hypothesis that problem wounds are hypoxic in nature (even when compared to the level of hypoxia seen in normal wounds). Animal models of hypoxic have shown retarded granulation tissue formation and epithelialization as well as reduced collagen synthesis (137, 154). Studies comparing the tissue oxygen pressure of normal and chronic wounds using transcutaneous and implanted probes found that the chronic wounds were markedly hypoxic (153, 155) and low oxygen and poor tissue perfusion was associated with decreased collagen synthesis and deposition (154). Clinical studies of wound healing show little or no correlation with moderate anaemia, blood loss, urine output, age, weight, or sex, (156, 157) although acute haemorrhage or delayed blood replacement, leading to hypovolaemia, does lead to impaired wound healing (158). This leads us to the conclusion that it is the delivery of oxygen at a tissue level that is clinically as well as experimentally most relevant.

Radiotherapy and chemotherapy in wound healing

Comparisons have been made between the proliferative events taking place during wound healing and those which occur during tumorigenesis (159–161). It is clear that these similarities include angiogenesis, stroma formation, and protease production, as well as the more general hypoxic nature of the microenvironment. Recent advances in the treatment of a variety of cancers have shown the benefit of combining radiotherapy and chemotherapy with surgical procedures. The increasing use of these modalities prior to or soon after operative procedures has led to concern about the deleterious effect that this might have upon wound healing.

The rationale behind the use of either chemotherapy or radiotherapy is that, though both techniques 'kill' dividing cells in an unselective way, their effect upon the tumour cells is greater than on other cell types due to the faster rate of division amongst the tumour cells (162, 163). This effect is achieved through disruption of genetic replication by high energy particles in radiotherapy, or the interference with cell metabolism by chemotherapeutic agents. Unfortunately, normal cells with a high mitotic rate, and hence a high proliferative rate, will also be affected. This is clearly illustrated by the leucopenia, anaemia, and thrombocytopenia that is often seen as a consequence of a variety of chemotherapeutic regimes (164). During the initial stages of wound repair there is a rapid proliferation of a host of cell types that would be vulnerable to cytotoxic treatments (165). Suppression of the haemopoietic tissues could also disrupt wound healing either by a lack of initiation of subsequent cascades due to decreased platelet degranulation or through an increased risk of infection secondary to the leucopenia.

Studies of low dose total body and local irradiation in mice have shown poor wound healing to be a consequence of myelosuppression, with local fibroblasts being relatively resistant to radiation damage (166). However, at higher doses there is evidence of decreased collagen production secondary to the adverse effects upon the local fibroblast population (167). In addition to the dose-related aspect of therapy it appears that the timing of treatment may be important. In the rat, low dose preoperative irradiation had little or no effect upon wound healing parameters (168) whilst the timing of preoperative abdominal irradiation prior to colonic anastomosis revealed an optimal period for treatment (169). Studies of preoperative radiotherapy in humans has shown an increased incidence of local wound complications such as lymphoedema, seroma formation, delayed wound healing, and infection (170, 171) whilst external irradiation leads to an increased risk of dehiscence of colorectal anastomoses (172). Delay in treatment until after the fifth postoperative day dramatically decreased the incidence of wound problems (173). Radiotherapy in the treatment of malignant disease will always represent a play-off between the advantages of tumour control and complications of therapy and in light of this, high dose intra-operative local treatment has been advocated for some advanced cancers (174). A study of pre- and postoperative chemotherapy with adriamycin in rats has shown a deficit in wound healing with preoperative treatment as well as with early (up to 28 days) postoperative regimens (175) though no impairment of human wound healing was seen when the drug was given 15 days postoperatively (176). Experimental results, however, may not always be clinically relevant. Despite a potentially deleterious effect upon wound healing from the chemotherapeutic agent 5-fluorouracil (177), it has now seen widespread use in randomized clinical trials for postoperative aduvant therapy in colorectal carcinoma without any significant effect upon wound healing. Combinations of chemotherapy and radiotherapy have shown varying effects on wound healing (176, 178) and are probably a result of the individual regimens used in each study.

Reconstructive procedures using either grafts or flaps are often employed to cover the defects created by radical surgical procedures for malignant disease. These techniques are particularly sensitive to local conditions such as ischaemia, infection, and the condition of the surrounding tissue. Late effects of irradiation include an obliterative endarteritis leading to atrophic and avascular tissues. Postoperative irradiation may compromise the vascularity of the flap whilst preoperative treatment will devascularize the tissue bed as well as the surrounding skin precluding a local rotation flap. There is evidence from both human and animal studies that flaps are at particular risk from radiation-induced damage (179, 180). Reconstruction of previously irradiated tissue can be managed successfully using either myocutaneous flaps or omental transpositions, though this is not without wound complications (181, 182).

Attempts have been made to reverse the impairment of wound healing produced by these treatment modalities using supplemental vitamins and growth factors in experimental models using rats. Platelet derived growth factor (PDGF), vitamin A, and vitamin E have all led to a reversal of radiation-induced poor wound healing (174, 183, 184) whilst the administration of transforming growth factor beta (TGFβ) produced similar effects upon adriamycin-induced damage (185). However, evidence of similar effects in humans is lacking.

Chemotherapy and radiotherapy both produce deleterious effects upon wound healing that are dependant on a variety of factors and are therefore difficult to predict. The timing and dose of both modalities relative to the surgery seem to be important in experimental situations, but in clinical practice the possible side-effects must be weighed against the potential benefits of such therapy in control of the disease. Difficulties encountered during surgery on areas of previously irradiated tissue once again emphasize the importance of ischaemia and local hypoxia in all aspects of wound healing.

Obesity in wound healing

The precise role of obesity in wound repair remains uncertain despite the conviction of many surgeons that it does have a detrimental effect. It is probable that the relationship is not a straightforward one but is associated with related problems which are responsible for the observed outcome. One clinical study found no relationship between patient weight and wound problems (156) whilst others have shown that wound infection and incisional hernia are both significantly more common in obese patients (186, 187) but the underlying mechanism remains obscure. However, a number of appealing hypotheses have been put forward. Obesity itself makes surgical procedures technically more difficult and blood vessels within the fat, lacking support, require more delicate handling if they are not to be torn. This tendency, combined with the difficulty of obliterating the dead space at the end of an operation, increases the chance of haematoma formation. Over-aggressive haemostasis with either diathermy or ligature can lead to areas of devitalized tissue within the wound. The end result in either case is to provide a nidus for infection to become established. Wound infection and its subsequent breakdown will then be almost inevitable.

References

1. Eaglestein, W. H. (1986). Wound healing and aging. *Dermatologic Clinics*, **4**, 481–4.
2. Hardy, M. A. (1989). The biology of scar formation. *Phys. Ther.*, **69**, 1014–24.
3. Lauker, R. M., Zheng, P., and Dong, G. (1986). Morphology of aged skin. *Dermatologic Clinicas*, **4**, 379–89.
4. Grove, G. L. (1982). Age-related differences in healing of superficial skin wounds in humans. *Arch. Derm. Res.*, **272**, 281–9.
5. Muehlman, C. and Rahimi, R. L. (1990). Aging integumentary system. *J. Am. Pod. Med. Assoc.*, **80**, 577–82.
6. Gilchrist, B. A., Stoff, J. S., and Soter, N. A. (1982). Chronological aging alters the response to ultraviolet-induced inflammation in human skin. *J. Investig. Dermat.*, **79**, 11–15.
7. Lober, C. W. and Fenske, N. A. (1991). Cutaneous aging: effect of intrinsic changes on surgical considerations. *South. Med. J.*, **84**, 1444–6.
8. Reichle, F. A., Rankin, K. P., and Shuman, C. R. (1979). The elderly patient with severe arterial insufficiency of the lower extremity. *Circulation*, **60**, 124.
9. Czerniecki, J. M., Harrington, R. M., Wyss, C. R., Sangeorzan, B. J., and Matsen, F. A. (1990). The effects of age and peripheral vascular disease on the circulatory and mechanical response of skin to loading. *Am. J. Phys. Med. Rehab.*, **69**, 302–6.
10. Bennett, P. H. (1984). Diabetes in the elderly: diagnosis and epidemiology. *Geriatrics*, **37**, 39.
11. Bell, E. T. (1957). Atherosclerotic gangrene of the lower extremities in diabetic and nondiabetic persons. *Am. J. Clin. Path.* **28**, 27.
12. Levin, M. E. and O'Neal, L. W. (1988). *The diabetic foot.* C. V. Mosby Co., St Louis.
13. Levin, M. E. (1983). Diabetes mellitus. In *Care of the geriatric patient*, (ed. F. Steinberg), (6th edn). C. V. Mosby Co., St Louis.
14. Boulton, A. S. M., Franks, C. I., Betts, R. P., Cuckworth, T., and Ward, J. D. (1984). Reduction of abnormal foot pressures in diabetic neuropathy using a new polymer insole material. *Diabetes Care*, **7**, 42.
15. Knatterud, G. L., Klimt, C. R., Levin, M. E., Jacobson, M. E., and Goldner, M. G. (1978). Effects of hypoglycemic agents on vascular complications in patients with adult-onset diabetes. *J. Am. Med. Assoc.*, **240**, 37.
16. Pecoraro, R. E., Ahroni, J. H., Boyko, E. J., and Stensel, V. L. (1991). Chronology and determinants of tissue repair in diabetic lower-extremity ulcers. *Diabetes*, **40**, 1305–13.
17. Arend, W. P., Collier, D. H., and Harmon, C. E. (1990). Musculoskeletal diseases. In *Geriatric Medicine*, (ed. R. W. Schrier), W. B. Saunders, Philadelphia.
18. Hunt, T. K. and Dunphy, J. E. (1979). *Fundamentals of wound management.* Appleton-Century-Crofts, New York.
19. Radl, J., Sepers, J. M., and Skuar, L. F. (1975). Immunoglobulin patterns in humans over 95 years of age. *Clin. Exper. Immun.*, **22**, 84.
20. Klinman, N. (1981). Antibody specific immunoregulation and the immunodeficiency of aging. *J. Exp. Med.*, **154**, 547–51.
21. Kay, M. B. (1990). Immunologic problems. In *Geriatric medicine*, (ed. R. W. Schrier), W. B. Saunders, Philadelphia.
22. Kay, M. B. (1979). Effect of age on human immunological parameters including T and B cell colony formation. *Recent Advances in Gerontology*, 442–3.
23. Weksler, M. E. (1981). The senescence of the immune system. *Hosp. Prac.*, **10**, 53–64.
24. Mendoza, C. B., Postlethwait, R. W., and Johnson, W. D. (1970). Veterans administration cooperative study of surgery for duodenal ulcer, II. Incidence of wound disruption following operation. *Arch. Surg.*, **101**, 396–8.
25. Flower, R. J., Moncacia, S., and Vase, J. (1980). Analgesic antipyletics and anti-inflammatory agents: drugs employed in the treatment of gout. In *Goodman and Gilman's, pharmacologic basis of therapeutics*, (ed. A. G. Gilman, I. S. Goodman, and A. Gilman), pp. 718–20. MacMillan, New York.
26. Alvarez, O. M., Levendorf, K. D., Smerbeck, R. V., Mertz, P. M., and Eaglestein, W. H. (1984). Effect of topically applied steroidal and non-steroidal anti-inflammatory agents on skin repair and regeneration. *Federation Proceedings*, **43**, 2793–8.
27. Corball, M., O'Dwyer, P., and Brady, M. P. (1985). The interaction of vitamin A and corticosteroids on wound healing. *J. Med. Sci.*, **154**, 306–70.
28. Ehrlich, H. P. and Hunt, T. K. (1986). The effects of cortisone and vitamin A on wound healing. *Ann. Surg.*, **167**, 3224–8.
29. Van Story-Lewis, P. E. and Tennenbaum, H. S. (1986). Gluccocorticoid inhibition of fibroblast contraction of collagen gels. *Biochem. Pharm.*, **35**, 1283–6.
30. Priestley, G. C. (1978). Effects of corticosteroids on the growth and metablism of fibroblasts cultured from human skin. *Br. J. Derm.*, **96**, 253–61.
31. Ponec, M., Dettaras, C., and Bachra, R. N. (1977). Effects of glucocorticoids on primary human skin fibroblasts. *Arch. Derm. Res.*, **259**, 117–23.
32. Eaglestein, W. H. (ed.) (1984). Current wound management: a symposium. *Clinical Dermatology*, **2**, 113–4.
33. Nemlander, A. (1983). Effect of cyclosporine on wound healing. *Transplantation*, **36**, 1–6.
34. Fischel, R. (1983). Cyclosporine A impairs wound healing in rats. *J. Surg. Res.*, **34**, 572–5.
35. Eisinger, D. and Sheil, A. G. R. (1985). A comparison of the effects of endosporin and standard agents on primary wound healing in the rat. *Surg. Gynae. Obstet.*, **160**, 135–8.
36. Lipschitz, D. A. (1982). Protein calorie malnutrition in the hospitalized elderly. *Primary Care*, **9**, 531–43.
37. Sava, T. M. (1983). Nutrition and fibronectin mediated phagocytic function. *Clinical Consults of Nutritional Supplementation*, **3**, 8.
38. Levenson, S. M. and Seifter, E. (1977). Dysnutrition, wound healing and resistance to infection. *Clin. Plas. Surg.*, **4**, 375.
39. Devin-Pinchcofsky, G. (1990). Nutritional assessment and intervention. In *Chronic wound care: a clinical source for health care professionals*, (ed. Diane, Krasner). Health Management Publications Inc., King of Prussia.
40. Goode, P. S. and Allman, R. M. (1989). The prevention and management of pressure ulcers. *Med. Clin. N. Am.*, **73**, 1511–24.
41. Taylor, T. V., Rimmer, S., and Day, B. (1974). Ascorbic acid supplementation in the treatment of pressure sores. *Lancet*, **ii**, 544–6.
42. McDermott, F. T., Galbraith, A. J., and Corlett, R. J. (1975). Inhibition of cell proliferation in renal failure and its significance to the uraemic syndrome: a review. *Scot. Med., J.*, **20**, 317–27.
43. Mott, T. J. and Ellis, H. (1967). A method of producing experimental uraemia in the rabbit with some observations on the influence of uraemia on peritoneal healing. *Br. J. Urol.*, **39**, 341–5.
44. McDermott, F. T., Nayman, J., and de Boer, W. G. R. M. (1968).

The effect of acute renal failure upon wound healing: histological and autoradiographic studies in the mouse. *Ann. Surg.*, **168**, 142–6.

45. Castrup, H. J. and Lennartz, K. J. (1972). Einfluss der uramie auf die proliferationskinetik des stratum basale der haut. *Beitraege Zur Pathologie*, **145**, 204–10.

46. Eriksen, H. O., Tranebjaerg, L., Clemmensen, I., Kjersem, H., and Skjoldby, O. (1983). Plasma fibronectin concentration in patients with chronic renal failure and treated with haemodialysis. *Scan. J. Clin. Lab. Invest.*, **43**, 723–6.

47. Yue, D. K., Swanson, B., McLennan, S., Marsh, M., Spaliviero, J., Delbridge, L., *et al.* (1986). Abnormalities of granulation tissue and collagen formation in experimental diabetes, uraemia and malnutrition. *Diabetic Medicine*, **3**, 221–5.

48. Yue, D. K., McLennan, S., Marsh, M., Mai, Y. W., Spaliviero, J., Delbridge, L., *et al.* (1987). Effects of experimental diabetes, uraemia, and malnutrition on wound healing. *Diabetes*, **36**, 295–9.

49. Colin, J. (1977). MS. Thesis, University of London.

50. Grande, L., Garcia-Valdecascas, J. C., Fuster, J., Visa, J., and Pera, C. (1990). Obstructive jaundice and wound healing. *Br. J. Surg.*, **77**, 440–2.

51. Armstrong, C. P., Bates, G. J., and Balderson, G. (1984). Wound healing in obstructive jaundice. *Br. J. Surg.*, **71**, 267–70.

52. Irvin, T. T., Vassilakis, J. S., Chattopadhyay, D. K., and Greaney, M. G. (1978). Abdominal wound healing in jaundiced patients. *Br. J. Surg.*, **65**, 521–2.

53. Taube, M., Elliot, P., and Ellis, H. (1981). Jaundice and wound healing: a tissue culture study. *Br. J. Exp. Path.*, **62**, 227–31.

54. Greaney, M. G., Van Noort, R., Smythe, A., and Irwin, T. T. (1979). Does obstructive jaundice adversely affect wound healing? *Br. J. Surg.*, **66**, 478–81.

55. Ellis, H. (1977). Wound healing. *Ann. Roy. Coll. Surg. Eng.*, **59**, 382–7.

56. Askew, A. R., Bates, G. J., and Balderson, G. (1984). Jaundice and the effect of sodium taurocholate taken orally upon abdominal wound healing. *Surg. Gyn. Obstet.*, **159**, 201–9.

57. Taube, M., Elliott, P., and Ellis, H. (1988). Toxicity of bilirubin and bilirubin diglucuronide to rat tissue culture fibroblasts. *Euro. Surg. Res.*, **20**, 190–4.

58. Zieve, L. (1986). Conditional deficiencies of ornithine or arginine. [Review.] *J. Am. Coll. Nut.*, **5**, 167–76.

59. Bayer, I. and Ellis, H. (1976). Jaundice and wound healing: an experimental study. *Br. J. Surg.*, **63**, 392–6.

60. Lee, E. (1972). The effect of obstructive jaundice on the migration of reticulo-endothelial cells and fibroblasts into early experimental granulomata. *Br. J. Surg.*, **59**, 875–7.

61. Takahashi, S. (1984). The influence of obstructive jaundice on wound healing of pancreatico-jejunostomy with reference to the function of the pancreas as assessed by glucose tolerance and pancreozymin-secretin test. [Japanese.] *J. Jap. Surg. Soc.*, **85**, 1332–43.

62. Than, T., McGee, J. O., Sokhi, G. S., Patrick, R. S., and Blumgart, L. H. (1974). Skin prolyl hydroxylase in patients with obstructive jaundice. *Lancet*, **ii**, 807–8.

63. Terranova, A. (1991). The effects of diabetes mellitus on wound healing. *Plastic Surgical Nursing*, **11**, 20–5.

64. Hamilton, A. I. and Blackwood, H. J. (1977). Insulin deficiency and cell proliferation in oral mucosal epithelium of the rat. *J. Anat.*, **124**, 757–63.

65. Yue, D. K., Swanson, B., McLennan, S., Marsh, M., Spaliviero, J., Delbridge, L., *et al.* (1986). Abnormalities of granulation tissue and collagen formation in experimental diabetes, uraemia and malnutrition. *Diabetic Medicine*, **3**, 221–5.

66. Goldstein, S., Niewiarowski, S., and Singal, D. P. (1975). Patho-

logical implications of cell aging *in vitro*. [Review.] *Federation Proceedings*, **34**, 56–63.

67. Kranz, D., Hecht, A., Fuhrmann, I., and Keim, U. (1977). The influence of diabetes mellitus and hypercorticism on the wound healing of experimental myocardial infarction in rats. *Experimentelle Pathologie*, **14**, 1–8.

68. Castrup, H. J. and Lennartz, K. J. (1972). Einfluss der uramie auf die proliferationskinetik des stratum basale der haut. *Beitraege Zur Pathologie*, **145**, 204–10.

69. Eriksen, H. O., Tranebjaerg, L., Clemmensen, I., Kjersem, H., and Skjoldby, O. (1983). Plasma fibronectin concentration in patients with chronic renal failure and treated with haemodialysis. *Scan. J. Clin. Lab. Investig.*, **43**, 723–6.

70. Caenazzo, A., Pietrogrande, F., Polato, G., Piva, E., Sartori, D., and Girolami, A. (1991). Decreased platelet mitogenic activity in patients with diabetes mellitus. *Haematologica*, **24**, 241–7.

71. Hennessey, P. J., Black, C. T., and Andrassy, R. J. (1990). EGF increases short-term type I collagen accumulation during wound healing in diabetic rats. *J. Ped. Surg.*, **25**, 893–7.

72. Spanheimer, R. G. (1988). Direct inhibition of collagen production *in vitro* by diabetic rat serum. *Metabolism: Clinical and Experimental*, **37**, 479–85.

73. Spanheimer, R. G., Umpierrez, G. E., and Stumpf, V. (1988). Decreased collagen production in diabetic rats. *Diabetes*, **37**, 371–6.

74. Sharma, C., Dalferes, E. R. Jr, Radhakrishnamurthy, B., Rosen, E. L., and Berenson, G. S. (1986). Nonenzymatic glycosylation of proteins and protease activities in granulation tissues in experimental diabetes. *Inflammation*, **10**, 403–11.

75. Di Girolamo, N., Underwood, A., McCluskey, P. J., and Wakefield, D. (1993). Functional activity of plasma fibronectin in patients with diabetes mellitus. *Diabetes*, **42**, 1606–13.

76. Tengrup, I., Hallmans, G., and Agren, M. S. (1988). Granulation tissue formation and metabolism of zinc and copper in alloxan-diabetic rats. *Scan. J. Plas. Recon. Surg. Hand Surg.*, **22**, 41–5.

77. Fahey, T. J. 3rd, Sadaty, A., Jones, W. G. 2nd, Barber, A., Smoller, B., and Shires, G. T. (1991). Diabetes impairs the late inflammatory response to wound healing. *J. Surg. Res.*, **50**, 308–13.

78. Hatchell, D. L., Magolan, J. J. Jr, Besson, M. J., *et al.* (1983). Damage to the epithelial basement membrane in the corneas of diabetic rabbits. *Arch. Ophthal.*, **101**, 469–71.

79. Sternberg, M., Grigorova-Borsos, A. M., Guillot, R., Kassab, J. P., Bakillah, A., Urios, P., *et al.* (1993). [Changes in collagen type IV metabolism in diabetes; in French.] (Review.) *Comptes Rendus des Séances de la Société de Biologie et de Ses Filiales*, **187**, 247–57.

80. Yue, D. K., McLennan, S., Marsh, M., Mai, Y. W., Spaliviero, J., Delbridge, L., *et al.* (1987). Effects of experimental diabetes, uraemia, and malnutrition on wound healing. *Diabetes*, **36**, 295–9.

81. Underwood, B. A. (1984). Vitamin A in animal and human nutrition. In *The retinoids*, (ed. M. B. Sporn, A. B. Roberts, and D. S. Goodman), Vol. 1, pp. 281–392. Academic Press, Orlando.

82. Fell, H. B. and Mellanby, E. (1953). Metaplasia produced in cultures of chick ectoderm by high vitamin A. *J. Physiol.* (London), **119**, 470–88.

83. Petkovich, M., Brand, N. J., Krust, A., and Chambon, P. (1987). A human retinoic acid receptor which belongs to the family of nuclear receptors. *Nature*, **330**, 444–50.

84. Glick, A. B., Flanders, K. C., Danielpour, D., Yuspa, S. H., and Sporn, M. B. (1989). Retinoic acid induces transforming growth

factor-β2 in cultured keratinocytes and mouse epidermis. *Cell Regul.*, **1**, 87–97.

85. Tokura, Y., Edelson, R. L., and Gasparro, F. P. (1992). Retinoid augmentation of bioactive interleukin-1 production by murine keratinocytes. *Br. J. Dermatol.*, **126**, 485–95.

86. Bailly, C., Drèze, S., Asselineau, D., Nusgens, B., Lapière, C. M., and Darmon, M. (1990). Retinoic acid inhibits the production of collagenase by human epidermal keratinocytes. *J. Invest. Dermatol.*, **94**, 47–51.

87. Brandaleone, H. and Papper, E. (1941). The effect of the local and oral administration of cod liver on the rate of wound healing in vitamin A-deficient and normal rats. *Ann. Surg.*, **114**, 791–8.

88. Gerber, L. E. and Erdman, J. W. (1982). Effect of retinyl acetate, β-carotene and retinoic acid on wound healing in rats. *J. Nutr.*, **112**, 1555–64.

89. Hung, V. C., Lee, J. Y.-Y., Zitelli, J. A., and Hebda, P. A. (1989). Topical retinoin and epithelial wound healing. *Arch. Dermatol.*, **125**, 65–9.

90. Herrmann, J. B. and Woodward, S. C. (1972). An experimental study of wound healing accelerators. *Am Surg.*, **38**, 26–34.

91. Salmela, K. and Ahonen, J. (1981). The effect of methylprednisolone and vitamin A on wound healing. I. *Acta Chir. Scand.*, **147**, 307–12.

92. Watcher, M. A. and Wheeland, R. G. (1989). The role of topical agents in the healing of full-thickness wounds. *J. Dermatol. Surg. Oncol.*, **15**, 1188–95.

93. Kim, R. Y. and Stern, W. H. (1990). Retinoids and butyrate modulate fibroblast growth and contraction of collagen matrices. *Invest. Ophthalmol. Vis. Sci.*, **31**, 1183–6.

94. Fisher, G. J., Esmann, J., Griffiths, C. E. M., Talwar, H. S., Duell, E. A., Hammerberg, C., *et al.* (1991). Cellular, immunologic and biochemical characterization of topical retinoic acid-treated human skin. *J. Invest. Dermatol.*, **96**, 699–707.

95. Smolin, G., Okumoto, M., and Friedlaender, M. (1979). Tretinoin and corneal wound epithelial healing. *Arch. Ophthalmol.*, **97**, 545–6.

96. Ubels, J. L., Edelhauser, H. F., and Austin, K. H. (1983). Healing of experimental corneal wounds treated with topically applied retinoids. *Am. J. Ophthalmol.*, **95**, 353–8.

97. Ehrlich, H. P. and Hunt, T. K. (1968). Effect of cortisone and vitamin A on wound healing. *Ann. Surg.*, **167**, 334–8.

98. Seifter, E., Rettura, G., Padawer, J., Stratford, F., Kambosos, D., and Levenson, S. M. (1981). Impaired wound healing in streptozotocin diabetes. Prevention by supplemental vitamin A. *Ann. Surg.*, **194**, 42–50.

99. Weinzweig, J., Levenson, S. M., Rettura, G., Weinzweig, N., Mendecki, J., Chang, T. H., and Seifter, E. (1990). Supplemental vitamin A prevents the tumor-induced defect in wound healing. *Ann. Surg.*, **211**, 269–76.

100. Phillips, J. D., Kim, C. S., Fonkalsrud, E. W., Zeng, H., and Dindar, H. (1992). Effects of chronic corticosteroids and vitamin A on the healing of intestinal anastomoses. *Am. J. Surg.*, **163**, 71–7.

101. Barbul, A., Thysen, B., Rettura, G., Levenson, S. M., and Seifter, E. (1978). White cell involvement in the inflammatory, wound healing, and immune actions of vitamin A. *J. Parent. Enter. Nutr.*, **2**, 129–38.

102. Salmela, K. (1981). The effect of methylprednisolone and vitamin A on wound healing. II. *Acta Chir. Scand.*, **147**, 313–5.

103. Hodges, R. E., Baker, E. M., Hood, J., Sauberlich, H. E., and March, S. C. (1969). Experimental scurvy in man. *Am. J. Clin. Nutr.*, **22**, 535–48.

104. Padh, H. (1991). Vitamin C: newer insights into its biochemical functions. *Nutr. Rev.*, **49**, 65–70.

105. Franceschi, R. T. (1992). The role of ascorbic acid in mesenchymal differentiation. *Nutr. Rev.*, **50**, 65–70.

106. Thomas, W. R. and Holt, P. G. (1978). Vitamin C and immunity: an assessment of the evidence. *Clin. Exp. Immunol.*, **32**, 370–9.

107. Anderson, R., Oosthuizen, R., Maritz, R., *et al.* (1980). The effects of increasing weekly doses of ascorbate on certain cellular and humoral immune functions in normal volunteers. *Am. J. Clin. Nutr.*, **33**, 71–6.

108. Lanman, T. H. and Ingalls, T. H. (1937). Vitamin C deficiency and wound healing: an experimental and clinical study. *Ann. Surg.*, **105**, 616–25.

109. Abercrombie, M., Flint, M. H., and James, D. W. (1956). Wound contraction in relation to collagen formation in scorbutic guinea-pigs. *J. Embryol. Exp. Morph.*, **4**, 167–75.

110. Gould, B. S. and Woessner, J. F. (1957). Biosynthesis of collagen. The influence of ascorbic acid on the proline, hydroxyproline, glycine, and collagen content of regenerating guinea pig skin. *J. Biol. Chem.*, **226**, 289–300.

111. Liotti, F. S., Bruschelli, G., and Mariucci, G. (1983). Stimulating effect of ascorbic acid on human skin fibroblast multiplication *in vitro*. *IRCS Med. Sci. (Pharmacol.)*, **11**, 502–3.

112. Phillips, C. L., Combs, S. B., and Pinnell, S. R. (1994). Effects of ascorbic acid on proliferation and collagen synthesis in relation to the donor age of human dermal fibroblasts. *J. Invest. Dermatol.*, **103**, 228–32.

113. Bartlett, M. K., Jones, C. M., and Ryan, A. E. (1942). Vitamin C and wound healing. I. Experimental wounds in guinea pigs. *New Engl. J. Med.*, **226**, 469–73.

114. Abt, A. F. and von Schuching, S. (1961). Catabolism of L-ascorbic-1-C^{14} acid as a measure of its utilization in the intact and wounded guinea pig on scorbutic, maintenance, and saturation diets. *Ann. NY Acad. Sci.*, **92**, 148–58.

115. Yu, R., Kurata, T., Kim, M., and Arakawa, N. (1991). The behavior of L-ascorbic acid in the healing process of dorsal wounds in guinea pigs. *J. Nutr. Sci. Vitaminol. (Tokyo)*, **37**, 207–11.

116. Irvin, T. T., Chattopadhyay, D. K., and Smythe, A. (1978). Ascorbic acid requirement in postoperative patients. *Surg. Gynecol. Obstet.*, **147**, 49–55.

117. Taylor, T. V., Rimmer, S., Day, B., Butcher, J., and Dymock, IW. (1974). Ascorbic acid supplementation in the treatment of pressure-sores. *Lancet*, **ii**, 544–6.

118. Pfister, R. R., Anderson, Hayes, S., and Paterson, C. A. (1981). The influence of parenteral ascorbate on the strength of corneal wounds. *Invest. Ophthalmol. Vis. Sci.*, **21**, 80–6.

119. Woolfe, S. N., Kenney, E. B., Hume, W. R., and Carranza, F. A. (1984). Relationship of ascorbic acid levels of blood and gingival tissue with response to periodontal therapy. *J. Clin. Periodontol.*, **11**, 159–65.

120. Goode, H. F., Burns, E., and Walker, B. E. (1992). Vitamin C depletion and pressure sores in elderly patients with femoral neck fracture. *Br. Med. J.*, **305**, 925–7.

121. Vallee, B. L., Coleman, J. E., and Auld, D. S. (1991). Zinc fingers, zinc clusters, and zinc twists in DNA-binding protein domains. *Proc. Natl. Acad. Sci. USA*, **88**, 999–1003.

122. Hicks, S. E. and Wallwork, J. C. (1987). Effect of dietary zinc deficiency on protein synthesis in cell-free systems isolated from rat liver. *J. Nutr.*, **117**, 1234–40.

123. Ågren, M. S., Franzén, L., and Chvapil, M. (1993). Effects on wound healing of zinc oxide in a hydrocolloid dressing. *J. Am. Acad. Dermatol.*, **28**, 221–7.

124. Iriyama, K., Mori, T., Takenaka, T., Teranishi, T., and Mori, H. (1982). Effect of serum zinc level on amount of collagen-hydroxyproline in the healing gut during total parenteral nutrition: an experimental study. *J. Parent. Enter. Nutr.*, **6**, 416–20.

125. Ågren, M. S. (1990). Studies on zinc in wound healing. *Acta Derm. Venereol.* (Suppl.), **154**, 1–36.

126. Ågren, M. S. and Franzén, L. (1990). Influence of zinc deficiency on breaking strength of 3-week-old skin incisions in the rat. *Acta. Chir. Scand.*, **156**, 667–70.

127. Watanabe, T., Arakawa, T., Fukuda, T., Higuchi, K., and Kobayashi, K. (1995). Zinc deficiency delays gastric ulcer healing in rats. *Dig. Dis. Sci.*, **40**, 1340–4.

128. Strömberg, H-E. and Ågren, M. S. (1984). Topical zinc oxide improves arterial and venous leg ulcers. *Br. J. Dermatol.*, **111**, 461–8.

129. Jin, L., Murakami, T. H., Janjua, N. A., and Hori, Y. (1994). The effects of zinc oxide and diethylthiocarbamate on mitotic index of epidermal basal cells of mouse skin. *Acta Med. Okayama.*, **48**, 231–6.

130. Ågren, M. S., Chvapil, M., and Franzén, L. (1991). Enhancement of re-epithelialization with topical zinc oxide in porcine partial-thickness wounds. *J. Surg. Res.*, **50**, 101–5.

131. Tarnow, P., Ågren, M. S., Jansson, J-O., and Steenfos, H. H. (1994). Topical zinc oxide treatment increases the endogenous gene expression of insulin-like growth factor-1 (IGF-1) in granulation tissue from porcine wounds. *Scand. J. Plast. Reconstr. Surg. Hand Surg.*, **28**, 255–8.

132. Ågren, M. S., Krusell, M., and Franzén, L. (1991). Release and absorption of zinc from zinc oxide and zinc sulfate in open wounds. *Acta Derm. Venereol.*, **71**, 330–3.

133. Ågren, M. S., Söderberg, T. A., Reuterving, C-O., Hallmans, G., and Tengrup, I. (1991). Effect of topical zinc oxide on bacterial growth and inflammation in full-thickness skin wounds in normal and diabetic rats. *Eur. J. Surg.*, **157**, 97–101.

134. Sunzel, B., Söderberg, T. A., Reuterving, C-O., Hallmans, G., Holm, S. E., and Hänström, L. (1991). Neutralizing effect of zinc oxide on dehydroabietic acid-induced toxicity on human polymorphonuclear leukocytes. *Biol. Trace. Elem. Res.*, **31**, 33–42.

135. Reed, B. and Clark, R. A. F. (1985). Cutaneous tissue repair: practical implications of current knowledge. II. *J. Am. Acad. Dermatol.*, **13**: 919–41.

136. Madden, J. W. and Arem, A. J. (1986). Wound healing: biologic and clinical features. In *Textbook of surgery*, (ed. D. C. Sabiston), Vol. 1, p. 207. W. B. Saunders, Philadelphia.

137. Niinikoski, J. (1969). Effect of oxygen supply on wound healing and formation of experimental granulation tissue. *Acta Physiol. Scan.*, **334**, 1–72.

138. Silver, I. A. (1969). The measurement of oxygen tension in healing tissue. In *Progress in respiration research, III*, (ed. H. Herzog), pp. 124–35. S. Karger, Basel.

139. Gottrup, F., Firmin, R., Rabkin, J., *et al.* (1987). Directly measured tissue oxygen tension and arterial oxygen tension assess tissue perfusion. *Crit. Care Med.*, **15**, 1030–6.

140. Hunt, T. K. and Pai, M. P. (1972). Effect of varying oxygen tensions on healing of open wounds. *Surg. Gynecol. Obstet.*, **135**, 561–7.

141. Stephens, F. O. and Hunt, T. K. (1971). Effect of changes in inspired oxygen and carbon dioxide tensions on wound tensile strength. *Ann. Surg.*, **173**, 515.

142. Niinikoski, J., Penttinen, R., and Kulonen, E. (1966). Effect of oxygen supply on the tensile strength of healing wound and of granulation tissue. *Acta Physiol. Scand.*, (Suppl.), **277** 146.

143. Sheffield, P. (1988). Tissue oxygen measurements. Chapter 2. In *Problem wounds: the role of oxygen*, (ed. J. C. Davis and T. K. Hunt), pp. 17–51. Elsevier, New York.

144. Babior, B. M. (1978). Oxygen-dependent microbial killing by phagocytes. *N. Engl. J. Med.*, **198**, 659.

145. Knighton, D. R., Halliday, B., and Hunt, T. K. (1986). Oxygen as an antibiotic. A comparison of the effects of inspired oxygen concentration and antibiotic administration on *in vivo* bacterial clearance. *Arch. Surg.*, **121**, 191–5.

146. Boerema, I., Meijne, N. G., Burmmelkamp, W. H., *et al.* (1960). Life without blood: a study of the influence of high atmospheric pressure and hypothermia on dilution of blood. *J. Cardiovasc. Surg.*, **1**, 133–46.

147. Krogh, A. (1919). The number and distribution of capillaries in muscle with calculations of the oxygen pressure lead recovery for supplying the tissue. *J. Physiol.*, **52**, 409–15.

148. Niinikoski, J. (1977). Oxygen and wound healing. *Clin. Plast. Surg.*, **4**, 361–74.

149. Uhl, E., Sirsjo, A., Haapaniemi, T., *et al.* (1994). Hyperbaric oxygen improves wound healing in normal and ischaemic skin tissue. *Plast. Reconstr. Surg.*, **93**, 835.

150. Knighton, D., Silver, I., and Hunt, T. (1994). Regulation of wound healing angiogenesis. Effect of oxygen gradients and inspired oxygen concentration. *Surgery*, **90**, 262–70.

151. Hammarlund, C. and Sundbergt. (1981). Hyperbaric oxygen reduced size of chronic leg ulcers; a randomized double-blind study. *Plast. Reconstr. Surg.*, **93**, 829.

152. Champion, W. M., McSherry, C. K., and Goulian, D. (1967). Effect of hyperbaric oxygen on the survival of pedicle skin flaps. *J. Surg. Research.*, **7**, 583–6.

153. Sheffield, P. J. (1985). Tissue oxygen measurements with respect to soft-tissue wound healing with normobaric and hyperbaric oxygen. *Hyperb. Oxyg. Rev.*, **6**, 18–46.

154. Mustoe, T. A., Ahn, S. T., Tarpley, J. E., and Pierce, F. G. (1994). Role of hypoxia in growth factor responses: differential effect of basic fibroblast growth factor and platelet-derived growth factor in an ischaemic wound model. *Wound. Rep. Reg.*, **2**, 277–83.

155. Sheffield, P. J. and Workman, W. T. (1985). Noninvasive tissue oxygen measurements in patients administered normobaric and hyperbaric oxygen by mask. *Hyperb. Oxyg. Rev.*, **6**, 47–62.

156. Jonsso, N. K., Jensen, J. A., Goodson, W. H., Schevenstuhl, H., West, J., Hopf, H. W., and Hunt, T. K. (1991). Tissue oxygenation, anaemia and perfusion in relation to wound healing in surgical patients. *Ann. Surg.*, **214**, 605–13.

157. Heughan, C., Chir, B., Grislis, G., and Hunt, T. (1974). The effect of anaemia on wound healing. *Ann. Surg.*, **179**, 1673–6.

158. Nasution, A. and Taylor, D. (1987). The effect of acute haemorrhage and of delayed blood replacement on wound healing: an experimental study. *Br. J. Surg.*, **68**, 306–9.

159. Bucknall, T. E. (1984). Factors affecting healing. Chapter 3. In *Wound healing for surgeons*, (ed. T. E. Bucknall and H. Ellis), pp. 42–74. Bailliere Tindall, London.

160. Dvorau, H. F. (1986). Tumours: wounds that do not heal. Similarities between tumour strome generation and wound healing. *N. Engl. J. Med.*, **315**, 1650.

161. Connolly, J. L., Ducatman, B. S., Schnitt, S. J., Dvorak, A. M., and Dvorak, H. F. (1993). Principles of cancer pathology. In *Cancer medicine*, Vol. I, (3rd edn), (ed. J. F. Holland, E. Fret III, R. C. Bast, Jr, D. W. Kufe, D. L. Morton, and R. R. Weichselbaum), pp. 432–50. Lea and Febiger, Philadelphia.

162. Norton, L. and Surbone, A. (1993). Principles of chemotherapy-cytokinetics. In *Cancer medicine*, Vol. 1, (3rd edn), (ed. J. F. Holland, E. Fret III, R. C. Bast, Jr, D. W. Kufe, D. L. Morton, and R. R. Weichselbaum), pp. 598–617. Lea and Febiger, Philadelphia.

163. Weichselbaum, R. R., Hallahan, D. E., and Chen, G. T. Y. (1993). Principles of radiation oncology – biological and physical basis to radiation oncology In *Cancer medicine*, Vol. 1, (3rd edn), (ed. J. F. Holland, E. Fret III, R. C. Bast Jr, D. W. Kufe,

D. L. Morton, and R. R. Weichselbaum), pp. 539–66. Lea and Febiger, Philadelphia.

164. Herrimann, F., Schulz, G., Wieser, M., Kolbe, K., Nicolay, U., Noack, M., *et al.* (1990). Effect of granulocyte-macrophage colony-stimulating factor on neutropenia and related morbidity induced by mylotoxic chemotherapy. *Am. J. Med.*, **88**, 619.

165. Clark, R. A. F. (1993). Basics of cutaneous wound repair. *J. Dermtol.*, **19**, 693–706.

166. Vegesna, V., Withers, H. R., Holly, F. E., and McBridge, W. H. (1993). The effect of local and systemic irradiation on impairment of wound healing in mice. Journal **135**, 431–3.

167. Springfield, D. S. (1993). Surgical wound healing. *Cancer Treatment and Research*, **67**, 81–98.

168. Wang, Q., Dickson, G. R., Abram, W. P., and Carr, K. E. (1994). Electron irradiation slows down wound repair in rat skin: a morpholgoical investigation. *Br. J. Dermatol.*, **130**, 551–5.

169. Degges, R. D., Cannon, D. J., and Lang, N. P. (1983). The effects of pre-operative radiation on healing of rat colonic anastomosis. *Dis. Colon. Rectum.*, **26**, 598–600.

170. Badr el Din, A., Coibion, M., Guenier, C., Nogaret, J. M., Lorent, I., Van Houtte, P., *et al.* (1989). Local post-operative morbidity following pre-operative irradiation in locally advanced breast cancer. *Eur. J. Surg. Oncology.*, **15**, 486–9.

171. Powers, W. E. and Palmer, L. A. (1968). Biological basis of pre-operative radiotherapy. *Am. J. Roentgenol.*, **102**, 17.

172. Schrock, T. R., Deveney, O. W., and Dunphy, J. E. (1973). Factors contributing to leakage of colonic anastomosis. *Ann. Surg.*, **177**, 513–8.

173. Ormsbt, M. V., Hilaris, B. S., Nori, D., and Brennan, M. F. (1989). Wound complications of adjuvant radiation therapy in patients with soft tissue sarcomas. *Ann. Surg.*, **210**, 93–9.

174. Levenson, S. M., Gruber, C. A., Rettura, G., Gruber, D. K., Demetriou, A. A., and Seifter, E. (1984). Supplemental vitamin A prevents the acute radiation induced defect in wound healing. *Ann. Surg.*, **200**, 494–512.

175. Lawrence, W. T., Talbot, T. L., and Norton, J. A. (1986). Pre-operative or post-operative doxorubicin hydrochloride (adriamycin): which is better for wound healing? *Surgery*, **100**, 9–13.

176. Arbeit, J. M., Hilarix, B. S., and Brennan, M. F. (1987). Wound complications in the multimodality treatment of extremity and superficial truncal sarcomas. *J. Clin. Oncol.*, **5**, 480–8.

177. Staley, C. J., Trippel, O. H., and Preston, F. W. (1961). Influence of 5-fluorose on wound healing. *Surgery*, **41**, 450–3.

178. Morain, W. D., Richmond, R. C., Jacobs, N. J., Douple, E. B., and Coughlin, C. T. (1986). Pre-operative irradiation potentiation with cisplatin: effect on rate of wound infection. *Am. J. Surg.*, **152**, 446–50.

179. Arnold, P. G., Lovich, S. F., and Palrolero, P. C. (1994). Muscle flaps in irradiated wounds: an account of 100 consecutive cases. *Plast. Reconstr. Surg.*, **93**, 324–8.

180. Kane, W. J., McCaffrey, T. V., Wand, T. D., and Koval, T. M. (1993). The effect of tissue exposantion on the random flap viability and wound tensile strength of previously irradiated rabbit skin. *Archives of Otolaryngology – Head and Neck Surgery*, **119**, 417–22.

181. Rudolph, R. (1982). Complications of surgery for radiotherapy skin damage. *Plast. Reconstr. Surg.*, **70**, 179–83.

182. Arnold, P. G. and Pairolero, P. C. (1986). Surgical management of the radiated chest wall. *Plast. Reconstr. Surg.*, **77**, 605–12.

183. Mustoe, T. A., Purdy, J., Gramates, P., Devel, T. F., Thompson, A., and Pierce, G. F. (1989). Reversal of impaired wound healing in irradiated rats by platelet-derived growth factor-BB. *Am. J. Surg.*, **158**, 345–50.

184. Taren, D. L., Chvapil, M., and Weber, C. W. (1987). Increasing the breaking strength of wounds exposed to pre-operative irradiation using vitamin E supplementation. *Int. J. Vit. Nut. Res.*, **57**, 133–7.

185. Curtsinger, L. J., Pietsch, J. D., Brown, G. L., von Fraunhofer, A., Ackerman, D., Polk, H. C., Jr, and Schultz, G. S. (1989). Reversal of adriamycin-impaired wound healing by transforming growth bactor β. *Surg. Gynecol. Obstet.*, **168**, 577–22.

186. Cruse, P. J. E. and Foored, R. (1973). A five year prospective study of 23 649 surgical wounds. *Arch. Surg.*, **107**, 206–10.

187. Bucknall, T. E., Cox, P. J., and Ellis, H. (1982). Burst abdomen and incisional hernia – a prospective study of 1,129 major laparotomies. *Br. Med. J.*, **284**, 931–3.

7

Infection
N. A. WILLIAMS and D.J. LEAPER

Pathogenesis and host response

Introduction

In order to cause disease, microorganisms have to possess a number of attributes which allow them to (i) enter the host, (ii) multiply *in vivo*, (iii) interfere with host defence mechanisms, and (iv) cause damage to the host. Possession of strategies for all of these steps are found in those organisms which are associated with human infectious disease (termed 'primary pathogens'). However, such organisms are rare in the microbial world. The vast majority of microorganisms lack a means of overcoming one or more of these hurdles to infection of the normal human body. The major barrier to infection is provided by the physical and chemical environment at the body surfaces. In the case of the skin, the tough layer of dead cells and keratin, together with the secretions of the sweat and sebaceous glands, create a formidable barrier. The mucosal surfaces of the respiratory, gastrointestinal, and urogenital tracts as well as the eye have specialized physiological functions which rely on them being more permeable, and thus other mechanisms have evolved to protect these sites. Such mechanisms include physical factors – for example, the mucociliary escalator of the respiratory tract, the flushing action of the tears, mucus in the gastrointestinal tract; and chemical factors including lowered pH, the presence of antimicrobials including lysozyme and IgA surfaces circumvents these innate defense mechanisms. Consequently, proven opportunity is provided for a range of microorganisms, some of which may come from the normal flora, which lack a means of entry, to multiply and spread within the body, causing disease (termed 'opportunists'). The following sections review the mechanisms evolved by the body to prevent such diseases and the attributes which some microbes have acquired to overcome them.

Initial environment

The immune defences of the body can be divided into the specific (those that involve recognition of antigenic determinants of the invading organism) and the non-specific (those not directed against specific antigens). The specific immune response takes a number of days to become active, particularly when the incoming pathogen has not been encountered previously. Taken together with the observation that many bacteria have a doubling time *in vitro* of as little as 20 minutes, this clearly indicates an important role for the non-specific defences of the body in limiting the multiplication and spread of invading organisms. Non-specific immune mechanisms contribute substantially to the initial control of infection. The body effectively slows down the replication of invading bacteria by a combination of the presence of antibacterials (most tissues contain sufficient lysozyme to kill some Gram-positive bacteria) and restricted access to nutrients in the tissue fluid. As a result, multiplication times for bacteria *in vivo* are usually substantially slower than those *in vitro*. For example, *Salmonella typhi* doubling times *in vivo* are between 4 and 10 h compared with 20 min on suitable media *in vitro*. The major nutrient restriction to the growth of bacteria in the body tissues is the lack of free iron, brought about by the action of iron chelators of the body, transferrin and lactoferrin. Iron is an essential nutrient for bacteria and those that are able to secure sufficient for their growth possess their own high-affinity iron chelators, siderophores, which compete favourably for iron with transferrin and lactoferrin.

The flow of blood into the tissue, maintaining high oxygen tension, may also be restrictive for the growth of anaerobic bacteria. In addition, the flow of lymph to the local draining lymph nodes will carry invading microorganisms away to these sites of phagocytosis. It is noteworthy that the physical and physiological conditions within many wounds will compromise these mechanisms, for example by interfering with the local blood supply. Such alterations will tend to favour the growth of incoming bacteria, such as the establishment of *Clostridium perfringens* (the gas gangrene organism) or *C. tetani* (the tetanus organism) in areas with low oxygen tension. Once established, such organisms are capable of secreting toxins which lead to tissue necrosis and thus a further reduction in oxygen tension. The inflammatory response which quickly follows tissue damage has evolved in part to counteract the disruption to blood flow which occurs in these conditions. In addition, the inflammatory response serves to recruit non-specific and specific effector mechanisms of the immune system to the site of damage and thus prevent possible infection.

Non-specific immune responses

The immediate result of tissue injury is the release of a range of inflammatory mediators including histamine from mast cells, serotonin from platelets, and a range of lysosomal enzymes released by damaged tissue cells. The factors involved are dealt with in more detail in Chapter 3. The result of the inflammatory response is an increase in blood flow to the affected area, together with extravasation of blood cells and products. Of major importance in the early response is the movement of monocytes and polymorphonucleocytes (PMNs), primarily neutrophils (basophils and eosinophils being more important following the establishment of an antibody response), between the endothelial cells of the blood vessels and out into the tissue by a process known as diapedesis. The extravasation of such cells is markedly enhanced by the complement components C5a and C3a which may be present as a result of triggering of the alternative pathway of complement activation (chemotaxis). Incoming monocytes (which mature into macrophages in the tissue) and PMNs engulf (phagocytose) invading organisms together with cell debris and destroy them intracellularly following fusion of lysosomes with the phagosome. The processes by which phagocytes destroy foreign particles are listed in Table 7.1.

Table 7.1 Mechanisms of intracellular killing by phagocytes

Oxygen independent	Acid pH
	Lysozyme: breaks down the peptidoglycan cell wall of Gram-positive bacteria
	Lactoferrin: restricts the presence of free iron (bacteriostatic)
	Vitamin B_{12}-binding protein (bacteriostatic)
	Proteases: cell digestion
	Acid hydrolases: cell digestion
	Cationic proteins: bactericidal (not present in macrophages)
Oxygen dependent (not present in mononuclear phagocytes)	Superoxide (O_2^-)
	Hydrogen peroxide (H_2O_2)
	Hydroxyl radicals (OH)
	Singlet oxygen (O_2)
	Halide (OCl^-)

The respiratory burst of neutrophils generates a range of very unstable oxygen-based molecules making these cells considerably more potent killers than the macrophages. However, the toxicity of these substances also leads to the rapid death of the PMNs. The release of lysosomal enzymes into the tissues as PMNs die contributes to the tissue damage and inflammation, producing pus. Macrophages, while less effective killers, are able to resynthesize their lysosomes and continue their activity over a number of days. Later in the response, when a specific antibody is present, the classical pathway of complement activation will be triggered on the surfaces of invading bacteria, and their killing by phagocytes will be greatly enhanced since such cells possess receptors for complement components and the Fc portion of antibody molecules. In addition, activated macrophages release interleukin (IL)-1 and tumour necrosis factor (TNF) which act both locally, to enhance the process of inflammation, and systemically to stimulate haemopoiesis (and hence the production of new monocytes and neutrophils) and increase body temperature via activity on the hypothalamus (fever). Relatively minor increases in body temperature can dramatically reduce the replicative rate of some microorganisms (1).

Successful opportunist pathogens have in many cases developed means of avoiding these initial immune reactions. In some cases microbial products interfere with the process of inflammation (e.g. Staphylococcal glycopeptide), disrupt the complement cascade (e.g. complement destruction by elastase produced by *Pseudomonas aeruginosa*), or disrupt the activity of incoming phagocytes. Examples of the latter include interference of chemotaxis by the α-toxin of *Staphylococcus aureus*, and preventing uptake by the phagocyte such as that caused by the M protein of *Streptococcus pyogenes*. In addition, the possession of coagulase enzyme by *S. aureus* converts fibrinogen to fibrin, forming a clot around the bacteria, which is difficult for incoming phagocytes to penetrate. Other bacteria, including *Streptococcus pyogenes*, *Staphylococcus aureus*, *P. aeruginosa*, and *C. perfringens*, actively attack the phagocytes by producing toxins (leucocidins).

A further consequence of the increased flow of lymph is that antigen-bearing cells are taken from the periphery to the local draining lymph nodes where they may be involved in the induction of specific immunity.

Antigen-specific immune responses

Antigen presentation

Most peripheral tissues contain a population of cells with dendritic morphology. The relationship between these cell types (termed non-lymphoid dendritic cells), the veiled cells present in afferent lymph, and the dendritic cells found in the lymphoid organs, lymph nodes, spleen, and thymus (termed lymphoid dendritic cells) remains unclear (2). To a large extent this is a problem of defining cell populations on the basis of their morphology. Nevertheless, they all share the common properties of being poorly phagocytic and expressing high levels of class II products of the major histocompatibility complex (MHC). Strong evidence suggests that the non-lymphoid dendritic cells form a system whose function is to sample the periphery for foreign material. Following administration of antigen, or immune complexes (3, 4) to the skin, the local dendritic cell population, the Langerhans cells (LC), have been shown to take up antigen and are found within 2 h in draining lymph nodes (4). Antigen-bearing cells are subsequently seen in the T cell-dependent areas of the draining lymph nodes. When isolated, these cells are strong stimulators of T lymphocyte proliferation in antigen-specific responses (5, 6). In the case of LC, their ability to present antigen to T cells appears to alter with the activation state of the T cells themselves. Thus, while freshly isolated LC are potent stimulators of antigen-specific responses of primed T cells, they are unable to present antigen to T cells from animals which have not previously encountered the antigen (7, 8). However, *in vitro* data suggest that maturation of the LC may be induced by culturing LC with granulocyte macrophage-colony stimulating factor (GM-CSF) (9) and is associated with changes in phenotype and morphology which make the LC indistinguishable from lymphoid dendritic cells (9, 10). *In vivo*, such maturation may occur during migration to the lymph nodes such that they acquire the ability to prime during or following transit. Whether similar maturation is necessary for other non-lymphoid dendritic cells to be able to stimulate a primary T cell response is not clear. Indeed, experiments suggest that class II-bearing cells from the small intestine stimulate naïve T cells, giving reactions with similar anamnestic characteristics to those which follow antigen presentation by cells from lymphoid organs (11). The significance of these observations for initiation of immune responses in the skin is unclear. It seems probable that the immaturity of LC serves to centralize the immune response to new foreign antigens, increasing the chances of interaction with antigen-reactive T cell clones and preventing the induction of a purely local reaction. Clearly, in all but minor abrasions, foreign material is introduced into deeper tissues than the epidermis, in which case dendritic cells and macrophages other than LC will also become involved in antigen uptake and presentation. Precise information about the relative capacity of these cells to present antigen to T cells is not known. Nevertheless, it is clear that

antigenic challenge at the periphery results in the migration of antigen-bearing class II-bearing cells to the lymph nodes in the afferent lymph.

Antigen which is endocytosed by antigen presenting cells (APC) is broken down (processed) in endosomes where it may associate with class II MHC molecules arriving from the trans-Golgi reticulum (12). It appears that the peptide binding groove of the class II molecule is open ended and binds peptides approximately 14 amino acids in length (13). These molecular complexes are transported to the cell surface to act as receptors for antigen-reactive T cells.

T cell activation

T lymphocytes which come into contact with the APC may in some cases possess a T cell receptor which binds to the peptide–MHC complex. As well as this antigen-dependent interaction between the two cells, antigen-independent interactions occur, mediated by a range of cell surface adhesion molecules. The complete range of such molecules involved in this way is not clear, however, a number have been identified (14). Figure 7.1 illustrates some of the important molecules involved in the interaction between the T cell and the APC. Some of the interactions are probably primarily involved in physically holding the cells together. This is probably the case for LFA-1 and its ligands ICAM-1 and ICAM-2. The avidity of the interaction between LFA-1 and ICAM-1 is markedly increased following cross-linking of the T cell receptor (15). This alteration is caused by a reversible change in LFA-1, which therefore favours strong interaction between the two cells if the T cell recognizes the antigen–MHC

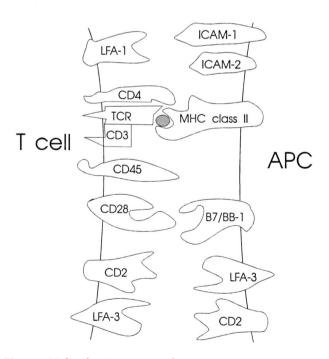

Fig. 7.1 Molecular interactions during antigen presentation to CD4-bearing T lymphocytes. APC, antigen-presenting cell; LFA, ICAM, inter-cellular adhesion molecule.

complex. However, in the absence of recognition, the equilibrium favours dissociation of the cells and interaction with other cells. Other adhesion molecules may be involved in stimulation of the cells since they have cytoplasmic tails associated with intracellular signalling mechanisms (14). Of particular interest in this respect is the interaction between CD28 and its ligand on the APC, B7/BB-1. Recent evidence suggests that in the absence of this interaction T cells may be rendered anergic, that is to say they may be unable to react to subsequent stimuli (16). T cell stimulation in the absence of this 'costimulus' may occur when non-professional APC, such as resting B cells, become involved in antigen presentation (17).

Interaction of APC and T cells result in the stimulation of the T cell into proliferation and maturation. Discussion of the precise intracellular signals which lead to T cell proliferation following antigen presentation are beyond the scope of this chapter, but for a review see that of Janeway (18). The events which follow depend on the type of T cell which is activated. Historically, T cells were divided into subsets on the basis of the expression of either CD8 or CD4 antigens. Since CD4 is a coreceptor for class II MHC molecules then antigen presentation of extracellular antigen, as described in the previous discussion, would stimulate predominantly CD4-bearing cells (T helper cells). Conversely, CD8 is a coreceptor for class I MHC products, which in general combines with peptides derived from intracytoplasmic processing. As a result, CD8-bearing T cells (cytotoxic cells) are of major importance in the response to intracytoplasmic parasites such as viruses. More recently, studies of cytokine secretion by CD4-bearing T cell clones have revealed the existence of different subsets of T helper cells. Initial observations in the mouse suggested the existence of two types, termed Th1 and Th2 (19). For some time these observations were difficult to transfer to studies in humans, but it now appears that the same broad distinctions exist, although many T cell clones are intermediate between the two types, termed Th0 (20). The range of cytokines produced by these subtypes of T helper cell may have a major effect on their function. Further, preferential stimulation of one type as opposed to another can result in biasing of the immune response in a particular direction, which, if appropriate, will result in more effective immunity; but if inappropriate, can exacerbate disease.

The major products of Th1 cells are gamma interferon (γ-IFN), IL-2, and IL-3. As a result, such cells are primarily involved in providing help for cellular responses such as cytotoxic T cells (for which IL-2 is a major growth factor) and enhancing the activation of macrophages and natural killer (NK) cells. Conversely, Th2 produce IL-4, IL-5, IL-6, IL-10, and IL-3. IL-4 acts as an autocrine growth factor and, together with IL-5 and IL-6, stimulates the activation and differentiation of B cells, thus providing help for antibody production and, in particular, IgE synthesis. IL-3 stimulates mast cells and haemopoiesis in the bone marrow. Interestingly, Th1 and Th2 cells are mutually antagonistic, in that Th1 cytokines, particularly γ-IFN, inhibit the activity of Th2 cells; and IL-10, produced by Th2, inhibits the activation of Th1 cells, probably via an effect on the APC (21, 22). These recent observations probably serve to explain many of the observations which

have suggested the existence of T suppressor cells. The implication of this antagonism is that there is potential for the immune response to be biased toward either cell-mediated or humoral responses. That this can occur *in vivo* is evident from studies of a murine model for *Leishmania donovani* infection in which it has been shown that prognosis for different mouse strains is dependent on the nature of the T cell response. Fatality is common in strains which exhibit a predominantly Th2 reaction and hence secrete high levels of IgE, whereas the infection is self-limiting in those where Th1 cells dominate, augmenting the ability of their macrophages to kill the parasite (23). It appears that similar biasing of the immune response can occur in humans, and may explain the spectrum of disease states found in infections such as leprosy. In the majority of instances, the immune response following invasion of the body by pathogens is probably balanced with respect to T cell subsets, but it is possible that minor deviations may affect the course of a whole range of infections. Of interest is the recent observation of the effects of environment on influencing the balance between Th1 and Th2 cells (24) which suggests that the nature of opening inflammatory reactions may have an important effect. In this model it is suggested that in the presence of activated NK cells, Th1 will dominate, whereas in the presence of activated mast cells and basophils, Th2 may predominate.

Effector systems

The role of the T helper cell subsets described above is to control and promote the effector function of the immune response. This is achieved primarily by the secretion of cytokines. Activated T cells provide help locally, following recirculation and extravasation into inflamed tissue, as well as in the lymphoid tissues. As described above, B cell help is provided primarily by IL-4, 5, and 6, although other cytokines are involved. IL-5 is of major importance in stimulating the differentiation of B cells into antibody-producing cells, and IL-6 is the major stimulator of antibody secretion by differentiated B cells. Interestingly, many cell types secrete IL-6, including fibroblasts, keratinocytes, endothelial cells, and macrophages. Its secretion by these cells at the site of trauma is likely to promote the release of antibody in the area where it is needed.

The major properties of the different classes of antibody molecules are summarized in Table 7.2. In the early response to challenge, IgM antibodies are of major importance, but as the response matures, IgG takes over as the dominant class. This shift in the class of antibody produced is paralleled by an increase in the affinity of the antibody for antigen. IgG is of major importance in clearing invading pathogens. There are four subclasses of IgG in the human, all with slightly different properties (Table 7.2). An antibody acts the enhance the clearance of invading microorganisms in a number of ways (summarized in Fig. 7.2). Alone it can agglutinate bacteria, restricting their spread within the tissues. However, it is its ability to trigger other immune effectors via the Fc portion of the molecule which make it such an important antimicrobial system. An antibody acts as a trigger for the activation of the complement cascade (classical pathway) which, as described

Table 7.2 Properties of different classes of human immunoglobulins

Immunoglobulin	IgG1	IgG2	IgG3	IgG4	IgM	IgA1	IgA2	IgE	IgD
Mean serum concentration (mg/ml)	9	3	1	0.5	1.5	3	0.5	5×10^{-5}	0.03
Complement fixation	++	+	+++	−	+++	−	−	−	−
Macrophage binding	++	+	++	−	−	−	−	−	−
Neutrophil binding	++	++	+++	+	−	+	+	−	−
Mast cell/basophil binding	−	−	−	−	−	−	−	+++	−
Platelet binding	+	+	+	+	−	−	−	−	
Transepithelial transfer	+/−	+/−	+/−	+/−	+/−	++	++	−	−
Placental transfer	+	+/−	+	+	−	−	−	−	−

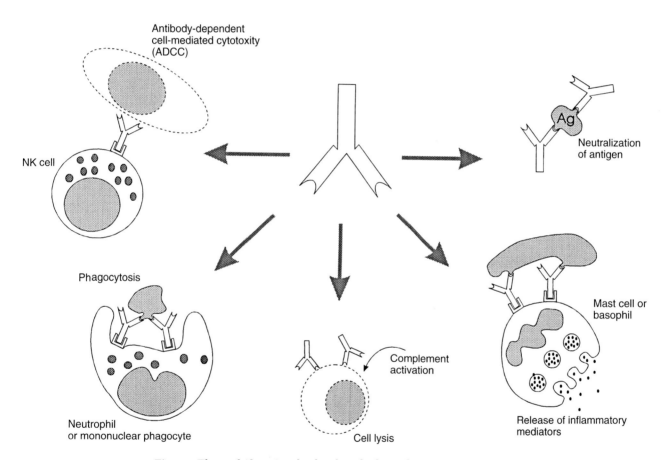

Fig. 7.2 The multifunctional role of antibody in the immune response.

above, leads to the production of important anaphylatoxins. In addition, complement components are deposited on the surface of the foreign particle; these may lead to the assembly of the membrane attack complex which can lead to target cell lysis (although many bacteria are resistant to this). Mononuclear phagocytes and neutrophils possess receptors both for the Fc portion of antibody and for the complement components C3b and C5b and thus are able to take up antibody-coated particles more effectively. IgE is particularly important in the control of inflammation since it acts as an antigen receptor for tissue mast cells and incoming basophils via binding to specialized Fc receptors on these cells.

In addition to helping B cells to produce antibody, activated T helper cells may migrate and enter peripheral sites of inflammation. Once in these sites, the production of Th1-type cytokines is important in stimulating the cell-mediated effector mechanisms of the immune response. γ-IFN leads to upregulation in the expression of class II MHC molecules on APC and induces its expression on a range of cell types which do not normally express class II. Such 'non-professional' APC include the keratinocytes of the skin, keratocytes of the cornea, resting B cells, and endothelial cells. As a result of these changes, the range of cells which may be involved in the local presentation of antigen may be increased, leading to more efficient triggering of the local immune reaction. Gamma-interferon also enhances the killing capacity of macrophages. The release of IL-2 by T helper cells results in their own further proliferation as well as the activation of cytotoxic T cells, which may themselves produce IL-2 and γ-IFN (25). Since cytotoxic T cells recognize antigen in the context of class I MHC antigen they will recognize and kill cells which have become infected with intracellular pathogens such as viruses. A further role of IL-2 is in the activation of NK cells. NK cells were first described by their ability to kill certain tumour cell targets *in vitro*, but they may be important in a range of inflammatory situations. NK cells kill in an antigen-independent manner and when treated with IL-2 they become further activated. The usefulness of these cells is probably greatest in infections with intracellular parasites, such as viruses, where indiscriminate cell killing, providing it is carefully controlled, may halt the replication of the pathogen prior to the onset of, and during a phase when it is hidden from, the specific immune response.

Microbial resistance to specific immunity

Avoidance of the specific immune response by opportunist pathogens can involve three major strategies:

(1) avoid invoking a response;
(2) suppress the response;
(3) keep one step ahead.

Examples of organisms which employ one or more of these strategies for survival *in vivo* are evident. Avoidance of invoking a response can occur if the organism possesses an intact non-immunogenic capsule, enters host cells where it is hidden from the immune system, or possesses surface antigens which mimic host antigens. An example of the latter is provided by the hyaluronic acid capsule of streptococci which mimics a major component of mammalian connective tissue. The host has evolved to be immunologically unresponsive to self-antigens and therefore fails to react to the pathogen. A further strategy of avoidance is the shedding of surface antigens which will bind antibody and may also block T cells, thus preventing them being able to bind to the pathogen itself. This mechanism is used by a wide range of organisms, including *Candida albicans*, *P. aeruginosa*, meningococcus, and many eukaryote parasites. There are a number of examples of pathogens which are able to suppress the immune response.

In the case of a number of viruses, suppression is antigen-specific, in that the immune response to antigens other than those of the virus is unaffected. Bacterial pathogens which suppress the immune response in general do so non-specifically, for example by the production of leucocidins (discussed above) which kill cells of the immune system. In addition, there is evidence that *P. aeruginosa* lipopolysaccharide stimulates T cell suppression of immunity. The third major strategy of immune avoidance that of keeping one step ahead is of less relevance to infections of wounds. General examples are, however, provided by agents such as *Borrelia recurrentis* and parasites such as trypanosomes, which can vary their surface antigens during an infection such that the targets of the cellular and humoral response are no longer present. Such organisms are able to avoid clearance for long periods in this way and hence lead to chronic infections. In general, the resistance mechanisms of opportunist pathogens are only partially effective and the infection is cleared as the immune system becomes more and more activated. Particular difficulties can clearly arise if other factors of health weaken the immune system, compromising its effective destruction of incoming pathogens.

Clinical aspects and wound infection

We live in harmony with an estimated 1×10^{14} organisms contained within us (26). Many of these organisms are commensals, but others can give rise to infection (invasion of tissue) if conditions are favourable. True pathogens tend to cause infection when normal defence mechanisms are breached; they may be commensals but are often transient in their colonization of tissues or tissue surfaces. Opportunists are organisms normally considered to be harmless but become pathogenic when host defence is modulated, as in the presence of a prosthetic graft, for example.

The size of an inoculum of microorganisms and the degree of their pathogenicity determine the establishment of infection. Host defences normally resist all but the most pathogenic organisms, but are materially depressed by systemic factors such as shock, immunosuppression, and poor nutrition and local factors such as ischaemia, trauma, or implantation of foreign material.

Infection causes delay of healing and in hospital practice this is particularly important. Hospital acquired (nosocomial) infections are associated with more virulent organisms and are a greater cause for concern (27). Misuse or over-use of antibiotics lead to resistance and emergence which may be carried on and potentiated by, for example, extrachromosomal plasmid mediation (28).

Bacteria involved in wound infections

The organisms of interest are listed in Table 7.3. Normal skin is colonized by many commensals and residents such as proprionibacteria or *Staphyloccus epidermidis*. The latter is now regarded as an important opportunistic pathogen, particularly in its multiply-resistant form in hospital practice (multiply-resistant coagulase-negative staphylococcus,

Table 7.3 Organisms encountered in wound management

Organism	Microbiological characteristics	Source	Effect
Staphylococci S. aureus S. epidermidis	Gram-positive cocci; form clumps Coagulase positive Coagulase negative	Present in nasopharynx of 15%	Causes suppuration in wounds Causes opportunistic infection – particularly prosthetic vascular and orthopaedic grafts
Streptococci	Gram-positive cocci; form chains Lancefield A–G groups	Pharynx group A (S. pyogenes) Bowel group D (S. faecalis)	Cellulitis through release of proteases In synergy with others in wound infections and abscesses, particularly after GI surgery
Clostridia	Gram-positive bacilli; anaerobic spore being	C. perfringens present in faeces and soil C. tetani	Gas gangrene through release of exotoxins and proteases Tetanus through release of exotoxin
Bacteroides	Anaerobic non-spore bearing	Large bowel, vagina, oropharynx	In synergy with AGNB cause wound infections, particularly after GI surgery
Aerobic Gram- negative bacilli (AGNB)	E. coli; klebsiella; proteus, etc. Pseudomonas	Present in faeces	Synergistic with bacteroides in wound infection Colonize burns, tracheostomy, and catheters

MRCNS). Prosthetic surgery involving vascular grafts or orthopaedic implants is vulnerable to this organism. Its more pathogenic relative, S. aureus, has also been associated with resistant hospital strains (methicillin-resistant S. aureus, MRSA). S. aureus wound infections are most common after 'clean' surgery (see below). True pathogens such as Streptococcus pyogenes (the β-haemolytic, Lancefield group A Streptococcus) and the enterobacteriaceae (such as E. coli) are usually transient on skin, but can cause infection when skin, or mucosal, integrity is lost for any reason.

There are many factors in skin (and mucosal) surfaces which resist invasion; both physical and chemical (29, 30). Rapid cell turnover and surface desquamation keep epithelial surfaces intact and dryness of skin and extremes of pH (for example the stomach) prevent bacterial penetration. Skin also has a high salt and lipid content and permits interbacterial competition. Measurement of colonization by impression plates or harvesting with moistened cotton buds is inaccurate: only cultured biopsies can give a true estimate of bacterial numbers and types.

Open viscus surgery and bacterial contamination

It is now widely accepted that the potential for infection in wounds can be estimated by the degree of contamination which occurs during surgery (31–34) (Table 7.4).

In clean wounds the incision is made through uninfected or uninflammed tissue and no viscus is opened. The organisms cultured from infected wounds following this type of surgery are Gram-positive staphylococci and streptococci (35). The less pathogenic S. epidermidis is important as an opportunist in prosthetic surgery including vascular, orthopaedic, and mesh-repair hernia surgery.

Table 7.4 Wound classification system

I	Clean	Wounds are non-traumatic (i.e. elective surgical) with no break in surgical technique, without any septic focus or viscus being opened
II	Clean–contaminated	Wounds are non-traumatic (i.e. elective surgery), with only a minor break in technique being allowed, or entry into a viscus without significant spillage
III	Contaminated	Wounds are traumatic, from a relatively clean source, or with a major break in technique or significant spillage from an open viscus, or when acute non-purulent infection in encountered
IV	Dirty	Wounds are traumatic, from a dirty source, or following delayed treatment, or when acute bacterial contamination or release of pus occurs

Potentially contaminated (clean–contaminated) wounds involve surgery in which a viscus is opened but with minimal spillage of material. Elective biliary surgery falls into this category. The organisms most likely to be responsible for infection are staphylococci and Gram-negative rods such as E. coli (35).

Contaminated operations involve surgery for inflammatory conditions such as appendicitis where there is significant spillage of organisms. Coliforms and anaerobes such as the Bacteroides species, usually acting in synergy, are the main cause of infection (35).

Dirty operations are those in which pus is encountered or when there is a free perforation. Faecal peritonitis following perforated sigmoid colon diverticulitis is an example. The organisms cultured from wound infections are similar to those encountered in contaminated operations.

This measurement of contamination should be based on largely hypothetical grounds, but matches the risk of wound infection quite well. Comparison between operations in audit is facilitated but the accurate definition of contamination is based on wound sampling at the end of operations. Irrigation and biopsy methods are better than the use of moistened cotton swabs (36). The harvesting of microorganisms is minimized by effective prophylaxis (37) but in clean wounds, where antibiotic prophylaxis is not generally used, contamination measured at operation correlates well with later infection rates (38). Cruse and Foord (39), in their large audit of surgical wounds, found the following rates of infection in relation to wound classification: clean (1.5 per cent); clean–contaminated (9 per cent); contaminated (20 per cent); and dirty (43 per cent). Another non-randomized audit has revealed that even lower rates can be achieved provided rigorous protocols are in place (40). In this second audit the respective figures were 4.5 per cent; < 3 per cent; 3 per cent; and < 10 per cent. The higher figure found in clean wound surgery reflects an in-depth follow-up of patients back into the community and primary health care setting. As patients are returned home earlier, particularly after day case surgery, it is critical that infections are not missed. High rates of clean wound infection also suggest the need for prophylactic antibiotics, particularly when any prosthetic material is implanted. However, clinical trials of antibiotic prophylaxis in clean, non-prosthetic surgery are clearly required because the risk of infection, although mostly minor in nature, is probably higher than most audits reveal.

The infective inoculum of microorganisms required to cause an infection is greatly reduced in numbers if a foreign body is present. It has been estimated that 5×10^6 pathogens per gram of tissue are required to cause an infection, but this can be reduced logarithmically if a suture, such as silk, is present (41). The final outcome of wound infection risk is, of course, dependent on many factors (other than contamination) and include host defence, tissue perfusion and shock, or presence of the systemic metabolic factors.

In some classical experiments performed over 30 years ago it was realized that the physiological determinant of wound infection was the delay in mobilization of host defences after a surgical or traumatic challenge (including an incision) (42). This delay lasts about 4h after wounding, when the acute inflammatory response is being mounted, and has been called the 'decisive period'. When antibiotic prophylaxis is used this is the time of greatest efficacy to support host resistance to wound infection.

Definition of wound infection

In audit of wound infection or trials of antibiotic prophylaxis the definition of wound infection (or other postoperative infection) may be critical. A wound infection is obvious when there is spontaneous discharge of pus, or discharge after removal of sutures, or opening of a wound. When a non-purulent discharge contains pathogens such as a coliform or *S. aureus*, again an infection may be counted. Spreading cellulitis (Fig. 7.3) following implantation of a pathogenic streptococcus, for example, is a clear infection but when minimal may be difficult to separate from the inflammation of healing.

Wounds should be inspected continually for up to six weeks after trauma or surgery to be sure an infection has not occurred. The time for most wound infections to develop is 7–9 days. With the increasing trend to day case surgery, wound inspection must be continued.

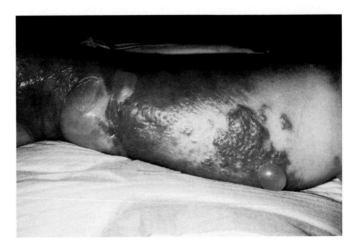

Fig. 7.3 Spreading cellulitis from a puncture wound of the ankle. (See plate section.)

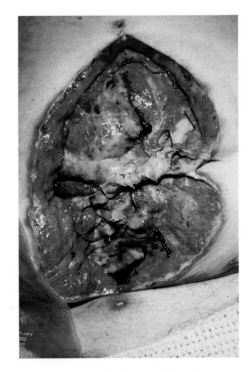

Fig. 7.4 Major wound infection. (See plate section.)

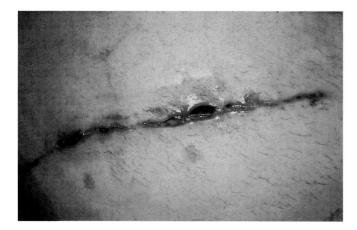

Fig. 7.5 Minor wound infection. (See plate section.)

A major wound infection (Fig. 7.4) is characterized by systemic toxicity (pyrexia and tachycardia) with local pain, wound breakdown, or extensive cellulitis which delays the patient's return home. Minor wound infection is not so complicated (Fig. 7.5).

Endogenous infections are usually community acquired-where an infection is caused by the patient's own organisms (skin or viscus)-whereas exogenous infection is nosocomial and acquired by poor theatre discipline or postoperative wound care. It is in this latter category that resistant organisms, such as MRSA, may be encountered with the additional risk of an epidemic (ERSA). Surveillance and audit have much to commend them in helping to recognize and prevent such infections. Imaging techniques may be required to recognize deep infections. Intra-abdominal abscesses may be identified by several modalities (e.g. ultrasound, CT scanning, isotopic scanning) which also permit guided aspiration and avoidance of surgery (43).

Grading of wound infection is not easy, but has been attempted for clinical trials of antibiotic prophylaxis (44, 45). In this grading, account is taken of

- additional treatment
- serous discharge from the wound
- erythema
- purulent exudate
- separation of deep tissues
- isolation of bacteria from wound swabs, and
- inpatient stay

which has been given the acronym ASEPSIS. Although a useful system, there has been little general use reported.

Surgical and environmental factors influencing wound infection

Skin preparation

For aesthetic reasons, and to facilitate removal of adhesive dressings, it is conventional to shave patients prior to surgical procedures. When shaving is not required for these reasons it can be safely avoided. Shaving more than 12 h before surgery risks an increase in bacteria, mobilized from the deeper layers, on to the skin surface, particularly if the shave is inexpert (39). Shaving immediately prior to surgery negates this risk. Clipping or the use of depilatory creams (46) are alternatives to comply with a clean wound infection rate of < 1 per cent. General good hygiene of patients (and the surgical team) is common sense; if patient or surgeon has a coincident septic skin focus then they should not enter the operating theatre. Total body washes using antiseptics are popular in mainland Europe, but have not become standard in the UK. There are controversial reports – some profess an advantage (47), others do not (48).

Hand washing and skin preparation

The use of antiseptics in wound care is covered fully in the next section (see Table 7.5). They are widely used in skin preparation prior to surgery. However, social hand-washing with soap and water, and adequate drying of the skin with disposable paper towels is adequate for inspecting or changing wound dressings on the ward. In theatre, prior to surgery, aqueous 4 per cent chlorhexidine (Hibiscrub) or 7.5 per cent povidone-iodine (Betadine) are ideal for hand-washing, with a reduction for skin flora of over 95 per cent (49). Prolonged hand-washing is not necessary. Scrubbing of the finger nails is recommended for the first case only of an operating session. Scrubbing hands and forearms and prolonged washes between operations only releases more organisms to the skin surface.

Similar reductions of skin flora can be expected after preparing the patient's skin with either 2.5 per cent alcoholic chlorhexidine or 10 per cent alcoholic povidone-iodine. Repeated or prolonged skin preparation tends to damage skin and release organisms.

Operating theatre discipline and environment

It is logical to ban patients and operating theatre staff when they have open infective skin lesions. The flow of patients and instruments through a set plan (clean to dirty) is also logical: the patient from entrance corridor to anaesthetic room, operating theatre, to ward; and instruments from CSSD, theatre, to sluice. There is no need for sticky pads at the theatre entrance and the use of overshoes for attending ward staff bringing patients for operation simply contaminates hands.

Ventilation in operating theatres is aimed at reduction of air contamination, mainly of *S. aureus* and *S. epidermidis*. Settle plates or slit samplers are regularly used to ensure efficiency. All theatres now employ a positive pressure (plenum) system with 20 air changes per hour and 5 μm filtration. Ultra-clean air is required for prosthetic orthopaedic surgery in which air flow is vertical and laminar with 40 changes per hour. Full operator coverings, modular theatres, and exhaust suits have been used to achieve very low rates of infection (50), but similar results have been achieved with appropriate antibiotic prophylaxis (51). To achieve comfort in operating theatres for personnel is important, and a range of 40–60 per cent air humidity and 15–20°C in temperature should be achieved.

Gowns are made of light woven cotton or similar synthetic material, but these do little to prevent transfer of a marker organism, such as the staphylococcus. Disposable non-woven cellulose gowns are ideal when transfer is a risk (and for patients with a risk of hepatitis or HIV transfer) but are expensive and not as comfortable to wear.

Gloves are worn to protect the patient from the operating team's bacteria, which may remain on their hands. The risk of transfer to patients is small and probably only significant when prosthetic surgery is undertaken. Like gowns, gloves can also protect the operating team from risk of viral infection which might be acquired from the patient. It is of course aesthetic to wear gloves, but the risk of puncture can exceed 50 per cent in long, difficult access operations.

Masks are necessary in prosthetic surgery, particularly in conjunction with hoods for long hair or a beard. There is little evidence that discarding a mask in non-prosthetic general surgical operations increases the risk of wound infection. Again, the mask can protect the operator from infected body fluids, particularly blood.

Incise drapes and wound guards

Adhesive polyurethane transparent films were introduced to secure operative drapes, avoid towel clips, and to isolate stomas from a planned new wound. They are widely used as wound dressings to cover sutured wounds, but there is little evidence that they reduce wound infections (52). Incise drapes impregnated with antiseptics such as povidone-iodine may lower the bacterial count at the skin surface but do not affect colonization in the wound during an operation (53). Wound guards, intended to protect the wound edges during an operative procedure, also seem to offer little protection against infection (54).

Drains

Drains were designed and used to minimize dead space in the wound, and to evacuate haematomas or body fluids with the intention of reducing the risk of infection. There is no clear evidence that drains are effective (55), but they are probably used when there is a risk of wound breakdown or collection of fluid, more to appease a surgeon's conscience than anything else. Closed disposable suction drains are the most widely used (56). Their built-in valve prevents reflux of fluid and prevents the inflow of external organisms which may occur with open drains. All drains are foreign bodies which cause a tissue reaction and should be used with care.

Wound closure

Sutures, staples (clips), and tapes are used to close tissues after an operation and are described in Chapter 4. Adequate surgery should ideally leave no dead tissue (by avoiding excessive trauma or use of diathermy) or foreign material (which should be removed with non-viable tissue) unless it is a prosthetic implant or closure material. The balance of using suture material to hold tissues together until they are healed has to be made with these factors in mind. Too much effort to close the theoretical risk of dead space may increase tissue tension and still not prevent the collection of a haematoma or a later infection. Adequate perfusion to the wound, deter-

mined by local and systemic factors, is probably the best predictor of healing with reduction of infection (57, 58). Sutures used for wound closure must be placed outside the biochemically active zone of the wound edge (59), otherwise they fail in holding tissue together. This lytic zone is widened by infection but can be minimized by the use of the least reactive fine material (usually a synthetic, non-absorbable monofilament). No great strength is required in bowel anastomosis, just opposition, whereas great indefinite strength is required for vascular anastomosis. Appropriate sutures should be used for these tasks.

Antiseptics in wound care

The use of antiseptics in skin preparation has been outlined above. They are in widespread use for sterilizing instruments (e.g. glutaraldehyde) or for surface disinfection (e.g. hypochlorites). Their use in open wound management is currently controversial, there being no evidence that surface sterility of a wound is required in healing by secondary intention, and in any case their antimicrobial activity for this use is short lived (as antiseptics are rapidly inactivated in contact with body fluids or pus) (60). Lord Lister used a phenol spray intraoperatively and effectively reduced wound infection after compound fractures, but intraoperative wound lavage with antiseptics is questionable. There are proponents (61), but many more have found no benefit (62–64). Table 7.5 lists the antiseptics in common use and their effects and indications.

Historical background

Antiseptics of many origins have been used as wound salves for millenia, and the story has been unravelled extensively by Majno (65) and Forrest (66, 67). The use of plant resins, myrrh, and gums was probably based on a concept that sap fills defects in plants after damage and could therefore be useful in human wounds. Many of these materials, particularly resins, do not decay and were considered to have a preservative action. This is certainly true of honey and sugar. Some plant extracts have a pleasant aromatic or strong smell, which would be an added benefit in infected necrotic wounds. Perhaps the pungent smells (for instance, frankincense) were considered to have a preventive action against putrefaction. Certainly urine and dung were used, possibly because of their ammoniacal smell in combination, but more probably ritualistically. Urine has found a use as a wound irrigant in war surgery – certainly fresh urine is sterile and available in large quantities when more conventional antiseptics are in short supply!

There was widespread use of antiseptics in Assyrian, Egyptian, and Greek medical care. Salt was used for embalming and was used in an attempt to prevent putrefaction of living flesh. Many other metallic compounds were used: copper pigments doubled up as an eye adornment; lead and aluminium had their adherents; and it is interesting that relatively recently zinc has been recognized to be a cofactor in healing (see Chapter 5). Hippocrates described his treatment of open wounds healing by secondary intention. Vinegar and wine were used to clean wounds and were recognized as stimulants

Table 7.5 Antiseptics in use for skin preparation and instrument cleaning

Name	Presentation	Uses	Comments
Chlorhexidine (Hibiscrub)	Alcoholic 0.5% Aqueous 4% (biguanide)	Skin preparation Skin preparation; surgical scrub; in dilute solutions in open wounds	Has cumulative effect Effective against Gram-positive organisms and relatively stable in presence of pus and body fluids
Povidone–iodine (Betadine)	Alcoholic 10% Aqueous 7.5%	Skin preparation Skin preparation; surgical scrub; in dilute solutions in open wounds	Safe, fast-acting broad spectrum. Some sporicidal activity. Antifungal. Iodine is not free but combined with polyvinylpyrrolidine (povidone)
Cetrimide (Savlon)	Aqueous	Hand-washing; instrument and surface cleaning	*Pseudomonas* spp. may grow in stored contaminated solutions. Ammonium compounds have good detergent action (surface active agent)
Alcohols	70% ethyl, isopropyl	Skin preparation	
Hypochlorites	Aqueous preparations (Eusol, Milton, Chloramine T)	Instrument and surface cleaning. (Debriding agent in open wounds?)	Should be reserved for use as disinfectant
Hexachlorophane	Aqueous bisphenol	Skin preparation; hand-washing	Has action against Gram-negative organisms

to healing. Foodstuffs such as honey, sugar, butter, and milk have all been used in this field. In addition to cleaning wound surfaces and reducing bacterial colonization, they may also have a topical nutritive effect which has not been explored in any depth as yet.

The current use of antiseptics for healing by secondary intention has been the subject of reviews (68, 69). The large debate and controversy has centred on the use of the disinfectant hypochlorite solutions. The argument has been taken up fiercely by nurse practitioners and has led to the virtual ban of hypochlorites in many hospitals. There is no doubt that the hypochlorites are excellent disinfectants for working surfaces, lavatories, and sluices, and to sterilize baby feeding bottles but the experimental evidence suggests they should be used with caution on open wounds. Although no-one would deny their use as debriding agents, they are clearly toxic to healing tissues. As Alexander Fleming put it, 'it is necessary in the estimation of the value of an antiseptic to study its effect on the tissues more than its effect on the bacteria' (70).

Hypochlorites

EUSOL is an acronym for Edinburgh University solution of lime, and is a solution of chlorinated lime and boric acid with a pH of 7.5–8.5. The medical military need for an antiseptic for field use led to the development of Dakin's solution (71, 72). Milton is a similar hypochlorite solution with a higher pH. Clinical evidence of the efficacy of hypochlorite solutions remains anecdotal, but they nevertheless became an established part of wound care. It would be interesting to see if they passed the strict code for clinical trials if they were introduced now. When these antiseptics were introduced there clearly was a need for a cheap, effective topical antimicrobial and debriding agent. It is interesting to note that Trueta managed

compound fractures and open wounds by a closed method, without any antimicrobials at all, some 20 years later (73). The treatment was very effective.

The hypochlorites are unstable solutions which are easily inactivated in contact with organic substances. They clearly are effective debriding agents, although their action is probably through damage to surface layers of living tissue, and are widely used prior to skin grafting. There are, however, equally effective alternative methods to clean necrotic wounds. As antibacterials, the antiseptics which do not damage living tissue are effective with a wide spectrum. The clinical use of hypochlorites (and the continuing nurse and doctor confrontation) has been well reviewed and argued (74–77). The use of hypochlorites still awaits proper clinical trials.

The experimental evidence against hypochlorites is based on their cytotoxicity on fibroblasts, white blood cells, and endothelial cells in culture; delay in healing of open wounds healing by secondary intention (measured by levels of hydroxyproline or prolonged inflammation); and in the rabbit ear chamber where vasoconstriction, cessation of blood flow, and tissue death can be observed (78–83).

Povidone–iodine

Aqueous free iodine is corrosive and stains tissues. Povidone–iodine is a polyvinylpyrrolidine iodophor, presented with a detergent as Betadine, in various concentrations. The 10 per cent aqueous form is equivalent to 1 per cent free iodine. Its effect on thyroid function is probably overstated, but free iodine can be absorbed following the use of povidone–iodine in open wounds. Dilute solutions are probably effective as topical antimicrobials but without the risk of tissue damage.

There is some evidence that povidone–iodine reduces infection in lacerations (84) and it is an effective skin preparation and hand-washing agent (49). However, in open wounds it should be used with caution as it may actually increase infection and delay healing (85–87). In experimental studies it has been shown to inhibit white blood cell and fibroblast growth in cell culture and reduce the acquisition of tensile strength in healing wounds (80, 81, 88).

Chlorhexidine

Chlorhexidine is effective as a hand-washing agent and for skin preparation (49). It is widely used for preoperative bathing or showering but with no definite benefit. Chlorhexidine does, however, have a prolonged broad spectrum of activity against Gram-positive and Gram-negative organisms. It is a useful alternative to povidone-iodine in cases of hypersensitivity and cannot be absorbed through intact skin. Chlorhexidine is less affected by body fluids and has been shown to be superior to other antiseptics in terms of its antimicrobial action (89). It is not exempt from toxic effects in tissues but has not been as fully assessed as other antiseptics.

Hydrogen peroxide

Hydrogen peroxide is widely used as a wound irrigant. Oxygen bubbles are released in contact with tissue – they may damage tissue and risk bubble embolus. There is no evidence of antimicrobial activity, nor is it toxic in rabbit ear chamber evaluation (78). Although hydrogen peroxide does not appear to interfere with healing, it is toxic to fibroblasts (80).

Antibiotics and their use in wound care

This chapter has already reviewed surgeon and environment-related factors and wound contamination which relate to the risk of wound infection. In addition, there are several other systemic factors which predispose patients to the risk of infection. These include age and nutrition (obesity or undernourishment), immunosuppression therapy (but also related to cancer and its treatment, blood transfusion, steroids, and immunodeficiency diseases), metabolic disease (diabetes mellitus, jaundice, renal failure), shock of any cause, and prolonged operations. In the decisive period observed by Burke (42) prophylactic antibiotic therapy should be considered in these, at risk, diseases (90). When wound contamination is severe, or when there is established infection, the choice of antibiotics remains much the same as for prophylaxis only it is prolonged until there is evidence of cure of infection. The choice is an empirical one, but can be accurate when based on past experience and studies of antibiotic spectra and a knowledge of the likely organisms encountered (44, 91, 92). For therapy, there may be further guidelines based on culture and sensitivity analysis of infected material, but these should not be waited for. Equally, if there is a measurable obvious clinical response to antibiotics it is foolhardy to change an antibiotic regimen without good reason, even if culture and sensitivity suggest that organisms cultured are resistant.

Antibiotics achieve a response more quickly if given parenterally (IV or IM). For prophylactic use the IV route, with administration at induction of anaesthesia, is related to an optimal effect. The frequency and duration of an antibiotic course depends on the pharmacokinetics of an antibiotic and the clinical response. In prophylaxis it is valueless to prolong administration beyond 24 h and, in therapy, a lack of clinical response after five days questions whether the antibiotic is appropriate or whether there is an infected collection which needs surgical evacuation (an abscess). There is no evidence of complications following genuine prophylactic use but prolonged antibiotic therapy risks resistance (MRSA and MRCNS being of particular concern to surgeons) and emergence (such as *Clostridium difficile* and the syndrome of pseudomembranous colitis). Some antibiotics are associated with specific side-effects such as bleeding (those that carry the N-methylthiotetrazole ring), or renal and oto-toxicity (particularly the aminoglycosides). The cost of antibiotics and the need to monitor their use also needs consideration. See Table 7.6 for a list of the antibiotics used in wound management.

Sulphonamides

Derived from the Bohemian dye industry, this group of antibiotics has found success in treating urinary tract infection, particularly in combination with trimethoprim. They are inhibitors of folic acid metabolism with a broad spectrum of activity (mainly against Gram-negative bacilli). Sulphonamides have little part to play in managing wound infections but the poorly absorbed group have been used in large bowel preparation (as neomycin and kanamycin also have) to reduce the risk of wound infection after colorectal surgery. Topical sulpha-drugs (silver sulphadiazine) have widespread use in burns therapy.

Penicillins

These antibiotics have a relatively short half life, with a narrow spectrum, and carry a risk of sensitivity. They are bactericidal and are themselves organically derived. Benzyl penicillin is the antibiotic of choice for streptococcal or clostridial wound infections. β-Lactamases (bacterially produced enzymes which inactivate antibiotics like cephalosporins and penicillins by breaking up their central β-lactam ring) produced by resistant bacteria destroy the penicillin molecule, particularly staphylococci and the enterobacteriaceae. Derivatives, such as flucloxacillin, are active against *S. aureus*; but MRSA has developed resistance to methicillin and poses a threat of further resistance following antibiotic misuse. The acylureido-penicillins range between having a wide spectrum (and have been used for empirical prophylaxis and therapy) to a limited spectrum action (for use against *Pseudomonas* species, for example). Augmentin, another broad spectrum drug, is a combination of amoxycillin and clavulanic acid which prevents β-lactamase degradation.

Cephalosporins

Originally isolated from the cephalosporium mould in the 1950s these antibiotics have an established role in surgical practise. They have a greater resistance to β-lactamases.

Table 7.6 Antibiotics in use for wound management

Antibiotic	Modification; presentation	Spectrum	Use
Penicillins			
Benzylpenicillin	Original; IV, IM	Streptococci/anaerobes	Multidrug chemotherapy; clostridial infections (also in prophylaxis for vascular amputations)
Phenoxymethyl penicillin	Original	Streptococci/anaerobes	Mild strepococcal infections
Ampicillin	Original; IM, IV	Streptococci/anaerobes; AGNB*	Therapy and prophylaxis
Clavulanic acid; amoxycillin	β-lactamase inhibitor	*Staphylococcus aureus*; AGNB*	Wide spectrum prophylaxis and therapy
Flucloxacillin	β-lactamase stability	*Staphylococcus aureus*	Narrow spectrum staphylococcal infections
Acylureide penicillins		AGNB*; *Pseudomonas*	Some (e.g. mezlocillin) are broad spectrum; others (e.g. piperacillin) narrow for anti-pseudomonas therapy
Cephalosporins			
Second generation	e.g. Cefuroxime, cefoxitin	Wide range of Gram-positive cocci and AGNB*	Used in general prophylaxis and therapy of susceptible infections. Cefoxitin has some anaerobic activity
Third generation	e.g. Cefotaxime, ceftazidime	Lessened anti-staphylococcal activity. Varied anti-anaerobe and pseudomonal activity	Used in empirical therapy of serious infections usually in combination
Sulphonamides			Topical use in burns therapy, see text
Aminoglycosides	e.g. Gentamicin		See text
Tetracyclines			See text
Imidazoles	e.g. Metronidazole		Effective and non-toxic for anaerobic infections
Macrolides	e.g. Erythromycin		May be used as alternative to penicillin in cases of allergy
Quinolones	e.g. Ciprofloxacin		Wide spectrum antibiotics for empirical use in severe infections
Carbopenems	e.g. Meropenem		Wide spectrum antibiotics for empirical use in severe infections

* AGNB = aerobic Gram-negative bacilli (*E. coli*, etc.).

As this group has been developed, greater potency against specific organisms has resulted at the expense of a narrower spectrum. The appropriate antibiotics are most effective when given parenterally, which can limit their use and there may be cross-sensitivity and allergy with the penicillins.

Aminoglycosides

These are cheap, effective antibiotics, active against staphylococci and aerobic Gram-negative bacilli. They are safe in prophylaxis, with a prolonged post-antibiotic effect, but need close monitoring (peak and trough) to avoid renal and oto-toxicity, particularly when renal function is impaired.

Nitroimidazoles

The most well known of this group, metronidazole, is an effective antianaerobe (against *Bacteroides* species, mainly). It is an alternative to lincomycin or clindamycin because it has little toxicity and avoids the risk of pseudomembranous colitis.

Tetracyclines

Antibiotics of this group have little place in prophylaxis or treatment but have been shown, when used as a peritoneal lavage, to greatly reduce wound infection after abdominal surgery (40).

Topical antibiotics

See Table 7.7. These have the disadvantage of causing topical allergy and systemic sensitivity. If used inappropriately they may encourage the emergence of new bacteria or resistance. Their use seems logical when there are signs of infection within a chronic ulcer and a microbiological swab has revealed pathogens, but there is little in the way of controlled trials which confirm their effectiveness. When there is clear spreading infection then an appropriate antibiotic should be given orally or parenterally.

Table 7.7 Topical antibiotics

Agent	Uses/indications
Mupiracin (Bactroban)	Is a potent antistaphylococcal agent (MRSA in particular), unrelated to any other antibiotics, with low levels of resistance emerging provided it is not used longer than 10 days It is presented as an ointment or a tulle
Neomycin	Is one of the aminoglycosides but is poorly absorbed orally and too toxic for systemic use If ulcers are very large it may be absorbed enough to cause ototoxicity in elderly patients It can cross-sensitize to other aminoglycosides and cause resistance It is presented as an ointment or dusting powder (Cicatrin) Framycetin is similar, used as an ointment (Soframycin) or tulle (Sofratulle)
Polymyxins	Combinations of colistin and polymyxin B Again, ototoxicity is a hazard if large areas of skin are treated
Silver sulphadiazine	Has had widespread use as a topical prophylactic agent for burns and, more specifically, for treating pseudomonal infections Its use in infected leg ulcers and pressure sores is also popular but not clearly substantiated
Tetracyclines	Have been used for skin infections but not for infected chronic ulcers or pressure sores Emergence and resistance are risks with local hypersensitivity
Fucidic acid	Is an antistaphylococcal agent Because of its narrow spectrum it should be reserved for resistance, principally MRSA It may cause local hypersensitivity
Metronidazole	Applied as a gel, has been used in deep ulcers which are malodorous because of anaerobic colonization; particularly fungating tumours

Infection management and control

Audit and surveillance test our effectiveness and efficiency (use of resources). It is now part of all clinical and nursing care. Most hospitals have guidelines for collection and analysis of nosocomial infection. Once the definition of wound infection is made and is accepted it is very easy to count, assess, and act on. Recognition of infection risks allows implementation of change or an action that can 'close the loop' of audit. Most audit is based on process, in relation to outbreaks of infection, or outcome, which assesses the incidence of infection. The dissemination of data on wound infection rates to surgeons can lead to a decrease of infection without any other action (93). The identification of risk factors encourages extra support where it is needed; but equally, rituals which are unrelated to wound infection may be questioned, with obvious savings (the use of masks or overshoes for all types of surgery serves as an example). It has been suggested that 'clean wound' infection rates are the most valuable reflection of surgical care in any hospital (34). However, follow-up of surgical wounds must be adequate to establish accurate infection rates. In these days of day case and short-stay surgery, it must be remembered that most wound infections take 7–9 days to develop. Surveillance allows quality control, but anonymity of individual surgeon's infection rates should be respected (although they need action) and their use in 'league tables' is to be deprecated.

Specific important tissue infection

Abdominal infection

It has been suggested that the gastrointestinal tract is potentially an undrained abscess. It is true that in adverse circumstances (abdominal infection, multiple trauma, pancreatitis, burns, or multiple transfusion) the normally sterile small bowel and stomach can become colonized by aerobic Gram-negative bacilli (AGNB). Translocation through the bowel wall to mesenteric lymph nodes may precede bacterial death and release of bacterial cell wall lipopolysacchoride (endotoxin). Macrophages, involved in the host response, release a complex cascade of cytokines (such as interleukins 1 and 6 and tumour necrosis factors) accompanied by activation of complement and release of prostaglandins. There follows a systemic inflammatory response syndrome (SIRS) of systemic toxicity, pyrexia, and rigors. The systemic nature of sepsis distinguishes it from localized infection, which can also cause it, but infection may not be present.

Following SIRS and shock there may be a multiple organ dysfunction syndrome (MODS) which presents with adult respiratory distress syndrome (ARDS); renal failure (acute tubular necrosis); hepatic, brain, and myocardial failure (related to hypoxia or oxygen free radical release following reperfusion injury); disseminated intravascular coagulation (with severe bleeding complications); and ileus and stress gastritis (colonization may be worsened by high gastric pH caused by the use of histamine receptor antagonists).

SIRS and MODS are associated with appreciable morbidity and mortality on intensive therapy units and methods of decontaminating or preventing (using other organisms as antagonists) the colonization of the gut are still being evaluated (94). In abdominal infections it is clearly the onset of SIRS and MODS which determine outcome and survival, not the infection (95, 96). The use of physiological scoring systems helps to identify patients at risk and to institute early resuscitation and treatment (97, 98).

Clostridial and non-clostridial soft tissue infections

Clostridial gas gangrene is caused predominantly by *Clostridium perfringens*. It is well recognized in military surgery when there is widespread tissue damage with ischaemia, devitalization, and contamination by foreign bodies, particularly if primary closure of such a wound has been attempted. Local signs of cellulitis, necrosis, and crepitus of tissues are rapidly followed by profound systemic toxicity and cardiovascular collapse. Effective treatment must employ high-dose penicillin therapy, adequate surgical debridement of non-viable tissue, and hyperbaric oxygen. In civilian practice, clostridial gas gangrene is occasionally encountered in the face of a depressed immune response (such as diabetes mellitus, or cancer therapy).

Non-clostridial tissue infections involve a 'soup' of organisms (enteric Gram-negative bacilli, anaerobes, and Gram-positive cocci) acting in synergy. There are several synonyms such as Fournier's gangrene (involving the scrotum) and Meleney's synergistic hospital gangrene (involving the abdominal wall). Gas may be present in the tissues and the infection spreads rapidly subdermally so that superficially it does not seem very extensive. Life-saving aggressive debridement of all affected tissue and late skin grafting is required with intensive systemic support and wide spectrum antibiotic therapy.

References

1. Sweet, C., Bird, R. A., Husseini, R. H., and Smith, H. (1984). Differential replication of attenuated and virulent influenza viruses in organ cultures of ferret bronchial epithelium. *Archives of Virology*, **80**, 219–24.
2. Steinman, R. M. (1991). The dentritic cell system and its role in immunogenicity. *Annual Reviews in Immunology*, **9**, 271–96.
3. Silberberg-Sinakin, I., Fedorko, M. E., Baer, R. L., Rosenthal, S. A., Berezowsky, V., and Thorbecke, G. J. (1977). Langerhans cells: target cells in immune complex reactions. *Cellular Immunology*, **32**, 400–16.
4. Silberberg-Sinakin, I., Thorbecke, G. J., Baer, R. L., Rosenthal, S. A., and Berezowsky, V. (1976). Antigen-bearing Langerhans cells in skin dermal lymphatics and in lymph nodes. *Cellular Immunology*, **25**, 137–51.
5. Braathen, L. R., Berle, E., Mobech-Hansen, U., and Thorsby, E. (1980). Studies on human epidermal Langerhans cells: II. Activation of human T lymphocytes to Herpes simplex virus. *Acta Dermato Venerologica* (Stockholm), **60**, 381–7.
6. Inaba, K., Schuler, G., Witmer, M. D., Valinsky, J., Atassi, B., and Steinman, R. M.(1986). The immunologic properties of purified Langerhans cells: distinct requirements for the stimulation of unprimed and sensitized T lymphocytes. *J. Exp. Med.*, **164**, 605–13.
7. Williams, N. A., Hill, T. J., and Hooper, D. C. (1991). Murine epidermal antigen presenting cells in primary and secondary T cell proliferative responses to Herpes simplex virus *in vitro*. *Immunology*, **72**, 34–9.
8. Williams, N. A., Hill, T. J., and Hooper, D. C. (1990). Murine epidermal antigen presenting cells in primary and secondary T cell proliferative responses to a soluble protein antigen *in vitro*. *Immunology*, **71**, 411–16.
9. Heufler, C., Koch, F., and Schuler, G. (1988). Granulocyte/macrophage colony stimulating factor and IL-1 mediate the maturation of murine epidermal Langerhans cells into potent immunostimulatory dendritic cells. . *Exp. Med.*, **167**, 700–5.
10. Schuler, G. and Steinman, R. M. (1985). Murine epidermal Langerhans cells mature into potent immunostimulatory dendritic cells *in vitro*. *J. Exp. Med.*, **161**, 526–46.
11. Williams, N. A., Wilson, A. D., Bailey, M., Bland, P. W., and Stokes, C. R. (1992). Primary antigen-specific T-cell proliferative responses following presentation of soluble protein antigen by cells from the murine small intestine. *Immunology*, **75**, 608–13.
12. Neefjes, J. J. and Ploegh, H. L. (1992). Intracellular transport of MHC class II molecules. *Immunology Today*, **13**, 179–84.
13. Rudensky, A. Y., Preston-Hurlburt, P., Hong, S. C., Barlow, A., and Janeway, C. A. (1991). Sequence analysis of peptides bound to MHC class II molecules. *Nature*, **346**, 622–7.
14. Springer, T. A. (1990). Adhesion receptors of the immune system. *Nature*, **346**, 425–34.
15. Dustin, M. L. and Springer, T. A. (1989). T cell receptor crosslinking transiently stimulates adhesiveness through LFA-1. *Nature*, **341**, 619–24.
16. Jenkins, M. K., Taylor, P. S., Norton, S. D., and Urdahl, K. B. (1991). CD28 delivers a costimulatory signal involved in antigen-specific IL-2 production by human T-cells. *J. Imm.*, **147**, 2461–6.
17. Eynon, E. E. and Parker, D. C. (1992). Small B-cells as antigen-presenting cells in the induction of tolerance to soluble protein antigens. *J. Exp. Med.*, **175**, 131–8.
18. Janeway, C. A., Jr. (1992). The T cell receptor as a multicomponent signalling machine: CD4/CD8 coreceptors and CD45 in T cell activation. *Ann. Revi. Imm.*, **10**, 645–74.
19. Mossman, T. R. and Coffman, R. L. (1987). Two types of mouse helper T-cell clone – implications for immune regulation. *Immunology Today*, **8**, 223–8.
20. Maggi, E., Del Prete, G. F., Macchia, D., Parronchi, P., Tiri, A., Chretien, I., et al. (1988). Profiles of lymphokine activities and helper function for IgE in human T cell clones. *Eur. J. Imm.*, **18**, 1045–50.
21. Mosmann, T. R. and Moore, K. W. (1991). The role of IL-10 in crossregulation of TH1 and TH2 responses. *Immunology Today*, **12**, A49–53.
22. Fiorentino, D. F., Zlotnik, A., Vieira, P., Mosmann, T. R., Howard, M., Moore, K. W., and O'Garra, A. (1991). IL-10 acts on the antigen-presenting cell to inhibit cytokine production by TH1 cells. *J. Imm.*, **146**, 3444–51.
23. Locksley, R. M. and Scott, P. (1991). Helper T-cell subsets in mouse leishmaniasis: induction, expansion and effector function. *Immunology Today*, **12**, A58–62.

24. Romagnani, S. (1992). Induction of Th1 and Th2 responses: a key role for the 'natural' immune response. *Immunology Today*, **13**, 379–81.

25. Fong, T. A. T. and Mosmann, T. R. (1992). Alloreactive murine CD8-T cell clones secrete the Th1 pattern of cytokines. *J. Imm.*, **144**, 1744–52.

26. Williams, R. E. O. (1973). Benefit and mischief from commensal bacteria. *J. Clin. Path.*, **26**, 811–18.

27. Casewell, M. (1982). The role of multiple resistant coliforms in hospital acquired infection. In *Recent advances in infection*, Vol. 2 (ed. D. S. Reeves and A. M. Geddes), pp. 231–50. Churchill Livingstone, Edinburgh.

28. Mehtar, S. (1992). Action of abtibiotics and the development of antibiotic resistance. In *Infection in surgical practice*, (ed. E. W. Taylor), pp. 68–75. Oxford University Press, Oxford.

29. Selwyn, S. (1980). Microbial interactions and antibiosis. In *Skin microbiology. Relevance to clinical infection*, (ed. H. I. Maibach and R. Aly). Springer, New York.

30. Selwyn, S. (1980). Skin preparation, the surgical scrub and related rituals. In *Controversies in surgical sepsis*, (ed. S. Karran), pp. 23–32. Praeger Scientific, Eastbourne.

31. National Academy of Sciences: *ad hoc* committee of the Committee on Trauma (1964). Post-operative wound infections, the influence of ultraviolet irradiation of the operative room and of various other factors. *Ann. Surg.*, **160** (Suppl. 2), 1–92.

32. Christou, N. V., Nohr, C. W., and Meakins, J. L. (1987). Assessing operative site infection in surgical patients. *Arch. Surg.*, **122**, 165–9.

33. Bremmelgaard, A., Raahave, D., Beier-Holgersen, *et al.* (1989). Computer-aided surveillance of surgical infections and identification of risk factors. *J. Hosp. Infect.*, **13**, 1–18.

34. Cruse, P. J. E. (1992). Classification of operations and audit of infection. In *Infection in surgical practice*, (ed. E. W. Taylor). Oxford University Press, Oxford.

35. Keighley, M. R. B. and Burdon, D. W. (1979). *Antimicrobial prophylaxis in surgery*. Pitman Medical, Tunbridge Wells.

36. Raahave, D. (1992). Wound contamination and post-operative infection. In *Infection in surgical practice*, (ed. E. W. Taylor), pp. 49–55. Oxford University Press, Oxford.

37. Cooper, M., Billings, P., Turner, A., and Leaper, D. (1987). Intraoperative microbiological sampling is unhelpful after prophylactic antibiotics. Proceedings V Mediterranean Congress of Chemotherapy. *Chemioterapia*, **6** (Suppl. 2), 563.

38. Dillon, M. L., Postlethwait, R. W., and Bowling, K. A. (1969). Operative wound cultures and wound infections. A study of 342 patients. *Ann. Surg.*, **170**, 1029–34.

39. Cruse, P. J. E. and Foord, R. (1980). The epidemiology of wound infection: a ten year prospective study of 62 939 wounds. *Surg. Clin. North Am.*, **60**, 27–40.

40. Krukowski, Z. H. and Mathesen, N. A. (1988). 10 year computerised audit of infection after general surgery. *Br. J. Surg.*, **75**, 857–61.

41. Elek, S. D. and Conen, P. E. (1957). The virulence of *Staphylococcus pyogenes* for man. A study of the problems of wound infection. *Br. J. Exp. Pathol.*, **38**, 573–86.

42. Burke, J. F. (1961). The effective period of preventive antibiotic action in experimental incisions and dermal lesions. *Surgery*, **50**, 161–8.

43. Lucarotti, M. E., Virjee, J., Thomas, W. E. G., and Leaper, D. J. (1991). Intra-abdominal abscesses. *Surgery*, **1**, 2335–41.

44. Leaper, D. J. and Pritchett, C. J. (1989). Prophylactic antibiotics in general surgical practice. *Curr. Pract. in Surg.*, **1**, 178–84.

45. Wilson, A. P. R., Treasure, T., Sturridge, M. F., and Gruneberg, R. N. (1986). A scoring method (ASEPSIS) for post-operative wound infections for use in clinical trials of antibiotic prophylaxis. *Lancet*, **i**, 311–13.

46. Seropian, R. and Reynolds, B. M. (1971). Wound infections after pre-operative depilatory versus razor preparation. *Am. J. Surg.*, **121**, 251–4.

47. Hayek, L. J., Emersen, J. M., and Gardner, A. M. N.(1987). A placebo controlled trial of the effect of two pre-operative baths or showers with chlohexidine detergent on post-operative wound infection rates. *J. Hosp. Infect.*, **10**, 165–72.

48. Rotter, M. L., Larsen, S. O., Cooke, E. M., *et al.* (1988). A comparison of the effects of pre-operative whole-body bathing with detergent alone and with detergent containing chlorhexidine gluconate on the frequency of wound infections after clean surgery. *The UWPCHIN J. Hosp. Infect.*, **11**, 310–20.

49. Lilly, H. A., Lombury, E. J. L., and Wilkins, M. D. (1979). Limits to progressive reduction of resident skin bacteria by disinfection. *J. Clin. Path.*, **32**, 382–5.

50. Lidwell, O. M., Lowbury, E. J. L., White, W., Blowers, R., Stanley, S. J., and Lowe, D. (1982). The effect of ultra clean air in operative wounds on deep sepsis in the joint after total hip or knee replacement: a randomised study. *Br. Med. J.*, **285**, 10–14.

51. Meers, P. D. (1983). Ventilation in operating rooms. *Br. Med. J.*, **286**, 244–5.

52. Jackson, D. W., Pollock, A. V., and Tindall, D. S. (1971). The value of a plastic adhesive drape in the prevention of wound infection. *Br. J. Surg.*, **58**, 340–2.

53. Lewis, D., Leaper, D. J., and Speller, D. C. E. (1984). Prevention of bacterial colonisation of wounds at operation: comparison of iodine impregnated (Ioban) drapes with conventional methods. *J. Hosp. Infect.*, **5**, 431–7.

54. Alexander-Williams, J., Oates, G. D., Brown, P. P., *et al.* (1972). Abdominal wound infections and plastic wound guards. *Br. Med. J.*, **59**, 142–6.

55. Bartolo, D. C. C., Andrews, H., Virjee, J., and Leaper, D. J. (1985). A comparative clinical and ultrasonic trial of the new Reliavac drain after cholecystectomy. *J. R. Coll. Surg. Ed.*, **30**, 358–9.

56. Harland, R. N. L. and Irving, M. H. (1988). Surgical drains. *Surgery*, **1**, 1360–2.

57. Jonsson, K., Jensen, J. A., Goodson, W. H., West, J. M., and Hunt, T. K. (1987). Assessment of perfusion in post-operative patients using tissue oxygen measurements. *Br. J. Surg.*, **74**, 263–7.

58. Gote, H., Raahave, D., and Baech, J. (1990). Tissue oximetry as a possible predictor of lethal complications after emergency intestinal surgery. *Surg. Res. Comm.*, **7**, 243–9.

59. Adamson, R. J., Musco, F., and Enquist, I. F. (1966). The chemical dimension of a healing incision. *Surg. Gynecol. Obstet.*, **123**, 515–21.

60. Russell, A. D., Hugo, W. B., and Ayliffe, G. A. H. (1982). *Principles and practice of disinfection, preservation and sterilisation*. Blackwell Scientific Publications, Oxford.

61. Gilmore, O. J. A. (1977). A reappraisal of the use of antiseptics in surgical practice. *Ann. Roy. Coll. Surg. Engl.*, **59**, 93–103.

62. Crosfil, M., Hall, R., and London, D. (1969). The use of chlorhexidine antisepsis in contaminated surgical wounds. *Br. J. Surg.*, **56**, 906–8.

63. Pollock, A. V. and Evans, M. (1975). Povidine iodine for the control of surgical wound infection: a controlled trial against topical cephaloridine. *Br. J. Surg.*, **62**, 292–4.

64. Galland, R. B., Saunders, J. H., Moslen, J. G., and Darrell, J. H. (1977). Prevention of wound infection in abdominal operations by perioperative antibiotics or povidone iodine. *Lancet*, **ii**, 1043–5.

65. Majno, G. (1975). *The healing hand: man and wound in the ancient wound*. Harvard University Press, Cambridge.

66. Forrest, R. D. (1982). Early history of wound treatment. *J. Roy. Soc. Med.*, **75**, 198–205.

67. Forrest, R. D. (1982). Development of wound therapy from the dark ages to the present. *J. Roy. Soc. Med.*, **75**, 268–73.

68. Leaper, D. J. and Simpson, R. A. (1986). The effect of antiseptics and topical antimicrobials on wound healing. *J. Antimicrob. Chemother.*, **17**, 135–7.

69. Brantley, S. K., Starnold, P. A., and Das, S. K. (1990). Antiseptic use in wound management. *Infections in Surgery*, **9**, 33–9.

70. Fleming, A. (1919). The action of chemical and physiological antiseptics in a septic wound. *Br. J. Surg.*, **7**, 99–129.

71. Lorrain-Smith, J., Drennan, A. M., Rettie, T., and Campbell, W. (1915). Antiseptic action of hypochlorous acid and its application to wound treatment. *Br. Med. J.*, **2**, 129–36.

72. Dakin, H. D. (1915). On the use of certain antiseptic substances in the treatment of infected wounds. *Br. Med. J.*, **2**, 318–21.

73. Trueta, J. (1939). Closed treatment of war fractures. *Lancet*, **i**, 1452–5.

74. Morgan, D. A. (1989). Chlorinated solutions: (E) useful or (E) useless. *Pharm. J.*, **239**, 219–20.

75. Cunliffe, W. J. (1990). Eusol – to use or not to use? *Dermatology in Practice*, **8**, 5–7.

76. Moore, D. (1992) Hypochlorites: a review of the evidence. *J. Wound Care*, **1**, 44–53.

77. Leaper, D. J. (1992). Eusol, still awaiting proper clinical trials. *Br. Med. J.*, **304**, 930–1.

78. Brennan, S. S. and Leaper, D. J. (1985). The effect of antiseptics on the healing wound: a study using the rabbit ear chamber. *Br. J. Surg.*, **72**, 780–2.

79. Cotter, J. L., Fader, R. C., and Lilley, C. (1985). Chemical parameters, antimicrobial activities and tissue toxicity of 0.1% sodium hypochlorite solutions. *Antimicrob. Agents Chemother.*, **28**, 118–22.

80. Lineaweaver, W., McMorris, S., Soucy, D., *et al.* (1985). Cellular and bacterial toxicities of topical antimicrobials. *Plast. Reconstr. Surg.*, **75**, 394–6.

81. Lineaweaver, W., Howard, R., Soucy, D., *et al.* (1985). Topical antimicrobial toxicity. *Arch. Surg.*, **120**, 267–70.

82. Deas, J., Billings, P., Brennan, S. S., Silver, I. A., and Leaper, D. J. (1986). The toxicity of commonly used antiseptics on fibroblasts in tissue culture. *Phlebology*, **1**, 205–9.

83. Lucarotti, M. E., Morgan, A. P., and Leaper, D. J. (1990). The effect of antiseptics and the moist environment on ulcer healing. An experimental and biochemical study. *Phlebology*, **5**, 173–9.

84. Gravett, A., Sterner, S., Clinton, J. E., *et al.* (1987). A trial of povidone iodine in the prevention of infection in sutured lacerations. *Ann. Emerg. Med.*, **16**, 167–71.

85. Faddis, D., Damel, D., and Boyer, J. (1977). Tissue toxicity of antiseptic solutions. *J. Trauma.*, **17**, 895–7.

86. Viljanto, J. (1980). Disinfection of surgical wounds without inhibition of normal wound healing. *Arch. Surg.*, **115**, 253–6.

87. Rodeheaver, G. T., Bellamy, W., Kody, M., *et al.* (1982). Bactericidal activity and toxicity of iodine-containing solution in wounds. *Arch. Surg.*, **117**, 181–5.

88. Vanden Broek, P. J., Buys, L. F. M., and Vanfurth, R. (1982). Interaction of povidone-iodine compounds, phagocytic cells, and micro-organisms. *Antimicrob. Agents. Chemother.*, **22**, 593–7.

89. Peterson, A. F., Rosenburg, A., and Alatary, S. D. (1978). Comparative evaluation of surgical scrub preparations. *Surg. Gynecol. Obstet.*, **146**, 63–5.

90. Nystrom, P.-O. (1994). Wound infection and antibiotic prophylaxis: a critical review. In *Proceedings of a round table symposium on surgical infection*, (ed. D. J. Leaper), Vol. 15, pp. 99–119. Surg Res Comm.

91. Taylor, E. W. (1992). General principles of antibiotic prophylaxis. In *Infection in surgical practice*, (ed. E. W. Taylor). Oxford University Press, Oxford.

92. Leaper, D. J. (1994). Prophylactic and therapeutic role of antibiotics in wound care. *Am. J. Surg.*, **167**, 15S–20S.

93. Haley, R. W., Culver, D. H., White, J. W., *et al.* (1985). The efficacy of infection surveillance and control programmes in preventing nosocomial infections in US hospitals. *Am. J. Epidemiol.*, **121**, 182–205.

94. Ramsay, G. (1994). Nosocomial infection, sepsis and organ failure in intensive care. In *Proceedings of a round table symposium on surgical infection*, (ed. D. J. Leaper), Vol. 15, pp. 133–51. Surg Res Comm.

95. Goris, R. J. A., te Boekhorst, T. P. A., Nuytinck, J. K. S., *et al.* (1985). Multiple organ failure: generalised autodestructive inflammation? *Arch. Surg.*, **120**, 1109–15.

96. Marshall, J. and Sweeney, D. (1990). Microbial infection and the septic response in critical surgical illness: sepsis, not infection, determines outcome. *Arch. Surg.*, **125**, 17–23.

97. Elebute, E. A. and Stoner, H. B. (1983). The grading of sepsis. *Br. J. Surg.*, **70**, 29–31.

98. Knaus, W. A., Draper, E. A., Wagner, D. P., and Zimmerman, J. E. (1985). Apache II: a severity of disease classification system. *Crit. Care Med.*, **13**, 818–29.

Further reading: pathogenesis and host response

Mims, C. A. (1982). *The pathogenesis of infectious disease*. Academic Press, London.

Sherris, J. C. and Ray, C. G. (1990). Pathogenesis of bacterial and viral infections. Chapter 10. In *Medical microbiology*, (2nd ed), (ed. J. C. Sherris), pp. 149–69. Elsevier, New York.

Sherris, J. C. and Ryan, K. J. (1990). Skin and wound infections. Chapter 59. In *Medical microbiology*, (2nd ed), (ed. J. C. Sherris), pp. 801–8. Elsevier, New York.

8

Management of traumatic wounds
M. C. R. WHITESIDE and R. J. MOOREHEAD

Introduction

A traumatic wound occurs when the body is subjected to a force which exceeds the strength of the skin or the underlying supporting tissues (1).These wounds range from minor cuts or abrasions to extensive tissue injuries which can be life threatening. It is the extent and character of the force which determines the nature of the injury and in practical terms wounds can be classified as tidy or untidy (2). In general terms a tidy wound may present a clean incision or laceration, is uncontaminated, less than 6h old, and is caused by low-energy trauma. Conversely an untidy wound has an irregular ragged edge, is contaminated, more than 12h old, and is usually caused by high-energy trauma. These include wounds with crushed tissue or burns. The spectrum of untidy wounds that a surgeon may encounter is wide; in this chapter the management of the various wounds that may be seen is considered.

Initial management

Even a major wound is not immediately life threatening unless there is serious haemorrhage leading to exsanguination. More severe wounds must not distract the emergency team from the first priorities in treating a patient which involve the usual ABC measures of resuscitation protocol – ensuring an adequate airway (A) is present, optimizing ventilation (B for breathing), and restoring the circulatory volume (C) as required (3).

After resuscitation a good history is essential in determining how, when, and where the injury occurred. This will give a guide to the degree of force which caused the wound, the possibility and nature of any contamination, and the likelihood of coexisting injury to other regions. Information on the general condition of the patient along with medications should be sought. Careful, thorough examination is required to identify injuries, particularly those in which the acute management will influence the mortality or morbidity. Injuries which appear minor must not be neglected, however, as these can result in long-term disability or disfigurement.

General principles of management

Appraisal of a traumatic wound requires adherence to certain basic precepts if a successful outcome is to be achieved (4).

Blood supply

There must be an adequate blood supply to the injured tissue for the wound to heal (2). In limb injuries the adequacy of the circulation distal to a wound must be assessed. Local contusion, penetrating injuries, fractures, and major joint dislocations may occlude or divide blood vessels. If such an injury is suspected it must be investigated and treated promptly.

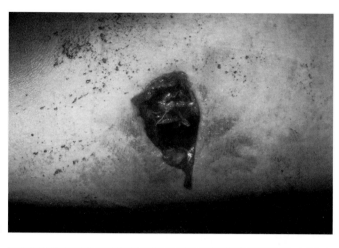

(a)

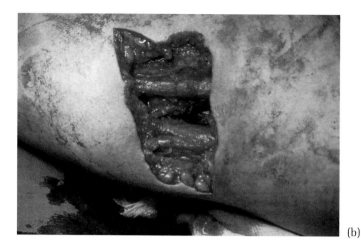

(b)

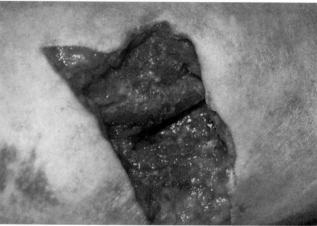

(c)

Fig. 8.1 Thigh wound (a) before and (b) after debridement; (c) clean and granulating. (See plate section.)

Debridement

All necrotic or devitalized tissue must be debrided (5) (Fig. 8.1). This is considered the most important single factor in the management of a contaminated wound (6). This has two benefits: it removes tissue that is heavily contaminated with dirt and bacteria, and protects the patient from invasive organisms. It also removes devitalized tissue, which improves the ability of the wound to resist infection. Host defences against invading bacteria are markedly reduced by foreign bodies present in the wound. It is also important to remove devitalized muscle as absorption of large amounts of myoglobin into the general circulation can lead to renal failure. Identification of all devitalized tissue in a wound can be difficult, particularly muscle. Viability of muscle can be assessed by contractility, bleeding, or colour and consistency (7).

There are several mechanisms by which devitalized soft tissue increases the likelihood of wound infection. The devitalized tissue acts as a culture medium which promotes bacterial growth. The anaerobic environment within the devitalized tissue will decrease leucocyte movement and phagocytosis (8) and also favours the growth of anaerobic organisms.

In certain sites complete excision of relatively small wounds may be possible, converting an untidy wound into a clean tidy wound. However, when the wound contains specialized tissues such as nerves, tendons, or vessels this is not feasible and selective debridement with irrigation should be performed.

Irrigation

Irrigation with saline is fundamental to the removal of contaminants and haematoma which provide an excellent culture medium for the proliferation of bacteria. Factors potentiating infection exist in soil and are characterized by high chemical reactivity (9) and interference with leucocyte function. Irrigation removes these and other contaminants, thereby decreasing the risk of infection. Manual scrubbing of a wound will cause a local increase in tissue oedema and therefore decrease host defences. However, vigorous cleaning with soap and water may be necessary to remove road grease, carbon, and dirt which, if left, can lead to unsightly tattooing.

Exploration

Wounds must be explored to allow adequate debridement and cleaning, and to identify damage to deep structures (10) (Fig. 8.2). This needs to be carried out under adequate anaesthesia, either local or general, depending on the extent of the wound. A bloodless field is usually necessary in treating limb wounds so the use of a tourniquet should be considered. The

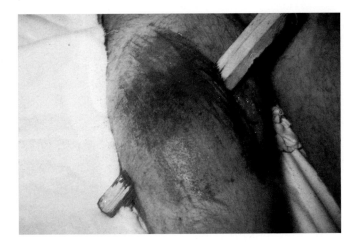

Fig. 8.2 Not all foreign bodies are as obvious as this length of wood embedded in the thigh from a bomb blast. (See plate section.)

importance of exploration has been emphasized in a study of forearm and hand lacerations explored in an Accident and Emergency department (11). Out of 100 lacerations explored, 49 deep injuries were discovered, including 33 tendon lacerations. All the deep injuries had been undetected clinically. Vessel, tendon, and nerve injuries are repaired as appropriate to restore function (12). In relatively tidy wounds, primary repair of tendons and nerves may be possible. In untidy wounds, however, it is advisable simply to identify the proximal and distal ends and mark them with a suture for repair at a later stage. Expert help should be sought at an early stage.

Antibiotics and tetanus

Antibiotic and tetanus prophylaxis are administered as appropriate (13). Prophylactic antibiotics are of value when the wound is heavily contaminated or if host resistance is compromised, for example, in patients with impaired circulation, diabetes, leukaemia, or who are taking immunosuppressive drugs. After major injury, parenteral antibiotic administration is advised as intestinal absorption is impaired. However, antibiotic treatment must not take the place of adequate debridement and cleaning. Tetanus, caused by *Clostridium tetani* (an anaerobic organism), is encouraged by the presence of devitalized tissue. Debridement of all dead tissue is therefore an important prophylactic measure against tetanus. The risk is very low in a clean or adequately debrided wound. The tetanus immunization state of the patient should be ascertained and if necessary a booster dose of toxin administered. Patients with heavily contaminated wounds may require passive immunization with human anti-tetanus globulin injection.

Wound dressings

Aseptic technique during wound examination is essential. If there is a delay in treatment a sterile dressing should be used to protect the wound from further contamination. Dressings should be porous to allow any serum and exudate to escape as they may provide a medium for bacterial growth. Contaminated wounds may be prepared for closure by frequent dressing changes of mesh gauze used in a 'wet to dry' fashion. This rapidly debrides the wound mechanically by removing loose and necrotic debris adhering to the gauze. Alternatively, low adherence absorptive or other debriding agents may be used together with surgical debridement.

Vascular injuries

Shunting a major arterial injury at an early stage can restore circulation and thereby limit further ischaemic injury whilst other injuries are dealt with (14). The duration of limb ischaemia following trauma to a major vessel is one of several factors which influence the incidence of compartment syndrome, ischaemic contracture, muscle necrosis, and amputation. If blood flow to a limb cannot be restored early, then these complications or even fatality may occur. The presence of severe concomitant injuries to veins, bone, or soft tissue will increase this risk. These complications are a consequence of vessel ligation, delayed repair, poor technique, raised compartment pressure, untimely fasciotomy, and infection. In an effort to avoid a long period of ischaemia and to expedite arterial reperfusion, accepted vascular and surgical practices may lapse with counterproductive results.

The effect of major vascular disruption is aggravated by hypovolaemic shock. The impairment of tissue perfusion and the corresponding fall in tissue p_{O_2} increases capillary permeability. This results in an increased exudation of fluid into the interstitial space which increases compartmental pressure and causes venous pressure to rise with further exudation of fluid (15). With a reduction in blood flow into the tissues, the extremity undergoes widespread small vessel thrombosis. Striated muscle will tolerate warm ischaemia for 4–8h, after which myonecrosis sets in (16–18). The limit to which warm ischaemia time is tolerated in an individual case will depend on the presence of collateral circulation and therefore cannot be predicted accurately. Even when circulation is promptly restored, the highly permeable capillary network may raise compartment pressures high enough to occlude large vessels. At this point, fasciotomy may be the only course available to prevent muscle necrosis, ischaemic contracture, or amputation (15).

The salvage rate in injured limbs falls sharply when long bone fractures accompany arterial injuries (19). In the past, in order to minimize ischaemic time, it was usual to repair the artery first (20, 21). However, such a vascular repair is susceptible to damage from long bone manipulation, bone fragments, and traction. In one series, amputation was required in most instances when stabilization of the bone did not precede vascular repair (23). Stabilizing bone first is logical (19, 24–27) as it minimizes further tissue damage by bone fragments and prevents interruption of the vascular repair. This, however, will result in a prolongation of ischaemic time and as a result the surgeon may compromise his fracture fixation. This can be overcome with vascular shunting. The advent of terrorism in

Northern Ireland has led to the acquisition of a large volume of experience in the management of vascular trauma (26–28). A routine policy of shunting arterial and venous injuries has favourably influenced the quality of surgical management, reducing complications and improving limb survival (15, 29–32). The advantage of shunts in the management of severe limb injury is evident (33–34). Their insertion at the outset allows the orthopaedic surgeon to work effectively to ensure accurate stable bone reduction and fixation without the concern over ischaemic time. The vascular repair can then be undertaken. Shunt reperfusion of severe traumatic wounds sharpens the demarcation between viable and devitalized tissue. This facilitates debridement and allows more time for thorough cleaning of a wound. Fasciotomy of the muscle compartments of the lower limb is often required after limb trauma, especially with coexisting vascular injury. Routine shunting of arteries and veins has significantly reduced the need for fasciotomy to be performed (29–31, 35).

Soft tissue infection

Traumatic wounds are particularly prone to the development of invasive bacterial infection due to the presence of devitalized tissue, foreign bodies, and bacteria. Cellulitis is an infection superficial to the investing fascia of the skeletal musculature. In traumatic wounds it is often a rapidly spreading infection caused primarily by haemolytic streptococci. Enzymes produced by the organism give rise to intense pain and a reddened appearance of the wound. Treatment with antibiotics is required (see Chapter 7).

Fasciitis is an infection of the fascial planes. Fascia is poorly suited for defence or localization of infection. It is sparsely vascularized tissue readily invaded by bacteria. When severe wound oedema, pain, and skin necrosis appear within 24–48h after injury, necrotizing fasciitis should be considered. The skin appearance may belie the severity of the infection, which may only be signalled by a sudden fever, hypotension, and confusion. Large amounts of extravascular fluid can be lost and debridement of the area can require extensive excision of tissue.

Myositis represents a bacterial infection that has penetrated and destroyed muscle bundles. The most important post-traumatic form is clostridial in origin and represents the classic gas gangrene most frequently encountered in war wounds. It is rapidly disseminated within muscles and frequently requires both radical debridement and amputation. Clostridial organisms are anaerobic Gram-positive spore-forming rods. When the spores are introduced into the appropriate anaerobic conditions they are activated and develop into toxin-producing bacteria. The requirement of an hypoxic medium implies that an open wound is less likely to allow favourable growth conditions. The recognition of myonecrosis is necessary for effective diagnosis and management of myositis. Such wounds are characterized by oedema and drainage of serous or serosanguinous exudate. Exposure of the muscle bundles in such wounds will disclose intense swelling of the muscle with discolouration of the fibres. This ranges from salmon pink to a gangrenous-like greenish blue colour.

Typically crepitus may be palpable. The affected muscle will not contract on stimulation and may bleed if incised. This bleeding is often persistent. Systemic toxaemia is manifested as tachycardia, fever, disorientation, and mild hypotension. Management requires correction of fluid deficit followed by full exposure of all tissues which may be infected, with debridement as indicated. If the abdominal wall is involved, full thickness excision with replacement by prosthetic mesh may be required. In extreme cases involving limbs, amputation is necessary by the guillotine method with the wound packed open.

Wound stability

Wound stability is essential to allow wound healing, as injured tissue heals most easily when rested and in a moist environment. Naturally, underlying fractures must be immobilized. After surgery on the arm or leg, even in the absence of fractures, the limb should be immobilized and elevated. This allows swelling to subside and provides the optimum conditions for healing.

Fasciotomy

Limb injuries result in swelling in the muscle compartments of the limb which, if severe, can lead to a 'compartment' syndrome. This occurs predominantly in crush or degloving injuries or, in cases with an associated vascular injury, after reperfusion. Untreated, it leads to ischaemia and necrosis within that compartment. Fasciotomy should be considered in any patient with undue pain of an extremity, pain with passive motion, or evidence of tightness in a compartment on examination (35). It should also be performed at an early stage in the management of patients with vascular or crush injuries (36). When necessary, it is performed by incising the skin and deep fascia along the whole length of the affected area, decompressing the underlying tissues (37). Fasciotomy wounds are later closed by direct suture or more often with a split skin graft.

Wound closure

See also Chapters 4 and 9. The decision to close a wound is based on judgement and experience. When in doubt, it is safer to leave a wound open and allow healing by secondary intention or close at a later stage by delayed primary suture. If the traumatic wound is tidy, contamination is minimal, and the time from injury to treatment is low the wound can be cleaned and closed primarily with minimal infection risk. If, however, the wound is untidy then delayed closure is essential to avoid infection. Small, untidy wounds with minimal tissue damage can be converted into tidy wounds by excision of the ragged wound edges and irrigation, allowing primary closure (38). When suturing a wound there should be no tension or dead space. The smallest size suture material practical for a wound should be used. In general, 3/0 monofilament is recommended for lower limbs, trunk, and scalp; 4/0 or 5/0 for hands and upper limbs; and 5/0 or 6/0 for face and neck.

Large wounds or those at high risk of developing sepsis should be debrided, then left open and dressed. Clean granulation tissue develops rapidly in a moist environment free from slough (1). If necessary, further debridement can be performed as doubtful tissue 'declares' itself. The wound can be closed by delayed primary suture (DPS), usually after five days, or, if small, may be left to heal by secondary intention, for example in a low velocity gun shot wound. Larger wounds unsuitable for DPS are covered with a split skin graft when clean. Alternatively, clean wounds can be covered with either a local or distant skin flap, but this does require expert help (8). The simplest cover in an emergency situation is a split skin graft, even if only used as a temporary dressing. It allows time for consultation and investigation in order to plan the definitive repair (1).

Errors in management

Some common errors occur in the management of traumatic wounds (6).

1. Failure to remove foreign material can lead to ugly traumatic tattooing which is very difficult to treat secondarily.

2. Closing a wound under tension can lead to wound breakdown or gross suture marks. Closing a wound in layers can be used to avoid dead space and reduce skin tension.

3. Failure to repair wounds accurately can result in unsightly scars or loss of function. For example, in a lip injury the mucocutaneous junction should be identified carefully and accurately reconstructed to avoid a 'step-like' deformity. Wounds involving eyelids require meticulous repair of the layers of conjunctiva, tarsal plate, muscle, and skin with careful approximation of the free margin to avoid notching.

4. Failure to recognize that a contaminated wound should be left for delayed primary suture will inevitably result in wound infection, breakdown, and prolonged healing time.

Management of different traumatic wounds

See also Chapter 4.

- *Abrasions* – these are areas of partial thickness skin loss which epithelialize spontaneously. Simple dressings only are suitable.

- *Cuts and incisions* – these are usually suitable for primary closure.

- *Stab wounds* – the presence of underlying injury or contamination must be excluded. If tidy they can be sutured primarily, otherwise debridement and delayed primary suture is necessary.

- *Shearing and degloving injuries* – the commonest cause is the entrapment of a limb between the road and a moving

vehicle tyre (4). Avulsion of the skin and subcutaneous tissues by a twisting mechanism ruptures the musculocutaneous and fasciocutaneous perforating vessels and devascularizes the outer tissues. A degloving injury should be suspected if pallor, loss of sensation, friction burn, tyre imprint, or abnormal skin mobility is present. Early recognition and treatment is the key to a satisfactory result. Ischaemic skin should be excised and the defect covered with a split skin graft. Harvesting the split skin graft from the degloved segment of skin is often possible. It has been shown that the immediate use of the degloved skin as a split skin graft gives satisfactory coverage (39). Primary reattachment of the skin by suture or compression is unsuccessful and should be avoided.

Lower limb injuries

Until this century, wounds to the lower limbs with skin loss and damage to underlying tissues, especially bone, frequently resulted in amputation (40). In recent years the treatment of such injuries has changed dramatically and has greatly improved the outcome for patients (41). The use of external fracture stabilization, radical debridement of devitalized soft tissue, 'second look' procedures, and early muscle flap closure has dramatically reduced the incidence of complications such as non-union and infection.

Injuries resulting from very high-energy forces (42) which result in loss of large amounts of soft tissue and bone remain a major problem (43). Success in the management of these wounds is best achieved through an aggressive collaborative effort between orthopaedic and plastic surgeons (44). The amount of energy expended in tissues determines the extent of the injury. In high-energy induced trauma, the real soft tissue injury is usually far more extensive than initially appreciated (41, 45, 46). It is usually impossible to predict the total extent of tissue injury on initial presentation. All devitalized tissue should be debrided before wound coverage is attempted. This includes devitalized soft tissue and bone. Serial debridement is often necessary as the real extent of the injury becomes apparent. Re-exploration of such a wound should take place 48 h after the initial debridement in the operating theatre and it should be repeated every 48–72 h until the wound is obviously viable (45).

Large defects resulting from adequate debridement of high-energy induced wounds require a large block of well vascularized, undamaged tissue to cover a wound and obliterate dead space. Free muscle transfers provide a good supply of undamaged, well vascularized tissue and are therefore reconstructive alternatives (Fig. 8.3). The rich vascularity of muscle flaps makes them effective in controlling subclinical infection (47), and their conformability gives the ability to fill dead space (48). These two factors have been responsible for the success in the management of such wounds. Because of their lack of bulk, cutaneous and fasciocutaneous flaps are not used in wounds with large amounts of dead space to fill. Bone defects should be grafted as soon as possible after the soft tissue wound is closed and stable.

Fortunately, flap cover of lower limb skin defects is only

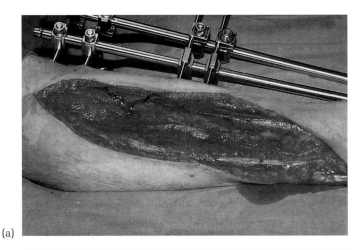

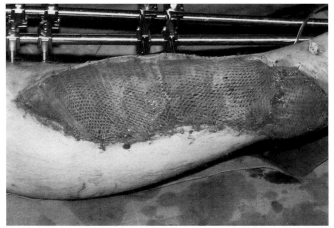

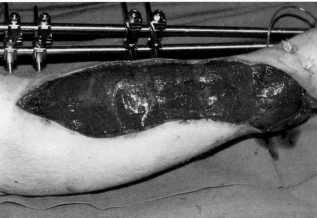

Fig. 8.3 (a) Large soft tissue defect over a fractured tibia and fibula; (b) the soft tissue defect covered with a free rectus muscle flap; and (c) the muscle flap covered with a meshed split skin graft. (See plate section.)

seldom needed. Split skin grafts are sufficient if there is a vascular recipient bed with no vital, exposed structures. The commonest cause of skin loss is the distally based pretibial traumatic skin flap, particularly if it has been sutured back into place (40). This wound commonly occurs in elderly women and is notoriously difficult to treat as there is little subcutaneous tissue with a poor blood supply (Fig. 8.4). Excision of non-viable tissue and split skin grafting is usually required. A common error is to attempt primary closure, which results in wound infection, thereby increasing the area eventually needing debridement.

Although skin grafting of lower limb defects is technically simpler than the use of flaps, expert care and attention to the wound is still required in the first few postoperative weeks. Reconstruction of lost skin will depend on the area of loss and its position. Flap cover is rarely required for skin loss of the groin or thigh due to the muscle covering the femur and the neurovascular bundle (40).

A frequent difficulty in the healed lower limb wound is the persistence of an atrophic, tight, adherent scar tethered to bone and often surrounded by discoloured, poor quality skin. The scar is vulnerable, often breaks down repeatedly, may lead to an osteomyelitis and, if left for years, may undergo malignant change (40). Treatment entails excising the scar and surrounding abnormal skin and covering the defect with a

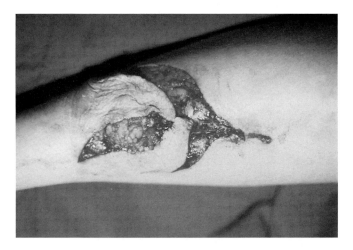

Fig. 8.4 A pretibial laceration. (See plate section.)

suitable flap. Chronic post-traumatic osteomyelitis of the tibia is a difficult condition to treat successfully and excision of infected bone and soft tissue is required with replacement with a bone graft (49) and a muscle flap which can provide a base for split skin grafting to provide skin cover. Such a muscle flap can allow healing of a difficult wound and is an ideal conduit for the delivery of antibiotics.

Missile injuries

Missile wounds represent a significant challenge for a surgeon who has to manage the great variety of injuries that can be inflicted. These injuries can cause widespread destruction to a variety of structures and organs, so a knowledge of anatomy is essential to anticipate injuries to soft tissue, bone, nerves, tendons, and vessels.

The wounding power of projectiles is an important subject which receives too little interest considering the frequency of missile injuries. An understanding of the ballistics of the various missiles encountered is also useful in predicting the amount of damage they may have caused (Fig. 8.5).

The nature of a bullet wound depends largely on the velocity of that missile. The wounding power is directly proportional to the bullet's kinetic energy (KE) at the time it strikes tissue (50). This is determined by the formula KE = $\frac{1}{2}mv^2$ where m is the missile mass and v its velocity. During the American civil war last century, large heavy missiles travelling at relatively slow speed caused massive tissue destruction. However, the velocity of the missile is more important in determining the impact energy, which is proportional to the square of the velocity. In the 20th century there has been a trend towards smaller, lighter missiles travelling at a higher velocity. This has therefore resulted in the development of higher energy missiles, as doubling the velocity will quadruple the energy imparted by the missile.

There is no sharp cut-off point between high and low velocity bullets (50). A low velocity bullet travels at around 200 m/s whereas a high velocity bullet from a rifle travels at over 650 m/s. Therefore a high velocity bullet has ten times the energy of one of equal weight at low velocity. Any factor that will retard the bullet's forward and rotary speed will cause a more rapid release of energy. Such factors are tissue

density, the bluntness of the point of the bullet, its yaw, and the degree of tumbling as it travels through tissue (51).

In low velocity bullet wounds, such as those caused by most handguns, the main injury is caused by the transit of the bullet through the tissues and damage is slight unless important structures are traversed (Figs 8.6, 8.7). Penetrating bullets crush and lacerate the tissues in their immediate path but at low velocity, bullets do not cause damage beyond the tract. The entrance wound of the low velocity bullet is usually circu-

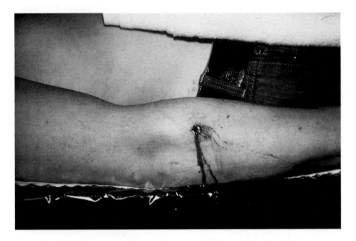

Fig. 8.6 A low velocity bullet wound to the arm. (See plate section.)

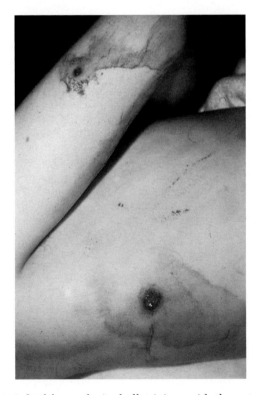

Fig. 8.7 A fatal low velocity bullet injury with the entrance in the arm and exit wound in the anterior chest wall. (See plate section.)

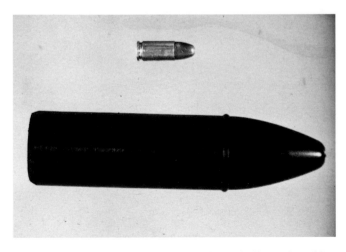

Fig. 8.5 Comparison in size of a low velocity bullet and a rubber bullet. (See plate section.)

lar and smaller than the bullet's diameter owing to tissue resilience at the point of entrance. The exit wound is usually a ragged slit, or star shaped, owing to the tumbling of the bullet as it passes through the soft tissues. If the gun was fired from close range there will be characteristic powder burns around the entrance wound.

Treatment of low velocity gunshot wounds will depend on the damage caused. If it is limited to soft tissue damage, minimal debridement may be all that is required. In a study from Belfast (52) it has been shown that simple low velocity wounds can be managed by local debridement of the entrance and exit wounds performed under local anaesthesia. The wounds are then closed in 4–5 days or allowed to heal by secondary intention.

High velocity bullet wounds present a considerably greater challenge to the surgeon than low velocity injuries (Figs 8.8, 8.9). They cause a temporary cavitation effect (53) which can be 30 times the size of the residual tract of the bullet. This is due to the retardation effect of tissues, causing a sudden release of an enormous amount of energy. The higher the velocity, the greater the cavity produced. The cavity is caused by movement being imparted to the tissue particles in front and around the nose of the bullet. The cavitation effect causes widespread tissue damage and in muscle results in an area of bloody, pulpy, or dead tissue due to rupture of capillaries between the muscle fibres. There will also be damage to adjacent structures which may not be immediately apparent at the time of initial debridement. Thrombosis to blood vessels and injury to stretched nerves occurs. Long bones can be fractured even though not struck directly. Various tissues react in different ways to missiles of the same size travelling at the same velocity. A missile has more wounding power and destroys more tissue against a solid organ such as liver than against an air filled structure such as the lungs.

If a high velocity bullet travels through soft tissue only, the perforating exit wound may be quite small and neither entrance nor exit wound gives an indication as to the enormous tissue damage that will have occurred internally. However, when there is a large amount of energy released, the tissues are unable to contain the force of the temporary cavitation and an explosive exit wound is produced, perhaps with tissue loss (Fig. 8.9).

High velocity wounds present a much more difficult management problem. The extent of tissue damage is usually considerable and injury to structures away from the track of the bullet must be considered. The same general principles of wound management apply, however (10). All high velocity injuries must be thoroughly explored and one should err on the side of a more radical excision (10, 54, 55). Two main factors determine the outcome of these wounds: the extent of tissue destruction and the amount of contamination. Following cavitation, a vacuum effect can suck in foreign material, including dirt, soil, and clothing, which greatly adds to contamination.

Following resuscitation, the skin over a large surrounding area is cleansed and shaved. Skin is remarkably viable and very resistant to damage by cavitation, and it should be treated as conservatively as possible. Rarely more than about 1 mm of the edge needs to be removed except when the skin is grossly damaged. The skin and subcutaneous tissues should be incised generously to get to the depths of the wound. Deep fascia must be incised along the length of the incision as this allows good exposure to the depths of the wound. Dead muscle, fat, and fascia are excised along with dirt, debris, missiles, and blood clot. Small metal fragments can be difficult to find

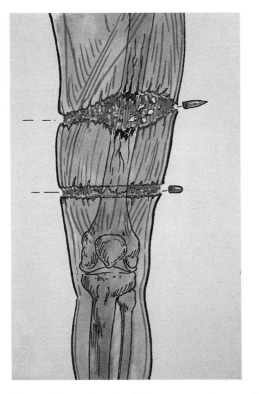

Fig. 8.8 Diagram illustrating the different wounding capabilities of a low and high velocity bullet in the lower limb. (See plate section.)

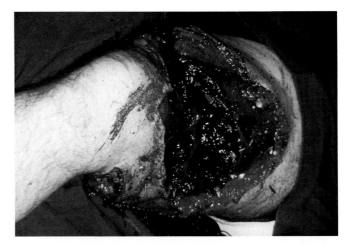

Fig. 8.9 Massive exit wound that can be created by a high velocity bullet. (See plate section.)

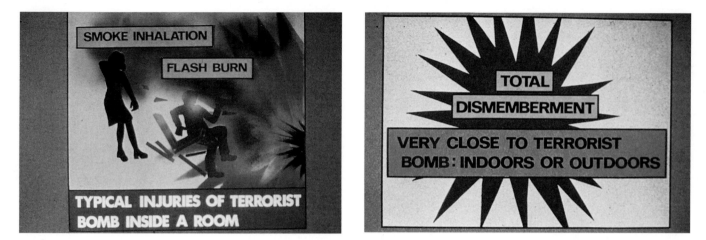

Fig. 8.10 The effect of a close proximity explosion.

and prolonged surgery looking for them is unnecessary. The foreign materials that must be removed because of a tendency to cause severe wound infection are mud, cloth, and extrinsic bone fragments (56). The last can be blown in from another person or another part of the patient and can be mistaken for a fracture on radiograph (57). The widely opened deep fascia which has been freely incised should be left open to avoid a compartment syndrome. All wounds are also left open without suture of skin or deep structures except with the following exceptions:

(1) facial wounds can be closed primarily after primary wound excision due to the excellent blood supply of this region;

(2) in chest wall wounds healthy muscle should be used to close sucking wounds, but the skin should be left open;

(3) blood vessels that have been repaired should be covered with viable muscle.

If a high velocity bullet wound has been thoroughly excised, it can be closed in 4–5 days by delayed primary suture. If there is excessive pain, oedema, or signs of infection, further examination of the wound under general anaesthetic is required. It usually means wound excision was incomplete and further debridement is necessary.

Bomb blast injuries (58, 59)

Exposure to explosive blast results in a well documented pattern of injury (60, 61). The components of the blast that cause injury are initially the shockwave, with its sharp leading edge of almost instantaneous pressure rise from ambient air pressure to the over-pressure created by the explosion, known as the shock front. This lasts a few milliseconds and is followed by a negative phase of low pressure of longer duration. Subsequently, the dynamic over-pressure or blast wind is the mass movement of the gaseous products of detonation away from the point of the explosion (Fig. 8.10).

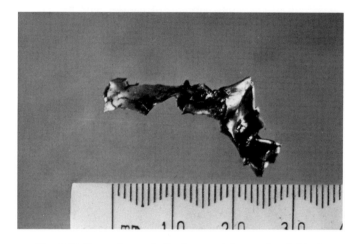

Fig. 8.11 Secondary missile fragment from a bomb blast.

The shock wave is responsible for the primary blast injury, blast lung, and tympanic membrane rupture. The dynamic over-pressure causes secondary injury from objects caught in the blast wave such as grit, stones, metal, masonry, and glass (Fig. 8.11). Nuts, nails, and bolts are often incorporated into antipersonnel mines. All these fragments can travel at over 2000 m/s and act as high velocity missiles producing severe tissue injury (Fig. 8.12). If these fragments strike bone, a shower of bone fragments causes further damage. The most frequent cause of injury in bomb blasts is due to these secondary missiles (60). Victims may also be injured by indirect violence as they are flung against surrounding objects. Traumatic amputation of limbs is rarely seen in survivors: reviews of bomb blast victims indicate that traumatic amputation is seen in only 1–2 per cent of those who survive to reach medical care (61, 62). Those who sustain such injury are likely to have other fatal injuries. A review of 1532 consecutive bomb victims (61) seen at the Accident and Emergency department of the Royal Victoria Hospital in Belfast at the height of the Troubles showed the majority (84 per cent) sustained only

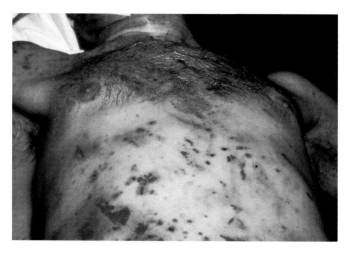

Fig. 8.12 Peppering due to secondary missiles from a bomb blast. (See plate section.)

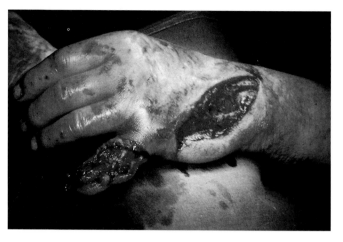

Fig. 8.13 Blast injury to the hand. (See plate section.)

minor injuries not requiring admission. In a review of fatalities in Northern Ireland between 1969 and 1977 it was shown that of 495 people killed, 50 per cent of the injuries were sustained in a building and 25 per cent of the subjects were in a vehicle (63). The vulnerability of the head and neck is emphasized by the fact that brain damage (66 per cent) and skull fracture (51 per cent) were the two single most commonly observed factors in the fatally wounded. Diffuse lung contusions (47 per cent), eardrum rupture (45 per cent), and liver lacerations (34 per cent) completed the five most commonly observed factors excluding serious soft tissue damage. Liver and other intra-abdominal organ laceration can best be explained through inertial considerations, whereby two organs of different mass and density are accelerated at different rates. Abdominal organ damage can also be caused by penetration fragments. Intestinal lacerations were usually multiple and commonly associated with fragment penetration but the liver and spleen were the two abdominal organs most frequently damaged.

Wounds caused by bomb blasts are often fatal or cause extensive damage (Fig. 8.13). In the initial management of bomb blast victims the usual resuscitation protocol is followed and life-threatening injuries are dealt with first. As the head and neck is subject to a disproportionate number of injuries in the form of fractures, lacerations, and burns, specific attention to the airway is vital. All wounds must be explored, no matter how trivial they seem on initial inspection. Primary amputation of injured limbs is often required. Penetrating wounds of the trunk carry a poor prognosis and must also be explored. Thorough debridement is necessary as there will be gross tissue damage and contamination. Following removal of all dead tissue and contaminants the wound is packed and closed by delayed primary suture.

High velocity fragments and falling debris pose the major hazard in bomb blasts and a predominance of head and neck injuries will be seen. Primary blast lung is rare except in the fatally wounded and orthopaedic and neurosurgical injuries will predominate in those requiring hospital admission.

Conclusion

The variety of traumatic wounds encountered is enormous. They vary from small clean incisions which can be closed primarily to grossly contaminated multiple tissue injuries which can be life threatening. The basic principles of wound management apply in every case. The importance of adequate wound debridement and exploration to exclude underlying injury must not be overlooked. If necessary, more experienced help should be sought at an early stage.

References

1. Whiteside, M. C. R. and Moorehead, R. J. (1992). *Traumatic wounds. Proceedings of the Second European Conference on Advances in Wound Management*, pp. 93–4. Harrogate, UK.
2. Batchelor, A. G. (1988). Wound management. *Surgery*, **54**, 1281–5.
3. Willett, K. M., Dorrell, H., and Kelly, P. (1990). ABC of major trauma, management of limb injuries. *Br. Med. J.*, **301**, 229–33.
4. Rosen, J. S. and Cleary, J. E. (1991). Surgical management of wound. *Clin. Podiatr. Med. Surg.*, **8**, 891–904.
5. Haury, B., Rodeheaver, G., Vensko, J., *et al.* (1978). Debridement: an essential component of traumatic wound care. *Am. J. Surg.*, **135**, 238–42.
6. Jones, R. C. and Shires, G. T. (1983). Principles in the management of wounds. In *Principles of surgery*, (4th edn), (ed. S. l. Schwartz), McGraw-Hill, New York, pp. 208–11.
7. Haury, B., Rodeheaver, G., Vensko, J., *et al.* (1980). Debridement: an essential component of wound care. In *Wound healing and wound infection, theory and surgical practice*, (ed. T. K. Hunt), pp. 229–41. Appleton-Century-Crofts, New York.
8. Mandel, G. L. (1974). Bactericidal activity of aerobic and anaerobic polymorphonuclear neutrophils. *Infect. Immun.*, **9**, 337–41.
9. Roberts, A. H., Rye, D. G., Edgerton, M. T., *et al.* (1979). Activity of antibiotics in contaminated wounds containing clay soil. *Am. J. Surg.*, **137**, 381–3.

10. Rautio, J. and Paavolainen, P. (1988). Afgan war wounded: experience with 200 cases. *J. Trauma*, **28**, 523–5.

11. McNicholl, B. P., Martin, J., and McAleese, P. (1992). Subclinical injuries in lacerations to the forearm and hand. *Br. J. Surg.*, **79**, 765–7.

12. Livingstone, R. H. and Wilson, R. I. (1975). Surgery of violence VI. Gunshot wounds of the limbs. *Br. Med. J.*, **1**, 667–9.

13. Ward, C. M. (1986). Soft tissue injuries. *Surgery*, **29**, 676–81.

14. Barros, D'Sa, A. A. B. and Moorehead, R. J. (1989). Combined arterial and venous intraluminal shunting in major trauma of the lower limb. *Eur. J. Vasc. Surg.*, **3**, 577–81.

15. Barros, D'Sa, A. A. B. (1988). How do we manage acute limb ischaemia due to trauma? In *Limb salvage and amputation for vascular disease*, (ed. R. N. Greenhalgh, C. W. Jamieson, and A. N. Nicolaides), Ch. 13, p. 135. W. B. Saunders, London.

16. Scully, R. W. and Hughes, C. W. (1956). Pathology of ischaemia of skeletal muscle in man. *Am. J. Pathol.*, **32**, 805–29.

17. Sanderson, R. A., Foley, R. K., McIvor, G. W. D., *et al.* (1975). Histological response of skeletal muscle to ischaemia. *Clin. Orthop.*, **113**, 27–35.

18. Miller, H. H. and Welch, C. S. (1947). Quantitative studies on the time factor in arterial injuries. *Ann. Surg.*, **130**, 428–38.

19. Smith, R. F., Szilagi, D. E., and Elliot, J. P. (1969). Fracture of the long bones with arterial injury due to blunt trauma. *Arch. Surg.*, **99**, 315–24.

20. Connolly, J. (1970). Management of fractures associated with arterial injuries. *Am. J. Surg.*, **120**, 331–4.

21. Hardy, J. D., Raju, S., Neely, W. A., *et al.* (1975). Aortic and other injuries. *Ann. Surg.*, **181**, 640–53.

22. O'Donnell, T. F., Brewster, D. C., Darling, R. C., *et al.* (1977). Arterial injuries associated with fractures and/or dislocation of the knee. *J. Trauma*, **17**, 341–4.

23. Doty, D. B., Treiman, R. L., Rothschild, P. D., and Caspae, M. R. (1967). Prevention of gangrene due to fractures. *Surg. Gynecol. Obstet.*, **125**, 284–5.

24. Sher, M. H. (1975). Principles on the management of arterial injuries associated with fractures/dislocations. *Ann. Surg.*, **182**, 630–4.

25. Koostra, G., Schippler, J. J., Boontje, A. H., *et al.* (1987). Femoral shaft fracture with injury of the superficial femoral artery in civilian accidents. *Surg. Gynecol. Obstet.*, **142**, 399–403.

26. Barros, D'Sa, A. A. B., Hassard, T. H., Livingston, R. H., *et al.* (1980). Missile-induced vascular trauma. *Injury*, 13–30.

27. Johnston, G. W. and Barros, D'Sa, A. A. B. (1981). Injuries of civil hostilities. In *Trauma*, (ed. D. C. Carter and H. C. Polk), p. 284. Butterworth, London.

29. Barros, D'Sa, A. A. B. Missile injuries of popliteal vessels. *Proceedings of the XVth Congress of the Latin-American Chapter of the International Cardiovascular Society, Acapulco, 1980.*

30. Barros, D'Sa, A. A. B. (1981). A decade of missile induced vascular trauma. *Ann. R. Coll. Surg. Engl.*, **64**, 37–44.

31 Barros, D'Sa, A. A. B. (1983). Vascular injuries. In *Lecture notes on trauma*, (ed. J. Templeton and R. I. Wilson), p. 107. Blackwell Scientific Publications, Oxford.

32. Elliot, J., Templeton, J., and Barros, D'Sa, A. A. B. (1984). Combined bony and vascular limb trauma: a new approach to treatment. *J. Bone Joint Surg.*, **66**B, 281.

33. Tachakra, S. G. and Smith, J. E. M. (1981). Severed limbs: the reattachment of major segments. *J. R. Coll. Surg. Edinb.*, **265**, 157–69.

34. Nunley, J. L., Koman, L. A., and Urganiak, J. R. (1981). Arterial shunting as an adjunct to major limb revascularisation. *Ann. Surg.*, **193**, 271–2.

35. Malsen, F. a III, Winquist, R. A., and Krugmire, R. B. Jr. (1980).

36. Diagnosis and management of compartmental syndromes. *J. Bone Joint Surg. Am.*, **62**, 286–91.

36. Du, Plessis, H. J., Marais, T. J., van Wyk, F. A., *et al.* (1983). Compartment syndrome and fasciotomy. *S. Afr. J. Surg.*, **21**, 193–206.

37. Mayer, J. R., Lim, L. T., Schuler, J. J., *et al.* (1985). Peripheral vascular trauma from close range shotgun injuries. *Arch. Surg.*, **120**, 1126.

38. Walker, C. C. (1984). *Surgical Handicraft Surgery*, **8**, 182–6.

39. Kudsk, K. A., Sheldon, G. F., and Walton, R. L. (1981). Degloving injuries of the extremities and torso. *J. Trauma*, **21**, 835–9.

40. Murry, D. S. (1990). Skin loss of the lower limb. *Injury*, **21**, 309–10.

41. Byrd, H. S., Cierny, G., and Tebbetts, J. B. (1981). The management of open tibial fractures with associated soft tissue loss; external pin fixation with early flap coverage. *Plast. Reconstr. Surg.*, **68**, 73–82.

42. Gustilo, R. B., Mendoza, R. M., and Williams, D. N. (1984). Problems in the management of type III (severe) open fractures: a new classification of type III open fractures. *J. Trauma*, **24**, 742–6.

43. Swartz, W. M. and Mears, D. C. (1985). The role of free tissue transfer in lower-extremity reconstruction. *Plast. Reconstr. Surg.*, **76**, 364–73.

44. Bosse, M. J., Burgess, a R., and Brumback, R. J. (1984). Evaluation and treatment of the high energy open tibia fracture. *Adv. Orthop. Surg.*, **8**, 3.

45. Yaremchuk, M. J., Brumback, R. J., Manson, P. N., *et al.* (1987). Acute and definitive management of traumatic osteocutaneous defects of the lower extremity. *Plast. Reconstr. Surg.*, **80**, 1–12.

46. Cierny, G., Byrd, H. S., and Jones, R. E. (1983). Primary versus delayed soft tissue coverage for severe open tibial fractures. A comparison of results. *Clin. Orthop.*, **178**, 54–63.

47. Chang, N. and Mathes, S. J. (1982). Comparison of the effect of bacterial inoculation in musculocutaneous and random pattern flaps. *Plast. Reconstr. Surg.*, **70**, 1–10.

48. May, J. W., Jr, Gallico, G. G., Jupiter, J., *et al.* (1984). Free latissimus dorsi muscle flap with skin graft for treatment of traumatic chronic bony wounds. *Plast. Reconstr. Surg.*, **73**, 641–51.

49. Papineau, L. J., Alfageme, A., Delcourt, *et al.* (1979) Chronic osteomyelitis: open excision and grafting after saucerization. *Int. Orthop.*, **3**, 165–76.

50. Rich, N. M. (1980). Missile injuries. *Am. J. Surg.*, **139**, 414–20.

51. Whitlock, I. H. (1981). Experience gained from treating facial injuries due to civil unrest. *Ann. R. Coll. Surg. Engl.*, **63**, 31–44.

52. Ritchie, A. J. and Harvey, C. F. (1990). Experience in low velocity gunshot injuries: a more conservative approach in selected cases. *J. R. Coll. Surg. Edinb.*, **35**, 302–4.

53. Cooper, G. J. and Ryan, J. M. (1990). Interaction of penetrating missiles with tissues: some common misapprehensions and implications for wound management. *Br. J. Surg.*, **77**, 606–10.

54. Marcus, N. A., Blair, W. F., Shuk, J. M., *et al.* (1961). Low velocity gunshot wounds to the extremities. *J. Trauma*, **1**, 354–60.

55. Coull, J. T. (1990). Military surgery. *Injury*, **21**, 270–2.

56. Coupland, R. M. and Howell, P. R. (1988). An experience of war surgery and wounds presenting after 3 days on the border of Afganistan. *Injury*, **19**, 259–62.

57. Coupland, R. M. (1989). Technical aspects of war wound excision. *Br. J. Surg.*, **76**, 663–7.

58. Maynad, R. L., Cooper, G. J., and Scott, R. (1988). Mechanism of injury in bomb blasts and explostions. In *Trauma-pathogenisis and treatment*, (ed. S. Westaby), pp. 30–41. Heinemann, London.

59. Mellor, S. G. (1991). Blast injury. In *Recent advances in surgery 14*, (ed. I. Taylor and C. D. Johnson), pp. 53–8. Churchill Livingstone, Edinburgh.

60. Hull, J. B. (1992). Traumatic amputation by explosive blast: pattern of injury in survivors. *Br. J. Surg.*, **79**, 1303–6.

61. Hadden, W. A., Rutherford, W. H., and Merrett, J. D. (1978). The injuries of terrorist bombing: a study of 1532 consecutive patients. *Br. J. Surg.*, **65**, 525–31.

62. Fryberg, E. R. and Tepas, J. J. (1988). Terrorist bombings: lessons learned from Belfast to Beirut. *Ann. Surg.*, **208**, 569–76.

63. Hill, J. F. (1979). Blast injury with particular reference to recent terrorist bombing incidents. *Ann. R. Coll. Surg. Engl.*, **61**, 4–11.

9

Clinical aspects of healing in specialized tissue

M. C. ROBSON, J. A. G. SAMPSON, C. J. VICKERY, D. J. LEAPER,
T. T. IRVIN, A. M. WAINWRIGHT, E. J. SMITH, R. J. WHISTON,
I. F. LANE, and R. C. L. FENELEY

Skin and burns

Anatomy, biochemistry, and physiology of skin

The skin of man is a large organ comprising a sheet-like investment of the whole body which adapts admirably to its contours and neatly conforms to its movements (1). However, it is more than just the physical exterior of the body being an interface with the environment. It serves as an organ of protection, controls the invasion of microorganisms, rations fluid gain or loss, regulates temperature, protects against injury from radiation and electricity, as well as providing immunologic surveillance (2). At the same time, the skin contains a vasculature and sweating system uniquely adapted to the thermoregulatory demands of the organism, and an extensive neuroreceptor network, which serves as a finely tuned array of complex transducers of environmental information. Each of these functions is specifically related to a cell or areas within the skin.

The skin is a highly specialized bilaminate structure resting on a layer of padding, the subcutaneous tissue. Its two layers, the outer epidermis and the inner dermis, are of varying thickness in different areas of the body, varying from 0.5 mm to 6 mm, but generally 1–2 mm thick. The outer, highly cellular epidermal layer measures 0.06–0.8 mm in thickness and is in close contact with the dermis through multiple irregular interpapillary ridges and grooves (2).

The outermost layer of the epidermis is the stratum corneum, composed of dry anucleate cornified cells (1). Its function is protective. The innermost or basal layer, the stratum germinativum, contains melanocytes as well as cells destined for keratin production, the keratinocytes. Between these two layers are keratinocytes in various stages of differentiation. The stratum spinosum, or spinous layer, constitutes the bulk of viable cells which are synthesizing keratin and precursor proteins for the granular layer cells. The stratum granulosum mainly synthesizes proteins (keratohyalin) related to the fully keratinized cell.

Cells derived from the neural crest (melanocytes) and mesenchyme (Langerhans cells), as well as cells of unknown origin (Merkel cells), migrate into the epidermis and become organized in specific association with specific keratinocytes (3). In addition, clusters of basal cells in the epidermis give rise to skin appendages (nails, the pilosebaceous apparatus, eccrine and apocrine sweat glands) during embryogenesis. The dermal–epidermal junctions undulate in most areas of the body, increasing surface contact between the two layers to provide the resistance of normal skin to shearing (4).

The dermis or inner, deeper layer of skin is 20–30 times thicker than the epidermis (3). It contains the nervous, vascular, lymphatic, and supporting structures for the epidermis as well as harbouring the epidermal appendages. The regions of the dermis, the papillary and reticular dermis, respond differently due to unique structural organization and biochemistry.

The dermis consists of fibrous molecules and a non-fibrous matrix. The fibrous proteins impart bulk, density, and tensile properties to skin, simultaneously allowing compliance and elasticity. Fibrous elements of the dermis consist mainly of collagen fibrils and elastic fibres which are synthesized and monitored by the dermal fibroblast. The collagen in the skin is primarily type I and III in a ratio of about 85 per cent to 15 per cent (1). The elastic fibres contain two components–aligned bundles of microfibrils which are believed to serve as a template, and a dense elastin matrix.

The non-fibrous portion of the dermis consists of glycosaminoglycans and glycoproteins of the amorphous ground substance. Glycosaminoglycans (GAGs) in the skin are polysaccharide chains. The most common are hyaluronic acid, dermatan sulphate and chondroitin 4- and 6-sulphate, and heparin. GAGs play a role in cutaneous permeability, allow cellular migration, and influence the polymerization of such fibrous matrix proteins as collagen (5).

The papillary dermis is only slightly thicker than the overlying epidermis. It is generally separated from the underlying reticular dermis by a horizontal plexus of vessels. This plexus provides the overlying papillary dermis with a rich blood supply. The majority of dermis is reticular dermis. It is distinguished by a relatively acellular, avascular dense collagenous and elastic connective tissue (1). Epidermal appendages either terminate in the lower levels of the reticular dermis or penetrate even deeper into the subcutaneous tissue. Vessels pierce the dermis, giving off supplying vessels to the hair follicles and sweat glands.

The blood supply to the skin is quite complex. There are two main anatomical patterns of blood supply. The first of these depends upon vessels from the aorta or its major branches which lie deep to the muscles. Perforating branches through the muscles or along fascial planes become the musculocutaneous and fasciocutaneous arteries. This vascular pattern forms the predominant blood supply to the skin of humans. In the other anatomical pattern, vessels from the aorta or its major branches form direct cutaneous arteries which lie superficial to the muscles and parallel to the skin for long distances, terminating in a distinctive small vessel plexus deep in the dermis at the interface with subcutaneous tissue.

The perforating arteries from the muscles ascend toward the papillary dermis. They send branches to other perforating arterioles in the mid-dermis to form a significant plexus before reaching the papillary dermis. When the ascending branches get to the papillary dermis, they branch into progressively smaller arterioles which develop a horizontal (papillary) plexus of interconnecting and looping microcirculatory elements in planes predominantly parallel to the skin surface (1). From these arterioles, simple or compound capillary loops are directed toward the epidermis.

The lymphatic system serves for transport of particulate and liquid matter from the extravascular compartment of the dermis (6). It arises as terminal bulbs in the papillary layer. The most superficial vessels are of a single cell thickness and often discontinuous. The larger collecting and transport channels have progressively thicker walls with no gaps in the endothelial lining. They descend to the hypodermis in pathways independent from those taken by the arterial and accompanying venous blood vessel components (1).

There are three nerve plexuses supplying sensibility to the skin. They are the subpapillary, intradermal, and subcutaneous plexuses, which roughly correspond to the vascular plexuses. Branches of filaments of these plexuses go to the dermal papillae of the papillary dermis, where the greatest concentration of receptors are located. The receptors are of three types: mechanoreceptors, thermoreceptors, and nociceptors; each of which is differently sensitive to certain types of stimuli (2).

Although all levels of the skin contribute to the various functions of the skin, the stratum corneum is most important (3). The stratum corneum prevents the loss of water, electrolytes, and plasma proteins. It also provides a good structural barrier against bacterial invasion and serves to maintain a normal balance of bacteria in the skin. There are normally two types of bacteria in the skin–the resident and the transient flora which are harboured in the hair follicles, particularly near the orifices of the sebaceous glands (2). These bacteria normally exist at levels of approximately 10^3 organisms per gram of tissue. Although resident organisms exist in a balanced state within the skin, the skin protects against invasion by the transient species by the dryness of the keratin layer and the antibacterial properties of the fatty acids in the sebum. Any break in the skin or any inflammation results in serum accumulation which inactivates sebum. In this situation, streptococci may rapidly colonize the skin (2). The stratum corneum thus serves as the rate-limiting barrier for most substances.

Although most melanin is in the basal layer of the epidermis, the stratum corneum does contain some melanin. Because melanin is the best absorber of ultraviolet light, skin devoid of stratum corneum can be injured by ultraviolet light at levels of one third to one fifth of that needed to injure normal skin (3).

Another important function of the skin is to provide a vehicle for temperature regulation. To maintain thermal equilibrium, body heat is dissipated by evaporation, conduction, radiation, convection, and via excreta (2). The rich dermal vascular network delivers blood to the body surface for heat dissipation. Normally, humans lose 70 per cent of the body heat load via conduction, 25 per cent by evaporation, and the remaining 5 per cent by convection or radiation (2).

Plastic surgery

This branch of medicine, which deals with reconstructive and plastic surgery, is broad and difficult to define. 'Plastic' means formative or capable of moulding (7). Surgeons working in reconstructive and plastic surgery mould the integument and musculoskeletal framework to correct deformity. Deformity can be real or imagined and may result from congenital, acquired, or psychological sources. Often, deformities include defects which must be covered or filled. Procedures in this field of surgery are often divided between reconstructive and aesthetic. In Sir Harold Gillies' definition: 'reconstructive surgery attempts to restore the individual to the normal, while aesthetic surgery attempts to surpass the normal' (8).

Although the origins of plastic surgery are difficult to trace in a direct line, it is customary to note that Susruta described operations for reconstruction of the amputated nose in the 6th and 7th centuries BC, that the Ebers Papyrus contained records of the reconstructive procedures in ancient Egypt, and that Celsus used advancement flaps at the beginning of the Christian era (7). In the 16th century, Gaspare Tagliacozzi wrote a milestone treatise on reconstruction of the nose using an arm flap. Modern plastic surgery as a coherent discipline can trace its roots directly to the 19th century work of Carpue, von Graefe, and Dieffenbach (7). Skin grafting was developed by Reverdin in France and by Lawson and Pollock in England.

War has always been a major stimulus to reconstructive surgery and many of these earlier developments were in response to war injuries. The modern specialty involving reconstructive and plastic surgical procedures really began in the wake of the First World War as a result of the leadership of Sir Harold Gillies in the United Kingdom, along with Kazanjian, Blair, and Ivy in the United States (7). The Second World War saw the emergence of numerous surgeons who devoted themselves entirely to the practice of reconstructive and plastic surgery and firmly established its place in modern medicine.

Whether a wound occurs as a result of surgical intervention or traumatic event, adherence to basic tenets of wound care will maximize the long-term results. Failure to adhere to these tenets will result in prolonged inflammation and healing time and a worse long-term result.

Cosmetic surgical techniques

In order to achieve an acceptable, aesthetically pleasing result following wound closure, steps must be taken to evaluate the wound adequately and prepare it for closure. For the intentional wound, made with a scalpel under aseptic conditions, these steps will be less involved than for a traumatic wound.

There is no substitute for a good history. A history can elicit the mechanism of injury and indicate the possible level of contamination of the wound. It can also raise the question of possible deeper injury and direct the course of the physical examination (9). Whether the patient is able to give an adequate history or not, a thorough physical examination is a necessity. Involvement of deeper structures must be investigated and the wound evaluated for possible foreign or necrotic debris. Facial lacerations should include the evaluation of the underlying sensory and motor nerves and their function. Extremity wound examinations should include distal testing of sensation, capillary refill, and joint mobility to rule out more proximal nerve, arterial, or musculotendinous injuries.

In order to eliminate further contamination of the wound, the skin should be scrubbed with a contact antimicrobial agent. The antiseptic agent should not be allowed in the depths of the wound because most of them are both bactericidal and cytotoxic (10). The depth of the wound itself is best cleansed by irrigation with a physiologic salt solution. For traumatic wounds, adequate debridement can be followed by irrigating with a pulsating jet lavage (11). Irrigation under pressure as high as 70 pounds per square inch (480 KN/m^2) is needed to remove small debris and bacteria adequately. The decrease in the bacterial counts and removal of small foreign bodies can help prevent wound infection after closure.

One of the first questions that must be asked when closing a traumatic wound is whether wound closure should be attempted at all. The history, revealing both the time since injury and the mechanism of injury, will determine whether a wound is appropriate for closure. If there is any question regarding the amount of bacteria in the wound, the wound can be biopsied and the bacterial level determined. If there are greater than 10^5 organisms per gram of tissue, bacterial contamination is too great to allow normal wound healing without infection (12). Such a wound will neither allow primary closure with sutures nor a more extensive technique such as skin grafting or flap formation (13). The beta-haemolytic streptococcus is more virulent than other species. The mere presence of the beta-haemolytic streptococcus in a wound will prevent adequate healing because of infection (12).

There has been much controversy and speculation regarding the proper timing of closure of wounds. Often heard are unattributed quotes of 'no closure after 24 hours' or 'no closure after 12 hours'. In a study of bacterial counts in wounds, it was found that the wounds with greater than 10^5 organisms per gram of tissue were, on average, over 5 h post-injury (14). These were the only wounds which developed infection. Wounds which occur in an area with greater vascularity will be able to minimize bacterial proliferation. Wounds which occur with a particularly high inoculum of bacteria will cause rapid bacterial proliferation. Clearly, the time from wounding is less important than the number of bacteria present in the wound.

Wound closure should exactly approximate anatomic planes. Technical closure not based on sound wound-healing concepts will have poor results. 'Skin sutures' placed merely for approximation serve little purpose. Depending upon the area of the body injured, these sutures are usually removed after 3–14 days. However, no wound will have enough collagen deposition at that point to resist dermal dehiscence. If

the dermis has too little tensile strength and dehisces, a widened scar with only an epidermal bridge will result.

The best technique for wound closure will be as atraumatic as possible. Wound edges should be co-apted to permit healing without a 'step' and yet not so tightly approximated that the oedema causes further ischaemia in the co-apted edges of the wound (9). The major strength in the skin is in the dermis. The collagen fibres present in the dermis will give the wound its tensile strength. Good approximation of the dermis will minimize the step between the two edges, and minimize the distance that the scar must bridge. Buried sutures should be placed in the dermis which will hold for approximately 42 days. This way, as the sutures are reabsorbed, the wound will have enough collagen deposition to give it adequate tensile strength to avoid disruption.

While fascia has a sufficient amount of collagen to permit approximation with sutures and promote collagen formation in the scar, the underlying muscle will not support sutures and may even necrose if the edges are tightly approximated. The best closure of a wound extending through muscle includes good apposition of the fascia and dermis. A buried dermal closure will place the knot in the depth of the wound and minimize the likelihood of their erosion to the surface of the skin or formation of stitch abscesses. A buried dermal suture performed with an absorbable material will be less likely to eventually erode or serve as a continous foreign body (9, 10). Sutures placed in fat will cause necrosis of this tissue, and serve simply as a foreign body and a nidus for infection (15).

The epidermis can be approximated with a running non-absorbable suture such as Nylon, which will best approximate the wound and give a polished effect to the eventual scar. These sutures should be placed only through the depth of the epidermis. If the dermis is included in the sutures, collagen bundles can invade the tracks and scar formation will occur when these stitches are left in place for as short a period as four days. This is more likely to occur in areas such as the face, where there is a high density of dermal appendages. The palmar or plantar surfaces have such a low density of dermal appendages that sutures may be left in place through both the dermis and epidermis for as long as 3 weeks without suture track scarring (9). A truly epidermal suture will fall out spontaneously in about 7 days as the epidermal cells are sloughed. When the sutures are removed, if desired, the surface of the wound may be further splinted for a time with paper tape strips.

Whenever possible, wounds should be closed primarily by edge approximation. If there is a true lack of tissue, occasionally the edges may be co-apted simply by undermining the adjacent edges of the dermis. When this is insufficient, placement of a graft or flap may be necessary to achieve closure.

A dressing serves several important functions to aid satisfactory wound healing. Acutely, it will protect the wound from further injury or additional bacterial contamination. A dressing of absorptive gauze with a wetting agent will allow exudate to be 'wicked' into the gauze away from the skin. Occlusive dressings will simply trap the exudate between the dressings and the wound, allowing bacterial proliferation and skin maceration. Wound oedema can be minimized by gentle compression with gauze wrappings. The oedema in the wound can, by neutralizing the sebum, make the wound more prone to infections (16). Finally, immobilization of the wound edges promotes healing and decreases pain. This is even more important over joints or in highly mobile areas.

Reconstruction with grafts and flaps

Closure of wounds by direct approximation and primary healing is desirable, whether dealing with a primary wound or a reconstructive procedure. When defects exist which cannot be sutured directly, grafts or flaps are required. Traditionally, closure by grafts is considered first, followed by the possibilities of local flaps and distant flaps. With the greater understanding of the safe use of axial and musculocutaneous flaps, these have assumed a more prominent place in the hierarchy of techniques. In addition, closure or reconstruction by the free transfer of composite tissue using microvascular anastomosis has become increasingly common. Direct closure, grafts, flaps, free tissue transfer, and scar rearrangement comprise the armamentarium of the reconstructive surgeon.

By definition, a skin graft is a segment of skin (epidermis and dermis) which has been totally separated from its blood supply and transplanted from its normal bed (donor site) to a new one (recipient site) (7). A split or partial thickness skin graft includes epidermis and part, but not all, of the dermis, whereas a full-thickness skin graft includes epidermis and the full thickness of the dermis.

Split skin grafts are best used to cover large denuded surfaces or on granulating wounds. They are also used when wound contraction is of minor consequence. A great advantage of these grafts is that their donor sites heal themselves from the remaining skin appendages, such as hair follicles and sweat glands.

Skin grafts which include the full thickness of the dermis tend to resemble normal skin better than split skin grafts. They provide more padding, a better colour match, a more nearly normal hair pattern, and they inhibit wound contraction in the recipient site (7). Because they require ideal conditions for survival they must be placed in a well-vascularized recipient site. The major disadvantage of full-thickness grafts is that their donor sites cannot heal spontaneously. Therefore, the size of the graft is limited to dimensions which will allow primary closure of the donor site. If this practice is not followed, the donor site from a large, full-thickness graft must be closed by a split skin graft.

A skin graft, like any graft, must obtain a blood supply from its recipient site to survive (7). Therefore, the recipient site must be capable of providing the necessary vascularity. Bare cortical bone, bare tendon, and bare cartilage cannot do this, and are unacceptable recipient sites for skin grafts. Heavily irradiated tissue, fibrotic long-standing granulation tissue, and ischaemic tissue with arteriosclerotic changes are relatively poor recipient beds.

Once a skin graft is transplanted to a recipient bed it has a limited time in which to become revascularized. During this plasmatic phase, a fibrin network is formed between the graft and the recipient bed which holds the graft in place. Within the first 48 h, connections are established between the bed and the empty 'ghost' vessels on the underside of the graft, due to neovascular budding into the empty vessels as a pathway of least resistance. As the vascular attachments are re-established, continuity of the lymphatic system is restored. Maturation of the skin graft occurs over a period of time as in any wound.

The leading cause of failure of the skin grafting procedure is prevention of good contact between the skin graft and its recipient bed by haematoma or seroma. Because of this, meticulous haemostasis of the bed is necessary before applying a graft. Inspection of the graft by the second or third day allows removal of any collection of fluid that is preventing contact of the graft with the bed.

Improper immobilization between the graft and the recipient site is another frequent cause of failure. Movement between the graft and the bed injures the budding capillaries and prevents vascularization.

Grafting on to an unacceptable or poor bed may also result in graft failure. Relatively avascular tissues and bacteria can make a bed unacceptable. If a potential graft bed contains greater than 10^5 organisms per gram of tissue or any beta-haemolytic streptococci, the chance of skin graft survival markedly decreases (17). Infection occurring after skin grafting used to be a common cause of graft failure, but is now a rare cause. If the recipient bed contains 10^5 or fewer bacteria per gram of tissue and no beta-haemolytic streptococci at the time of graft application, it is unusual to lose a graft because of infection. However, if a graft is not inspected until too late, the loss will be interpreted as having been caused by infection because a non-vascularized graft becomes a perfect pabulum for bacteria, and secondary infection intervenes.

Postoperative care of the skin graft is as important as the operative technique. Most grafts should be inspected by 48–72 h using an aseptic technique. Any fluid found beneath the graft should be aspirated or evacuated by making a small 'nick' in the graft to express it. If fluid is not removed by 96 h, evidence has been presented that the graft epithelializes on the undersurface, preventing satisfactory vascularization (18). The graft must be immobilized and protected for at least 5–7 days. Oedema should be prevented in the recipient bed for 4–6 months.

Deformities and defects are best corrected or closed by primary approximation whenever possible because skin grafting is usually thought of as a second choice. However, cases exist where skin grafting is either not possible or not desirable. When the area in need of reconstruction lacks the vascularity necessary to support a skin graft, tissue to reconstruct the defect must carry its own blood supply (7). When two surfaces must be reconstructed, an inherent blood supply is necessary. Sometimes, a skin graft may be able to correct a deformity or close a defect, but may not be the most desirable type of reconstruction. This is true if future surgery will be necessary beneath the reconstructed area, if near-normal sensation is required of the reconstructed tissue, or if the hoped-for aesthetic result cannot be achieved by a skin graft (7). In all of these circumstances reconstruction can be effected by a skin flap.

By definition, a skin flap is a segment of skin and subcutaneous tissue which is transferred from its original position on the body to another site while maintaining its own inherent vasculature for nourishment (7). In some cases, deeper tissue, such as muscle or bone, is carried with the skin flap. All flaps have a 'pedicle', which is their vascular base of attachment.

To understand skin flaps, a thorough knowledge of the blood supply of the skin and the flap is necessary. The vascular pattern that forms the predominant blood supply to the skin in humans is made up of perforating branches through the muscles or along fascial planes, becoming the *musculocutaneous* and *fasciocutaneous arteries*, and terminate by supplying the dermal–subdermal plexus of the skin. The other anatomical pattern forms the *direct cutaneous arteries* which lie superficial to the muscles and parallel to the skin for long distances, and supply the dermal–subdermal plexus directly.

A *cutaneous*, or *random pattern flap,* is a flap based on a blood supply from musculocutaneous arteries penetrating perpendicularly into its base, supplying the length of the flap through the longitudinal dermal–subdermal plexus (7). The surviving length of this flap is limited by the perfusion pressure in the vessels. An *axial*, or *arterial pattern flap*, receives its blood supply from a direct cutaneous artery which enters its base and runs longitudinally within the flap. The length of the flap is determined by the length of the direct cutaneous artery supplying it, plus an additional random portion at the termination of the artery supplied by the dermal–subdermal plexus.

A third type of flap, the *musculocutaneous* or *myocutaneous flap,* is based on a muscle which is adequately supplied with blood flow through a single dominant vascular pedicle. The muscle, with its overlying skin and subcutaneous tissue, is raised as a flap and transferred as a unit on the segmental vascular pedicle. This allows a large area of skin to be transferred on multiple muscle perforators fed by the pedicle without the limitations imposed on cutaneous or random flaps. Likewise, a fasciocutaneous flap may be raised by including the vascularized fascia in the same way. Any of these types of flaps can be transferred by dividing the vascular pedicle and re-anastomosing it in a recipient site (7). When this technique is used, the flap is classified as a *free flap*. A free flap is not considered a graft since vascularization and nourishment is immediately re-established through the pedicle.

Historically, most skin flaps were of the cutaneous or random pattern type. Since they lack an anatomically recognized arteriovenous system they have strict length limitations. The length cannot survive beyond the blood supply of the dermal–subdermal anastomotic plexus perfused by the perforating musculocutaneous arteries without special conditioning of the flap. The flap can be conditioned to survive to greater lengths by performing a preliminary 'delay' procedure on the flap to enhance the blood supply to a specific area of tissue. The purpose of the delay is to condition the extra length of the flap to survive in a state of relative hypoxia at the time of transfer.

Axial or arterial pattern flaps are supplied by a specific longitudinal arteriovenous network. Therefore, traditional length to base width ratios play no role in the designing of the flap. In fact, no skin is necessary at the base of these flaps, and the artery and vein alone can serve as the base of the pedicle (7). The key to the use of an axial flap is an exact knowledge of the anatomy of the direct cutaneous arteries. This type of flap is not universally useful because there are a limited number of direct axial arteries with known cutaneous vascular territories.

Since axial pattern flaps are limited by the small number of known cutaneous vascular territories and since the remainder of the body's skin is supplied by perforating musculocutaneous arteries, elevating the muscle with its longitudinal segmental artery to supply an overlying skin flap makes sense. Musculocutaneous vascular territories exist over all regions of the body. Using these known musculocutaneous vascular territories, compound flaps of skin, subcutaneous tissue, and muscle can be designed for almost any defect.

Microvascular surgical techniques make it feasible to anastomose arteries and veins of less than 1 mm in diameter. Therefore, skin flaps and skin–muscle flaps can be transferred as free flaps. Success rates of greater than 95 per cent for this type of flap transfer are now routinely reported. Free flaps are not justified when other means of reconstruction such as skin grafts, cutaneous, axial, or musculocutaneous flaps are *equally* satisfactory. However, the free flap frequently does provide the best solution for reconstructive problems and occasionally may be the only salvage for a particular patient.

All types of skin flaps have certain characteristics which help differentiate their reconstructive results from skin grafts. The skin of a flap tends to maintain its original colour and texture and preserve hair growth, sebaceous secretion, sweating, and sensation. Flaps tend to be more durable than skin grafts, especially over a bony prominence or other pressure point. Finally, flaps tend to grow in proportion to total body growth.

The single most important requirement for flap survival is adequate nutrient blood flow (7). The flap is planned and the transfer procedure executed so that sufficient inflow of arterial blood and outflow of venous blood for all of the tissue comprising the flap is maintained. If the arterial inflow to a flap can be predicted to be insufficient, it can be augmented by a delay procedure as discussed previously.

Once a flap has been properly designed and elevated, the flap should survive transfer. Failure can still occur in certain circumstances (7). Suturing a flap into place under excessive tension can interfere either with venous outflow or, if excessive, arterial inflow. Kinking of the flap at the time of transfer or postoperatively can similarly cause vascular compromise. Most frequently, kinking results in venous embarrassment. A mild to moderate degree of inflammatory oedema occurs in all flaps. If this is inhibited by a tight constricting dressing, vascular compromise will occur. However, often an even amount of compression is of aid to a flap to help prevent excessive kinking or to overcome the oedema of gravity.

Just as a haematoma will spell disaster for a skin graft, it may totally destroy a flap. Often the haematoma is difficult to diagnose in the flap because of the normal degree of postoperative oedema. Infection is not a common cause of flap failure because of the excellent blood supply of a flap with its accompanying cellular and humoral host defence factors. However, when infection does occur, it can destroy a flap.

Just as in skin grafting, donor site considerations are important in using skin flaps (7). When possible, an adjacent donor site is preferred to allow a local flap instead of a distant flap. As a general rule, axial pattern flaps are preferred to cutaneous or random flaps. Another important consideration is that the donor site must be able to spare the tissue to be transferred without serious loss of function. It is contraindicated to use a muscle with a critical function as a donor muscle for a musculocutaneous pattern flap.

Scar formation, contractures, and scar revision

Scar formation is the fundamental phenomenon of wound healing in most human tissues including the dermis. An understanding of normal wound healing, and insight into the factors which make a scar less than optimal, are both essential to planning scar revisions. All scars must proceed through the inflammatory, proliferative, and maturation phases of wound healing and will, therefore, require time to reach their final appearance. If the mature scar is not satisfactory, application of the basic principles of reconstruction can then be expected to result in an improved scar.

The most common reasons for unacceptable scars are an unfavourable direction of the original wound or incision with regard to the normal lines of skin tension, failure of proper dermal approximation, and a pathological extension of normal wound contraction which results in a contracture (19).

The simplest scar revision consists of excising the scar and reapproximating the wound edges. If the excessive scarring was due to an improper direction of the original wound, the wound direction should be realigned so that the new scar will fall in the lines of minimum resting tension (Kraissl's or Langer's lines) (20). As a general rule, these lines will run perpendicular to the fibres of the underlying muscle. Often, realigning a scar to the minimum resting skin tension lines will allow it to become almost invisible. Although a degree of wound contraction is a normal part of wound healing, contracture is preventable. Placing the direction in the lines of minimum resting tension will greatly help, as well as elongating the line of contracture by excising the old scar as an ellipse.

An unacceptable scar may be due to a deficiency in tissue (7). If the original wound was closed under excessive tension, a widened hypertrophic or depressed scar, or a contracture would be expected. When the scar is incised or excised, the edges retract widely and the tissue deficiency becomes apparent. A split or full-thickness skin graft will replace the deficiency and improve the scar. Skin grafts are useful for scar revision in areas where previous scars or skin grafts are of poor quality or have a poor colour match.

Skin flaps are sometimes indicated for scar revision. A depressed scar may require a flap for bulk. A scar may be atrophic due to ischaemia and a flap with its inherent blood supply may be required to increase the vascularity of the revision (7). Finally, just as with a skin graft, a flap may improve a scar by adding tissue to relieve tension.

The z-plasty is a technique by which two triangular skin flaps are interchanged in position to gain length along a scar or skin fold at the expense of the adjacent tissues (7). Understanding of the geometry and principles of the z-plasty allows the reconstructive surgeon to lengthen a contracted scar, obliterate a web contracture, add to an area of deficient tissue, and change the direction of a scar, thus providing an important technique of scar revision (21).

Proliferative scar formation

In the integumentary system, even though the processes of wound healing have apparently progressed normally, proliferative scar formation, either hypertrophic scars or keloid, may result. This can occur even though the physician understands normal wound healing and performs all steps correctly in wounds of the integument, tendons, nerves, joints, or tubular structures (19). Still, the balance between collagen synthesis and degradation appears to be upset, resulting in proliferative scar formation.

Hypertrophic scars are large masses of collagen which remain within the bounds of the original wound from which they are derived. This differs from keloid formation, where the collagen mass extends beyond the original bounds of the wound. At the extremes, keloid and hypertrophic scar are easily distinguishable. However, in many cases, there is considerable overlap in features, which may blur this distinction (19).

Clinically, a keloid appears raised, firm, and the overlying epithelium tends to be darker than normal. Microscopically, there are thick, homogeneous bands of collagen and a paucity of cellular elements. Hypertrophic scars are histologically similar to keloids, although the collagen tends to whorl about clusters of macrophages, fibroblasts, and vessels.

The keloid and hypertrophic scar are both the end result of collagen over-production. In many cases, the aetiology of this over-production in the hypertrophic scar is understood and, therefore, correctable. It appears that the normal wound healing process begins and seems to continue. It does not shut off, so normal wound contraction becomes contracture and ends up with a hypertrophic scar (19). Since contraction is a normal part of the physiology of wound healing, it is neither possible nor desirous to prevent wound contraction. However, one may be able to prevent the abnormal continuation of wound contraction leading to a contracture, hypertrophy, and deformity.

One way to reduce hypertrophic scar formation is to minimize the time in which normal wound contraction takes place. We can reduce the amount and the intensity of the inflammation. For instance, the burn wound can be excised and closed very early to decrease the inflammatory phase. It is desirable to reduce this time because it has been demonstrated that hypertrophic scars are related to the amount of time that the wound is allowed to remain in the inflammatory phase before it moves into the proliferative phase (22). The inflammatory phase should be reduced not only in wounds healing by secondary or tertiary intention, but also in those healing by primary intention.

Another technique to decrease hypertrophic scar is to minimize or eliminate a deficiency of tissue. In closing wounds it is important to make sure that an adequate amount of tissue is available for proper closure. Patients should not have wounds closed with undue increased tension, as this will result in a hypertrophic scar.

A less than ideal result can occur if the wound is lined up geometrically in the wrong direction. Electively, incisions are placed in Kraissl's lines or lines of minimum tension (20). These lines, which are perpendicular to the underlying muscle pull, allow the wounds to have less tension as muscles contract beneath the wounds. Wounds not in Kraissl's lines are under constant tension and result in a hypertrophic scar (19).

Another very effective treatment of hypertrophic scarring is the application of direct pressure. The mechanism of this modulation of collagen deposition is not certain. It may be related to a relative hypoperfusion of the area, as the external pressure required must exceed capillary blood pressure (22 mmHg or 3 kPa) in order to be effective (19). The results of long-term treatment with graded pressure garments have been particularly rewarding in burn patients, although the concept is generally applicable.

It is the authors' belief that hypertrophic scarring is not a true disturbance of normal physiology of wound healing, but basically a problem of tension due to either tissue deficiency or misdirection of a wound, resulting in uncontrolled wound contraction. Surgery is used to improve these scars because there is usually a normal healing mechanism.

A keloid is a disturbance that extends beyond the original wound boundaries. It is not the result of something done by the provider and no amount of surgery will correct it. Keloids are not the result of wound healing out of control because they do not occur in every wound. The aetiology of keloid formation has proven elusive and so has the treatment. Keloid formation appears to be unrelated to tension or other mechanical factors. A biochemical imbalance is most likely but to date no particular hormone or compound has been positively identified.

Keloids have a predilection to form over the butterfly area of the sternum, and the mandible and deltoid areas. The rate of collagen synthesis is increased in fibroblasts from keloids. The water content of the collagen of keloidal tissue seems to be higher than collagen from either normally healing wounds or hypertrophic scars. Similarly, the amount of acid-soluble collagen appears to be greater. The amount of glycosaminoglycans produced by fibroblasts is obviously high and there is a redistribution of the proteoglycans with chondroitin 4-sulphate being produced disproportionately (23).

The treatment of a keloid involves understanding the disturbance in the normal healing pathway and attempting to correct it. Initial treatment of keloids is not surgical. Although the temptation to excise keloids is great, this usually results in the return of an even worse keloid. The initial treatment should be by triamcinolone injections. If triamcinolone is injected into the wound every 3–4 weeks, the collagen can be manipulated and the amount of cross-linking in the collagen and the amount of collagenase can be modulated. If injections are continued until there is no excess abnormal collagen, then the lesion can be excised. If abnormal collagen build-up can be prevented during this wound healing phase, then

normal scar may result rather than another keloid. There are other experimental ways that collagen can be modulated. Lysyl oxidase inhibitors such as BAPN or penicillamine can control intracellular and extracellular collagen synthesis by changing the cross-linking. Colchicine can evaluate collagen kinetics. Retinoic acid and alpha and gamma interferon can reduce collagen production from keloid fibroblasts (24, 25).

There are many other types of abnormal wound healing. As the molecular basis for each of the processes in the wound healing scheme are being defined, oxygen, vitamin deficiencies, pharmacologic effects of steroids and chemotherapeutic agents can affect the normal processes. Similarly, genetic abnormalities of collagen synthesis, enzyme deficiencies, or elastin production cause abnormal wound healing.

Dermatological surgery

Techniques for excision and closure of skin lesions are the same as discussed earlier for the closure of wounds. Attention to elective incision lines and a biologically sound wound closure are important. However, two other techniques for skin lesion ablation deserve mention – cryosurgery and Mohs micrographic surgery.

Cryosurgery is the application of subfreezing temperature to living tissue to achieve selective tissue necrosis. The therapeutic temperature at the tissue level can range from −20°C to −170°C (26). These profound temperature changes produce rapid physical changes leading to cell death. These events are divided into direct cellular effects, vascular effects, and possible changes in the immunologic response (26).

The cellular effect is primarily due to the formation of intracellular ice crystals which lead to cell membrane rupture and/or cellular dehydration. The most important characteristic of the tissue determining its response to freezing is its vascularity, as flowing blood is an efficient means of heat convection. The vascular response to freezing has been studied by Zacarian (26). They noted that in a hamster cheek pouch model all circulation stopped within 30 min at −20°C. Thawing resulted in vasodilation, which produced a showering of emboli, occluding the distal vessels, and subsequent ischaemic necrosis.

The optimal lethal effect of this therapy is with a 'fast freeze–hold–slow thaw' cycle which is repeated at least twice for maximal response. The size and site of the tumour being treated influence the results of cryosurgery, as does the tumour histology. Well-differentiated lesions respond more completely than anaplastic lesions. Since water content of tissue also affects the result, bone and high density connective tissue are not easily treated.

The technique of cryosurgery is used to treat both malignant and non-malignant cutaneous lesions. Therapy for malignancies should include a 3–5 mm margin of normal tissue (26). Cryosurgery is a treatment modality for basal and squamous cell tumours, but it is not recommended for melanoma. It has also been found effective in uterine cervical cancer, and is being tested for treatment of breast, liver, and locally advanced rectal and tracheo-bronchial tumours.

Dr Frederic Mohs in the early 1940s developed the

technique of systematic microscopic tissue analysis after *in situ* fixation with zinc chloride application and serial resection of skin cancers (27). Tromovitch further advanced the science by using a fresh technique where the zinc paste was excluded as a chemical fixative (28). This fresh technique is currently the most popular method.

Mohs' technique is applicable to tumours that grow by contiguous cellular invasion of adjacent tissue, especially those with poorly defined borders, or tumours in an area where maximal preservation of normal tissue is sought, such as in the periorbital region.

Lesions to be treated should be biopsied by routine paraffin-embedded methods, to allow the most accurate diagnosis to be made. Treatment begins as the clinically visible tumour is curetted away, and the remaining tissue is excised in a saucer-like manner with 2–3 mm margin. The tissue thickness is usually 2–3 mm. The tissue slices are mapped and the 'surgeon–pathologist' examines the tissue microscopically. The location of malignant cells can be pinpointed and these steps repeated to remove all malignant tissue.

Using these techniques, Dr Mohs reported 9000 cases with a 99 per cent cure rate for basal cell carcinoma (29). In 3000 cases of epithelial squamous cell carcinoma he found a 94 per cent cure rate. Although the Mohs technique provides a controlled excision of malignancy with a very acceptable cure rate, it is not without complications. Wound infection, excessive wound haemorrhage, and cicatricial scarring in wounds left to heal by secondary intention may result.

Burns: clinical aspects of burn wound healing

Thermal injuries primarily injure the skin and its adjacent structures. Secondarily, all systems of the body may be deranged. The significance of intact skin cannot be overemphasized. The skin is by size and weight the second largest organ of the body, next to muscle. Although often not recognized as such, it is also a vital organ. Loss of large amounts of skin, if not replaced by autograft skin, is incompatible with life. Skin has very limited ability for regeneration and lacks much of the functional reserve characteristic of internal organs. Even without skin loss, invasive bacterial infection limited to the skin can lead to death without any sign of systemic invasion (30).

Even if the skin is not totally lost or if lost skin can be replaced, thermal injuries alter the skin and produce scar. This is why survival statistics are not the only measure of success in thermal injuries. Scar can yield unsightly deformities, function-limiting contractures, and change a person's identity and personality. Since intact skin is of such significance, it is obvious that prevention of thermal injuries is more important than their treatment.

Human skin is injured by heat in two ways. First is an immediate direct cellular injury, which is followed by a delayed injury due to progressive dermal ischaemia. The skin can tolerate temperatures up to 40°C for relatively long periods before injury. Temperatures above this level produce a logarithmic increase in tissue destruction (31). The degree of tissue destruction is related both to temperature and duration of exposure to the heat source.

Following thermal injury, changes continue to occur in the affected tissue for some time and significant tissue necrosis occurs after the initial insult. The idea that the progressive changes in the burn wound may be due to microvascular changes secondary to inflammation led investigators to study the possible role of mediators, specifically eicosanoids, free oxygen radicals, and vasoactive amines.

First aid for the burn wound

Successful treatment of the burn victim remains the effective treatment and ultimate healing of the burn wound. The multisystemic response of the burn patient, and his/her ultimate death or survival are closely related to the successful management of the burn wound (3). However, attention to the wound should be delayed until other life-saving measures have been instituted. The exceptions to this delay are cooling the wound and release of constricting eschar of limbs or chest. Although the exact pharmacologic manipulation to block various mediator production is still in the experimental phase and not yet determined for humans, cooling the burn wound not only prevents leucocyte sticking but actually increases wound perfusion (32). To be effective in preventing the microvascular changes, the cooling must occur within the first 30 min after injury. Cooling can have a direct cellular effect as well as decreasing the progressive changes. Heggers and colleagues postulate that cooling maintains the normal haemostasis between PGE_2 and $PGF_{2\alpha}$, thus preventing excess PGE_2 and the eventual production of excess thromboxane (33).

In addition to cooling, the other first aid measure for the burn wound is escharotomy. This may be necessary for the chest and/or the extremities. Acute respiratory distress seen early after burning is usually due to a deep burn with an unyielding eschar about the anterior and lateral aspects of the chest (3). An escharotomy releases the restriction of rib motion, increases thoracic excursion, and improves ventilatory function. Encircling eschar to the extremities can cause vascular embarrassment because of the development of obligatory oedema in the deep tissues. Repeated monitoring of capillary refill or blood flow with use of a Doppler flowmeter will determine the need for surgical escharotomy or enzymatic decompression.

Mechanisms to aid healing of the burn wound

All wounds, regardless of depth, are candidates for cooling and necessary escharotomy. Once these measures are completed, the burn wound management depends upon the depth of the injury. An algorithm or decision tree is helpful in determining management (3). Historically, burn wounds were divided into first, second, third, and fourth degree burns. For practical purposes today, wounds can be divided on admission into shallow wounds and deep wounds. Shallow wounds will heal by epithelialization within two weeks. Deep wounds include all other burns. This division allows burns to be divided between those requiring operative management (deep wounds) and those which can be managed non-operatively (shallow wounds).

To make the first decision, patients are cleansed and debrided of dead tissue and blisters, since blister fluid contains inflammatory mediators, such as thromboxane, known to be detrimental to the microcirculation (34). Since Zawacki has shown that sound desiccation converts the zone of stasis and deepens the burn, aspiration of the blisters, leaving the blister epithelium intact, is physiologically sound and may be advantageous (35). If the blister is totally debrided, prevention of desiccation is indicated.

After cleansing and debridement, a decision on burn depth is made. For those categorized as shallow wounds, temporary closure of the burn wound with a dressing which will not impede epithelialization is the authors' choice for patients presenting with fresh burns immediately after injury. Although biologic dressings have been the gold standard for temporary burn wound closure, synthetic dressings which prevent desiccation and allow epithelialization of shallow burns to occur are now more desirable. Two types of such dressings are available. The first is a transparent thin film dressing which prevents wound dehydration and desiccation. This type of occlusive dressing accelerates wound healing by maintenance of a moist environment, prevention of scab formation, and facilitation of epidermal cell migration through a fluid or semi-fluid environment (3). These dressings have not been as effective on burn wounds as they have on donor sites because the exudate contains thromboxane which is injurious to the microvasculature and serves as a culture medium for bacterial growth.

The second type of synthetic dressing is a bilaminate dressing which approximates the structure of skin. The most effective of these is Biobrane®, consisting of a knitted Nylon fabric bonded to a silicone membrane and coated with collagen peptides (36). This dressing can be applied to shallow wounds, covered with a compressive dressing to assure adherence, and then be left in place until epithelialization occurs.

Another approach to these shallow wounds is simply to protect them with a non-adherent dressing while epithelialization occurs. Finally, the shallow wound can be treated with an antibacterial cream. Usually, this is unnecessary for the truly shallow wound, unless it covers large amounts of the body. The antibacterial cream can be applied with or without a dressing, but the authors favour a dressing to keep the wound from desiccating and to help decrease the hypermetabolism of the burned patient (3).

Positioning and splinting must be incorporated into non-operative wound management. The burn wound will contract until it meets an opposing force (22). Therefore, any body parts capable of flexing will do so unless prevented. Since it has been stated that the position of comfort is the position of contracture, the patient must be positioned to prevent contracture immediately on admission. Proper positioning is not enough. The forces of contraction leading to eventual contracture must be opposed. Splints must be fashioned and used in non-operative management as well as in the postoperative phase.

Operative management of the burn wound

Non-operative treatment of the burn wound is reserved mostly for shallow wounds. Deep wounds will usually require operative management. These wounds include deep, partial thickness burns which will not heal efficaciously by epithelialization. The first decision for deep wounds is the timing of removal of the necrotic tissue. There is much debate on when to excise the burn wound (37). However, there is no debate that non-viable tissue must be removed. The authors believe this should begin as soon as the patient is stable. This can be accomplished by several techniques. The first is formal full-thickness excision, often down to fascia, which is most useful for small circumscribed full-thickness burn wounds or occasionally for larger burns in children. These wounds, though they may contain viable elements, usually are mostly full thickness and may be expeditiously managed by excision of suspected necrotic tissues and definitive wound closure.

As the burn wound involves a greater percentage of the total body surface area, it is more likely to be of non-uniform depth and full-thickness excision and autografting can create logistic problems (3). Available donor sites for coverage decrease as the size of the total burn wound in need of excision increases. In such cases, removal of viable cells which may occur in full-thickness fascial excision seems hard to justify.

An alternative to full-thickness burn wound excision is tangential or sequential excision of the non-viable portion of the burn wound. This is based on Jackson's description of concentric zones of injury (38). The idea is to remove the non-viable zone of coagulation. If this sequential excision is only in a deep, partial thickness wound, the technique is also called an intradermal debridement. Although sequential layered excision offers no advantages in the treatment of large full-thickness burns, it does allow early removal of non-viable tissue while preserving deep dermal viable tissue in deep, partial thickness injuries (3). The important feature of this technique is that immediate wound closure is important after excision, and desiccation must not be allowed to occur.

Once the necrotic tissue has been removed from the burn wound, closure can proceed. If, following removal of tissue, the wound appears to have an adequate dermal base, a decision must be made. If one feels the wound is superficial enough, a temporary closure can be performed as described in the non-operative management section. The authors' choice in this situation is to use Biobrane®. However, the deeper partial thickness and full-thickness defects require autograft closure. The approach to initial skin grafting is most important in the final rehabilitation of the patient and the prevention of future reconstructive procedures (39). The goal is not just to cover the wound with epithelium, but to obtain closure with a serviceable, functional, and aesthetically acceptable skin. Therefore, it is necessary that the initial definitive closure be made with an adequate amount of skin. This requires grafting with the patient's joints either in maximum extension and abduction, such as the axilla, or in maximum flexion such as the dorsum of the metacarpophalangeal joints of the hand (3).

When limited amounts of quality skin are available, priority areas exist for the best skin. These include the face and neck (especially the eyelids), the hands, and the flexion creases (e.g. axilla, popliteal fossa, and antecubital fossa). These priorities include function first and then aesthetics. When grafting the face, one should consider the aesthetic units and plan the grafts to include entire aesthetic units to prevent the 'patchwork quilt' effect of spot grafts (3). Sheet grafts are used whenever possible. Meshed grafts yield unacceptable results when spread beyond a ratio of 1:1.5. The interstices heal by epithelium devoid of dermis and thus the graft area is prone to contraction.

Even when wounds are quite massive, early permanent closure may be possible. Techniques such as tissue culture of autologous epidermis and immunosuppression of allograft skin are being reported with increasing success rates (37).

In large burn wounds, in which donor sites are insufficient and where such techniques as discussed above are not available, temporary closure of the burn wound is necessary. Both biologic and biosynthetic dressings can serve this purpose. As opposed to the shallow wounds, deep wounds, following excision of eschar, can be covered with dressings that allow vascularization. Allograft skin and amniotic membranes are more effective as biologic dressings in this situation than xenograft skin, since by allowing vascular ingrowth, they maintain more effective bacterial control of the burn wound (40). The authors have been using Biobrane® in place of biologic dressings after excision of deep wounds when donor sites are not available or if the excised wound is not acceptable for immediate autografting. Roberts and colleagues compared Biobrane® to porcine xenografts on excised wounds and found them equally efficacious for initial coverage (41). Similarly, Purdue and colleagues reported a multi-institutional prospectively randomized study comparing Biobrane® and allograft skin on excised wounds, showing no difference with respect to adherence, rejection, infection, autograft take, or final wound appearance (42).

If care is taken to assure the highest graft take possible and the best quality skin is transplanted, wound closure will occur in a way that will decrease future contractures and hypertrophic scars. However, functional and aesthetic results can be improved following wound closure. Function must be regained after the period of immobilization necessitated by skin grafting. Encouragement of an active range of motion within the first few days after grafting has no physiological basis for success (3). The graft must first survive on plasma followed by linking up and ingrowth of capillaries. During this phase, movement will result in shearing and a decrease in graft 'take'. Therefore, motion before 5–7 days is probably of no benefit.

By 10–14 days after grafting, skin grafts are stable enough to withstand pressure. Graded pressure garments will lead to a flatter, more uniform wound surface. The pressure will particularly aid the graft junctions and prevent immature collagen from producing hypertrophic scarring. In a randomized series, it was shown that the combination of pressure garments, oral penicillin, and topical antiprostaglandin cream was the most useful in decreasing pruritus, erythema, and hypertrophic scarring (3). The use of pressure garments should be maintained for six months to two years, depending on the age of the patient.

Skin grafts will effect wound closure in an overwhelming number of acute burn cases. Only when an unacceptable bed such as exposed bone or tendon is present does one have to resort to flaps for coverage in the acute situation. Therefore, the use of flaps will be discussed in the next section, under reconstruction.

Late management of burn wound scarring

Proliferative scar formation (either hypertrophic scar or keloid) may result following integumentary burns, even though the processes of wound healing have apparently progressed normally. Hypertrophic scars, the proliferative scars most frequently seen after burns, appear to be related to wound contraction just as discussed in the earlier skin section. Since one way to reduce hypertrophic scar formation is to minimize the time and the intensity of the inflammation, the burn wound can be excised and closed very early to decrease the length of the inflammatory phase. This emphasizes the need for successful skin graft 'take' at the time of initial excision and grafting during the acute care of the burn wound.

Another technique to decrease hypertrophic scar is to minimize or eliminate any deficiency of tissue. In closing burn wounds initially, it is important that an adequate amount of tissue is used. This means, whenever possible, that sheet grafts are used instead of meshed grafts or 'postage stamp' grafts.

Pressure is an effective adjunct in the control of scar maturation. Pressure garments customized to the individual patient should be applied as soon as possible after wound healing is completed to prevent further shortening of the collagen. Flexible elastomer beneath the garments aids in delivering uniform pressure in concave areas such as the axilla, clavicle, neck, hand, and inferior chest.

Despite improved aggressive acute care, healing of burns too frequently leaves residual deformities. Wound contraction, a normal and necessary part of healing, promotes distortions that produce visual disfigurement and functional limitation. If possible, reconstruction is postponed until wounds have matured. Frequently, postponement is not possible if the deformity is progressive or causing a functional deficit.

The first priority must always remain the prevention of deformity (43). Obviously this receives great emphasis in acute therapy, but the importance of postoperative splinting or pressure garments must be remembered after each reconstructive procedure. The next priority is reconstruction of active function. The final priority is restoration of passive function. Once the priorities of reconstruction have been determined, the techniques available are many and diverse. Simplicity is often a virtue, so closure of wounds by direct approximation and primary healing is desirable whenever possible (43). This is true both when dealing with the primary burn and with a reconstructive procedure. Often defects exist which cannot be sutured directly. In such situations grafts or flaps are required. Traditionally, closure by skin grafts has been considered first, followed by local and distant flaps. The simplest method which will produce the desired result is chosen. In burn reconstruction, the z-plasty, which is in reality two random flaps, is often considered before a skin graft (43).

More recently, with the better understanding of the safe use of axial and musculocutaneous flaps, these have assumed a more prominent place. In addition, closure or reconstruction by the free transfer of composite tissue using microvascular anastomosis has become increasingly common as its complication rate has become comparable to that of myocutaneous flaps.

Skin expansion techniques are also rapidly gaining popularity. These can now be performed to yield another type of flap tissue for reconstruction. Gradual stretching of the skin can theoretically occur without the risk of cell necrosis and dermal rupture. Epidermal cells appear to be essentially unaltered and the thickness of the epidermis remains unchanged. The dermis thins and there is an increase in the number of fibroblast and myofibroblasts. There is marked thinning of the subcutaneous tissue and atrophy of muscle both above and below the expander. Although none of these changes would seem to be detrimental in using expanded skin for reconstruction, Rees and colleagues demonstrated marked disruption of the reticular dermal collagen in expanded skin (44). This work might dampen the enthusiasm for the use of tissue expansion in the burn patient. Certainly in a situation of insufficient unburned skin, any chance of damaging the skin to be used for reconstruction must be viewed for the proper risk:benefit ratio (43). Despite this worry, there are areas in which burn scars cannot be reconstructed adequately with conventional means. These include areas of alopecia on the scalp and the male face, where expanded hair-bearing adjacent skin would seem ideal. Other burn deformities of the head and neck call for reconstruction with skin of similar colour, tone, texture, thickness, and composition.

Direct closure, grafts, flaps, free tissue transfer, and tissue expansion comprise the armamentarium of the reconstructive burns surgeon. All of the techniques useful to achieve satisfactory healing of unburned skin can be adapted for the burned patient. Understanding the anatomy, biochemistry, and physiology of skin and the various processes of the wound healing scheme allow one to arrive at a biologically sound plan to manage any injury to the skin from the simple incision or laceration to the most complex thermal injury.

The abdominal wall

Incisions

Access to the abdominal cavity requires a variety of incisions for the best exposure and minimal trauma. Most abdominal surgical wounds are closed at the time of surgery and heal by primary intention. Occasionally, particularly in dirty surgical operations or in contaminated military wounds (Chapters 7 and 8), some or all of the anatomical layers of the abdominal wall are left open, to be closed later (delayed primary suture, see Chapter 4; refs 45–47), or, more rarely, to heal completely by secondary intention. However, primary closure of the abdominal wall is usually undertaken after most emergency and elective abdominal surgical procedures and can be undertaken safely by most grades of surgical staff (including those in training). Surgeons use techniques which allow safe and reliable closure, are preferably straightforward and quick to make as well as close, and which leave the abdominal wall strong enough to resist postoperative distraction forces caused by coughing, retching, or ileus. At the end of a long and difficult procedure, it may be all too easy to close the abdomen without adequate concentration or attention to detail, or to delegate the task to inexperienced junior staff, the result being that the success of the operation is marred by postoperative wound failure.

Several incisions have been described for access to the abdominal contents (Fig. 9.1). The choice of incision must allow adequate access, be easily extended if required, and leave a cosmetically acceptable scar. Factors of importance in the siting of the scar include obesity and the build of the patient, previous abdominal incisions, the possibility or necessity for stoma formation, the required speed of access to the abdominal contents in an emergency situation, and the individual surgeon's preference. Cosmetic concerns with regard to the length and siting of the scar are of relatively secondary importance. Surgeons in training should be discouraged from undertaking abdominal surgery through tiny incisions (as if they were a mark of particular surgical ability). Care must be taken when siting an incision in the vicinity of a previous incision. There is a risk of skin bridge necrosis between closely adjacent scars and the resulting cosmetic result may be unacceptable (Fig. 9.2). Most surgeons favour reusing a previous

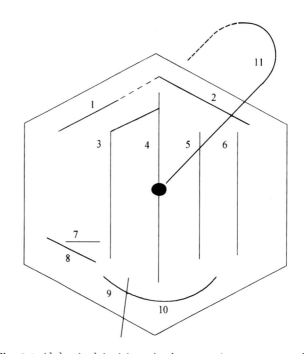

Fig. 9.1 Abdominal incisions (and appropriate surgery undertaken): 1, Kocher's (biliary tree); 2, continuation as 'rooftop' (upper abdomen–pancreas); 3, Rutherford–Morrison (gastroduodenal, biliary); 4, midline (laparotomy); 5, left paramedian (spleen–aorta); 6, left pararectal (spleen–aorta); 7, Lanz (appendix); 8, McBurney's (gridiron); 9, McEvedy (strangulated femoral hernia); 10, Pfannenstiel (pelvis); 11, left thoraco-abdominal (oesophagogastric).

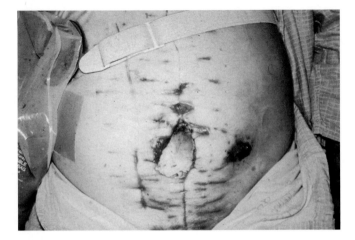

Fig. 9.2 Necrosis of skin bridge between two vertical incisions. (See plate section.)

incision, excising large unsightly scars in the process and resuturing the skin 'as new' at the end of the procedure. Direct comparison of abdominal incisions is difficult because many are not suited for emergency operations in patients who, coincidentally, have the highest complication rates. Traditionally it has been taught that oblique and transverse incisions result in stronger wounds than vertical incisions. This has not been confirmed in a randomized clinical trial, which compared incisional hernia rates after different abdominal incisions, but showed no statistically significant differences in complication rates following any particular incision (48, 49).

Second abdominal operations have inherent difficulties not present at the first procedure. Apart from the siting of the incision, on entering the abdominal cavity the surgeon will have to contend with the inevitable adhesions resulting from the original surgery. By incision and dissection to the deepest fascial layer of the abdominal wound it should be possible to find a plane laterally between the parietal peritoneum and adhesions. Alternatively, if the incision is extended slightly beyond the old scar, it may be possible to find an adhesion-free point of entry into the abdomen.

Vertical

These may be midline, paramedian, or pararectal. Paramedian and pararectal incisions provide access to more lateral abdominal structures (such as the spleen), but little extra length is required of a midline incision to provide similar exposure. These laterally placed vertical incisions are more technically demanding and time consuming than midline incisions to make, and are not appropriate for emergency abdominal surgery. During the period when catgut was the principle suture material used to close the abdominal wall, midline incisions were found to be more prone to wound failure (dehiscence or hernia formation) than lateral incisions. Subsequently, the paramedian incision found favour because a structured, layered closure could be performed, and there was a shutter effect after release of the laterally retracted

rectus muscle, which added to the integrity of the repair (50). Paramedian incisions, which split the rectus muscle, carry a risk of denervation and subsequent reduction in the function of an integral part of the anterior abdominal wall, which perhaps risks incisional herniation. With the development of modern suture materials with more predictable and dependable characteristics than catgut, the midline abdominal incision has become the most frequently used in major abdominal surgery. It is particularly suited to emergency procedures because it is made in a relatively bloodless plane, and is quick and straightforward, particularly in a 'virgin' abdominal wall. The paramedian incision is less commonly used as a primary approach to the abdomen, but it may be appropriate to reuse an old paramedian incision for a re-laparotomy, rather than risk necrosis of the intervening skin bridge if a midline incision is used (Fig. 9.2).

Midline incisions may be extended to any required length between the xiphisternum and the pubis as the situation demands; the umbilicus is skirted, incised, or excised. Further upward extension of the wound can be achieved by splitting or bypassing the xiphisternum and continued extension into the chest is an option for combined thoraco-abdominal procedures.

Transverse

These may be of any length, placed in any quadrant of the abdomen, or extend across the whole width of the abdomen, above or below the umbilicus. Transverse incisions are reputed to heal well, with acceptable cosmetic results, and many surgeons believe they are stronger than vertical wounds. They may be less painful than vertical incisions, and pain is more easily controlled than after vertical wounds; by using 'segmental' regional analgesia less spinal nerve territory is encroached on. Transverse incisions are generally muscle cutting and therefore slower to make, with more blood loss. Although they are not favoured for rapid access to the abdomen in an emergency (laparotomy), the Pfannenstiel incision (a transverse suprapubic incision, which separates rather than cuts the two rectus abdominus muscles) is widely used in gynaecology for both elective and emergency access to the pelvis. It gives limited access if unforeseen complications occur.

Oblique

Oblique incisions are used for access to particular abdominal structures; the most widely recognized being the right subcostal incision for cholecystectomy (Kocher's incision) and right iliac fossa 'gridiron' incision for appendicectomy. The scars in skin following oblique incisions often 'spread' and give poor cosmetic results. Kocher's incision (like many upper abdominal incisions) is associated with considerable postoperative pain. In thin patients with a narrow subcostal angle, an upper midline approach gives as good or better access than a right subcostal; but in obese patients with a wide subcostal angle, the latter approach is favoured. Prior to the advent of laparoscopic cholecystectomy, the transverse right upper quadrant 'mini-laparotomy' incision was popularized for cholecystectomy and is less prone to failure or wound pain, and gives a superior cosmetic result. The 'rooftop' incision is essentially an amalgamation of left and right subcostal incisions and provides good access for gastric, hepatobiliary, and pancreatic procedures. Despite being more difficult and longer to undertake, with division of both rectus abdominus muscles, these incisions heal well.

The classical (McBurney) right iliac fossa 'gridiron' incision for appendicectomy is an oblique, muscle-splitting incision in the direction of the fibres of the external oblique aponeurosis beneath. The skin incision for appendicectomy is now more often made in a cosmetic, more transverse direction (Lanz), by following a skin crease.

Some surgeons advocate an oblique modification of McEvedy's vertical incision for dealing with a complicated femoral hernia. An oblique or transverse groin incision is made in the skin, with the deeper layers being incised in a vertical fashion. This may improve healing with an acceptable cosmetic result because the wound avoids crossing the groin crease.

Types of abdominal surgery

Operations in the abdomen are subdivided into clean, clean–contaminated, contaminated, and dirty procedures (Chapter 7). Failure of wound healing and infection can be related directly to the degree of contamination. Wounds following clean abdominal surgery can be sutured primarily with a satisfactory result. At the 'dirty' end of the operative spectrum more complications of healing occur: contused or heavily contaminated wounds are possibly better left unsutured, to be closed by delayed primary closure or to heal by secondary intention and avoid problems of wound infection and dehiscence. Wounds in the intermediate contamination groups can usually be sutured primarily with appropriate antibiotic prophylaxis and surgical technique.

Choice of suture and techniques for wound closure

The correct choice of suture and suture technique employed to close wounds has been argued about since the earliest references to suture materials were made in the Caraka Samhita 3000 years ago and in the Susruta Samhita 2500 years ago, in which the use of plaited horsehair, cotton, leather strips, and tree bark fibres as materials for closing wounds was first described (Chapter 2; refs 51, 52). Closure of the abdomen involves both closure of skin and restoration of the integrity of the underlying musculo-aponeurotic layers. How to achieve sound, reproducible musculoaponeurotic closure without wound dehiscence, later herniation, stitch abscess, or sinus formation is the challenge.

Sutures are absorbable or non-absorbable and may be monofilament, multifilament, or braided. They come in a variety of diameters with an array of needles (usually swaged on to the suture to facilitate passage through tissue), designed to penetrate a range of different tissues. There are enthusiasts for all types of sutures and needles in all areas of surgery and abdominal wall closure is no exception. Abdominal wall closure may utilize either a layered (53, 54) or a mass closure (55–60) with absorbable or non-absorbable suture materials inserted in a continuous or interrupted fashion. 'Simple' over

and over continuous suturing is most commonly used, although there are enthusiasts for mass closure using the 'near and far' technique (61) first attributed to Smead in 1900, but published by Jones in 1941 (62). In modern surgical practice, the majority of midline abdominal incisions are closed using a continuous mass closure technique, whilst transverse and oblique wounds are closed in layers. The skin is closed according to surgical preference (63), but a subcuticular technique gives the best cosmetic results. There is no advantage in suturing subcutaneous fat as a separate layer as this in no way increases the strength of the wound and merely adds unnecessarily to the volume of implanted suture material (64). The most widely accepted suture materials for mass closure are non-absorbable monofilament sutures such as Nylon or polypropylene, which may be used as a single thread or a loop (to avoid a knot). A few enthusiasts use staples for abdominal wall closure (65).

Stitch sinuses may develop around non-absorbable suture materials (66), particularly in relation to large knots which can irritate and later erode through the skin after healing appears to be complete, especially in cachectic patients. The constant sawing motion of non-absorbable sutures on the rectus sheath may be partly responsible for late herniation and persistent wound pain (67). Synthetic absorbable sutures have been used for abdominal wall closure (including mass closure) to overcome the stitch-sinus problem. There is no evidence to date that the incidence of sinus formation is significantly reduced using absorbable materials; indeed in the presence of wound infection, suture absorption is delayed (68, 69) and sinuses form at least as frequently as with non-absorbable sutures (68, 70). Using absorbable suture materials to close abdominal wounds risks premature absorption of the suture and wound failure. This was certainly the cause of many wound failures when catgut was the suture used in abdominal closure (71). Subsequently, a variety of synthetic absorbable suture materials have been used with varying success (72). In essence, provided absorbable sutures are of large enough diameter and have suitable absorption profiles to preserve wound integrity whilst healing occurs, then they may be used for abdominal wall closure. However, those who advocate abdominal wall closure using non-absorbable suture materials would argue that the results of Jenkins' study of over 1500 abdominal wounds closed with Nylon (in which there was only one dehiscence) is the gold standard by which other techniques and suture materials should be measured (73). Jenkins pioneered the suture–wound length ratio which he established should be at least 4:1 for 'safe' wound closure. This can be achieved by taking 'one centimetre bites, one centimetre apart' with a continuous suture. Subsequent authors have suggested the optimum bite size be increased to 1.2–1.5 cm for maximum security in closing the linea alba (74). Wounds can lengthen up to 30 per cent when the tissues are congested and oedematous after surgery and in the presence of postoperative abdominal distension due to adynamic ileus. If the suture length is insufficient to absorb this increase in wound length then the repair may fail due to sutures breaking or cutting out (73). There are cogent arguments and trial results (58, 60, 66, 68, 75, 76) which proffer advantages to different combinations of sutures and suture techniques.

Personal preference borne out by audited results may be the final arbiter for each surgeon's practise.

The use of a subcuticular suture technique to close the skin improves the cosmetic outcome after surgery (77). It is also quicker and uses less suture material than interrupted methods and overall is associated with fewer wound complications (78, 79). This may be performed using absorbable or non-absorbable materials, although there is a small incidence of suture sinuses developing in relation to knots of absorbable material and probably the best cosmetic result is achieved with non-absorbable material which is removed after skin healing. For quick closures of long incisions, clips or staples may be used (80), but although these save time on insertion they are considerably more expensive than simple sutures (and more time consuming to remove).

For planned re-laparotomy a temporary abdominal wall closure using a polypropylene mesh or zipper has been advocated (81). This has been improved with the use of etappenlavage or second look surgery, which has been shown to have a low morbidity for re-laparotomy (82), although this is controversial.

Wound healing in the abdominal wall

Skin heals by regeneration (although specialized structures such as sweat glands are not regenerated) and the deeper connective tissues heal by repair with the laying down of collagen scar tissue (83). Epithelial regeneration occurs in wounds healing by secondary intention in the same manner as incised wounds healing by primary intention; the difference is one of magnitude. Connective tissue repair occurs in similar processes in incised, primarily sutured wounds as in those healing by secondary intention. Debridement of devitalized tissue with removal of foreign material and contamination with avoidance of systemic, or local, hypoperfusion and hypoxia is the basis for preventing wound infection (Chapters 4, 5, and 7) (84–92). Added to this is the undoubted benefit of prophylactic antibiotics and adequate skin and bowel preparation. If the peritoneum or subcutaneous tissues are heavily contaminated then lavage with saline or weak antiseptic or antibiotic solutions may help to prevent wound infection, although this is controversial (93). Antiseptics retard the formation of granulation tissue *in vitro* and in experimental wounds (Chapter 7) but the 'Listerian' approach of antiseptic lavage during wound closure has been shown significantly to reduce the incidence of infection of orthopaedic prostheses following major joint arthroplasties (94).

Effects of raised intra-abdominal pressure on abdominal wound healing

Raised intra-abdominal pressure (IAP) results in a reduced blood flow to the anterior abdominal wall which can impair wound healing. Doppler assessment of rectus sheath blood flow shows a more than 60 per cent reduction with IAP over 10 mmHg (1.3 kPa) (95). If abdominal wounds are closed under tension, this reduced blood flow may contribute to the increased incidence of wound infection and failure. Cardiac output may also be decreased by high IAP, because venous return is reduced (preload) and systemic vascular resistance is raised (afterload). IAP also reduces thoracic volume and increases intrathoracic pressure. The consequent decrease in lung functional residual capacity (FRC) may lead to hypoxaemia and hypercarbia. Positive pressure ventilation (PPV) is used to overcome this but PPV exacerbates IAP. Further rises in IAP reduces FRC, allowing direct compression of the pulmonary vasculature, increasing the pulmonary vascular resistance, and intensifying the ventilation–perfusion mismatch. Blood flow is also reduced to the renal and splanchnic vascular beds in the presence of high IAP. This results in impaired renal function and permits bacterial translocation from the bowel across a compromised intestinal mucosa.

Intra-abdominal pressure rises in response to severe intra- or retroperitoneal haemorrhage, including that from blunt or penetrating trauma, and after pelvic fractures. Haemorrhagic shock may be followed by significant fluid shifts exacerbated by therapeutic transfusion, which, particularly in association with abdominal injury or surgery, can result in marked peritoneal, visceral, and abdominal wall oedema with intestinal dilatation and 'third space' fluid losses into the bowel lumen. The net result will be a further rise in IAP, a reduction in abdominal wall compliance, and difficulty in closing an abdominal wound without excessive tension. The most common cause of difficult closure of the abdominal wall is intestinal dilatation due to mechanical obstruction or adynamic ileus. Surgery to relieve the obstruction or surgical deflation of distended bowel usually facilitates closure. When it is impossible to close the abdominal wall primarily then saline-soaked or weak antiseptic-soaked gauze packs may be used to cover the exposed viscera and are held in place by loose, all-layer retention sutures. When visceral dilatation and oedema have resolved, abdominal wall compliance may increase enough to allow secondary suture. Alternatively, abdominal wall integrity can be restored using a non-absorbable mesh.

Failure of wound healing

The most dramatic failure of abdominal wall healing, and most catastrophic for the patient, is the 'burst abdomen' (wound dehiscence, evisceration, or eventration – Fig. 9.3). This occurs after less than 1 per cent of all major abdominal incisions in modern surgical practice and this low incidence can be attributed to adoption of the technique of mass closure of the abdominal wall using modern material (58, 96). Dehiscence is the result of suture breakage, knot slippage, cutting out of sutures (97–99) or disruption remote from the site of wound closure. Although there are many mitigating factors for wound dehiscence, such as abdominal distension, infection, or poor wound healing in a compromised patient, the commonest cause is cutting out of sutures placed within the zone of collagenolysis (100–102) at the wound edge, and represents a technical failure of surgery. Wound dehiscence usually occurs 6–10 days following surgery, but has been reported 12 years after laparotomy (103). It carries a mortality of between 10 and 35 per cent (104–107). Dehiscence is frequently preceded by the 'pink sign', a discharge of

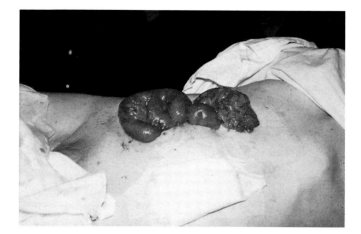

Fig. 9.3 Burst abdomen. (See plate section.)

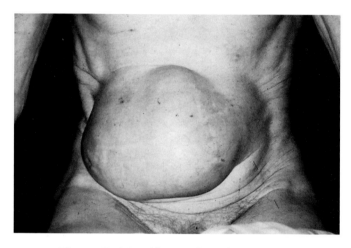

Fig. 9.4 Incisional hernia. (See plate section.)

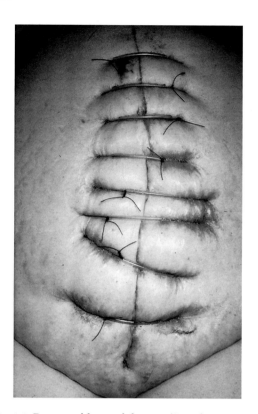

Fig. 9.5 Resutured burst abdomen. (See plate section.)

serosanguinous peritoneal fluid from the abdominal cavity through the wound. There is a complete failure of healing of the deeper layers of the wound and the skin sutures may be all that prevent complete dehiscence. This is rarely painful but the patient, who is often making progress after their surgery, may have an unwelcome surprise! The superficial layers of the wound may heal, despite dehiscence of the deeper layers, but an incisional hernia usually results (Fig. 9.4). If the patient is fit enough the abdominal wall should be resutured.

Alternative techniques to resuture after wound dehiscence have been tried, including packing the wound (to allow healing by secondary intention) and the use of restraining corsets, elastic hosiery, or the 'many-tailed bandage'. Most surgeons, however, opt for immediate resuture of the wound with full relaxation and general anaesthetic, provided gross contamination or infection is not present as an incisional hernia may be preventable. All-layers mass closure, including the skin, with interrupted non-absorbable monofilament suture material is the technique of choice (Fig. 9.5). Alternatively, the abdominal wall can be resutured by mass closure taking wider bites of musculoaponeurotic tissue using a continuous tech-

nique and suturing the skin separately. The routine use of all-layer 'deep-tension' sutures for primary closure of wounds at risk is controversial; some consider that they merely 'treat the surgeon' and in reality cause more pain, making the siting of stomas difficult, strangle the wound, impeding healing and risking enterocutaneous fistula formation (95, 108–111). Others maintain that the support given by such sutures is essential if difficult wounds are to heal (112). The usual material used for deep-tension sutures is a heavy nylon inserted with a large curved needle. Plastic splints are used to protect the skin wound. Other materials have been used, for example, lengths of plastic infusion tubing led through rubber corks to prevent slippage (113) and adjustable nylon ties, originally designed to hold electric wiring and close the top of rubbish sacks! (114).

Incisional hernias occur in up to 10 per cent of abdominal wounds (58, 70, 115) after ten years, with two thirds of these being evident within five years of surgery (116–119). Risk factors for hernia development include infection (58, 97, 120), obesity (121), metabolic disorders, hypoxia, immunosuppressive treatments, previous abdominal surgery (122), wound dehiscence, or a previous incisional hernia. However, the precise aetiology of many hernias appearing a year or more after surgery is unclear (123). Early incisional hernias tend to be larger than those appearing later, and a third of these are symptomatic (116). Whilst there is no need to contemplate repair if they are causing few symptoms, incisional hernias associated with pain or intestinal obstruction, particularly if large and loculated as a result of adhesions, require intervention. Repair of large incisional hernias can be difficult, both in the freeing of incarcerated bowel loops and in the definitive repair of the anterior abdominal wall defect. If the edges of the abdominal wall defect can be opposed and primarily sutured by mass closure, then this is the best method of repair (124). When the defect is large or if there is tissue loss (including that caused by the surgical raising of tissue flaps, for example the transverse rectus abdominus myocutaneous flap used for breast reconstruction), repair using a non-absorbable mesh may be required (125). Mesh closures have inherent risks, particularly related to wound infection, with extrusion of the mesh or the necessity for surgical removal of the mesh to allow resolution of infection. Omental interposition or peritoneal closure over the bowel should be attempted to prevent direct contact of bowel with the mesh. Various different types of mesh are available. Polytetra-fluoroethylene (PTFE) or polypropylene mesh are the most appropriate. Absorbable mesh, for example polyglycolic acid mesh, reduces the incidence of infection, extrusion, and enterocutaneous fistula formation, but the high incidence of late incisional hernias occurring after their use is unacceptable. Recurrence of incisional hernias after repair is common, reaching over 40 per cent in many series (116, 122, 126).

Incisional hernias have been recognized through the 5 and 10 mm port incisions of laparoscopic surgery (127). Although this is uncommon, formal sutured repair of laparoscopic abdominal wall incisions is recommended.

The gastrointestinal tract

Introduction

Wound healing assumes critical significance in the surgery of the gastrointestinal tract. Complications of healing, such as anastomotic dehiscence, are accompanied by serious morbidity and a significant mortality rate. Any of the factors known to influence wound healing may compromise healing of wounds of the abdominal viscera, but there is a growing body of evidence that the experience or expertise of the surgeon may be the most important determinant of success or failure after gastrointestinal surgery (128, 129). The dangers of the 'occasional' surgeon have been identified by Devlin (130) in an analysis of the findings of the confidential enquiry into perioperative deaths (131). According to Devlin, a significant problem in the UK is that surgeons are inclined to undertake procedures with which they are unfamiliar rather than refer such cases to specialists with greater experience. The problem areas for wound healing in the gastrointestinal tract are in the surgery of the oesophagus, large intestine (particularly low anterior resection and pouch operations), liver, biliary tract, and the pancreas. Such surgery should be undertaken only by surgeons who have a special interest and expertise in these fields.

Intestinal anastomoses

The fundamental requirements for successful anastomoses in the alimentary canal are a good blood supply to the anastomosis, avoidance of tension at the suture line, and secure inversion of the cut edges of the gut. These are simple technical factors but they require good judgement and surgical experience.

Careful inversion of the mucosal edges of the suture line is required for secure anastomosis of the intestine. Experiments with everting techniques of suture which deliberately allow the mucosa to pout through the suture line have proved to be unsuccessful in animals (132) and humans (133), and it appears that the absence of peritoneal or serosal continuity in the everting anastomosis is an important factor in the high incidence of dehiscence associated with this technique. Techniques of an inverting suture vary but many surgeons now use a single layer of sutures which includes all layers of the bowel wall except the mucosa (Fig. 9.6). This technique is referred to as a serosubmucosal suture and it may be regarded as the optimal technique for anastomoses in the large intestine (134, 135). The collagenous submucosal layer of the intestine is the only layer of the bowel wall with significant suture-holding capacity. The rationale for the single-layer anastomosis is that it causes less disturbance to the blood supply of the suture line and less narrowing of the lumen of the bowel than the two-layer method.

The choice of suture material in anastomosis of the intestine varies according to the preference of the surgeon. In recent years there has been a trend towards the use of synthetic absorbable materials such as polglycolic acid (Dexon®), polyglactin (Vicryl®), or polydioxanone (PDS®). However, there is little to choose between the various suture materials. Excellent results have been reported with a wide range of sutures, including stainless steel wire (136, 137). The intestinal wound or anastomosis requires the support of sutures for a relatively limited period assuming that there are no coexisting factors which may impair or delay intestinal healing. The normal pattern of wound repair is shown in Fig. 9.7. There is

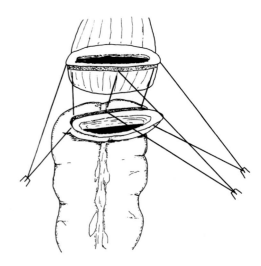

Fig. 9.6 The serosubmucosal suture in colorectal anastomosis. The suture incorporates the strong collagenous submucosal layer of the bowel.

Plate Section

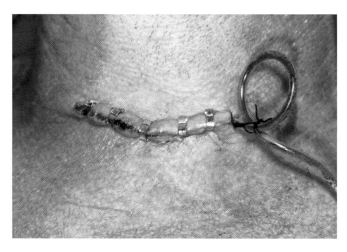

Fig. 2.6 Michel clips to close a collar incision after thyroidectomy.

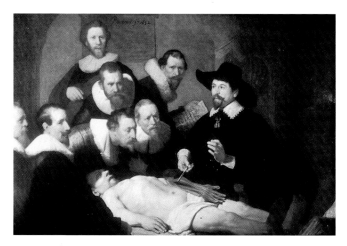

Fig. 2.7 The anatomy lesson of Dr Tulp (Rembrandt).

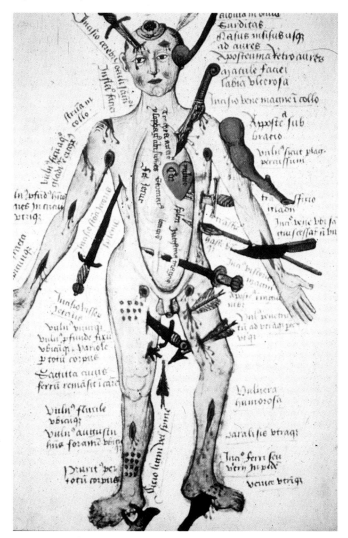

Fig. 2.8 The 'wound man'.

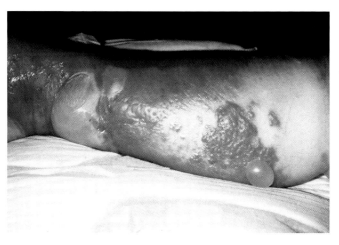

Fig. 7.3 Spreading cellulitis from a puncture wound of the ankle.

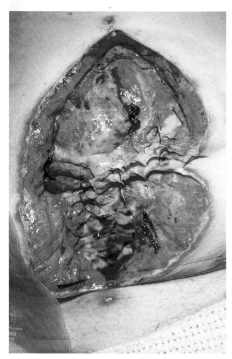

Fig. 7.4 Major wound infection.

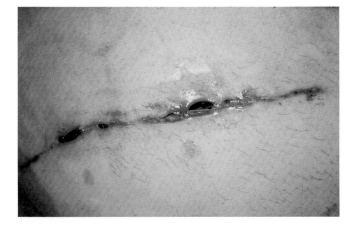

Fig. 7.5 Minor wound infection.

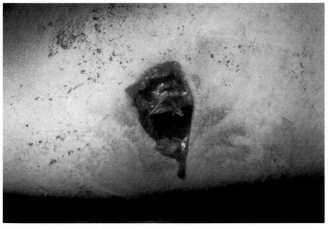

(a)

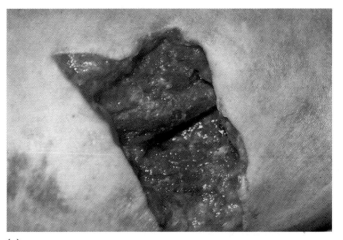

(c)

Fig. 8.1 Thigh wound (a) before and (b) after debridement; (c) clean and granulating.

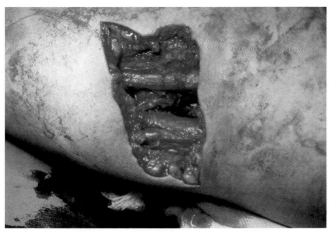

(b)

Fig. 8.2 Not all foreign bodies are as obvious as this length of wood embedded in the thigh from a bomb blast.

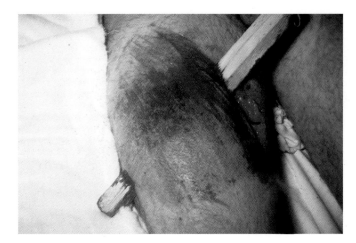

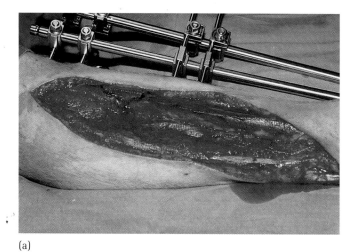

(a)

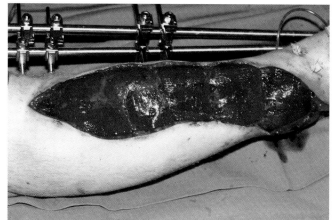

(b)

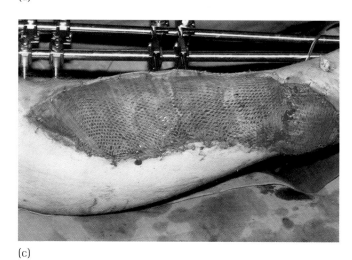

(c)

Fig. 8.3 (a) Large soft tissue defect over a fractured tibia and fibula; (b) The soft tissue defect covered with a free rectus muscle flap; and (c) the muscle flap covered with a meshed split skin graft.

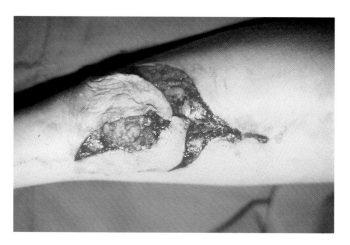

Fig. 8.4 A pretibial laceration.

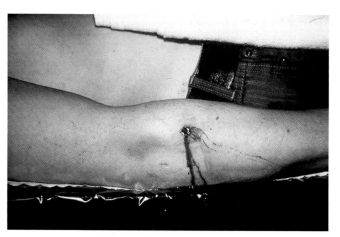

Fig. 8.6 A low velocity bullet wound to the arm.

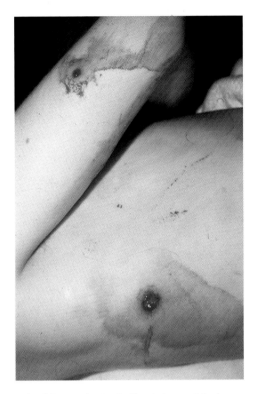

Fig. 8.7 A fatal low velocity bullet injury with the entrance in the arm and exit wound in the anterior chest wall.

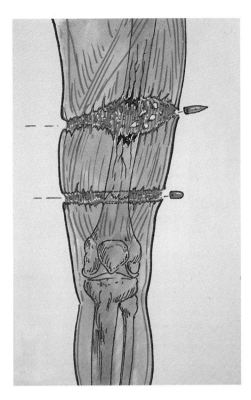

Fig. 8.8 Diagram illustrating the different wounding capabilities of a low and high velocity bullet in the lower limb.

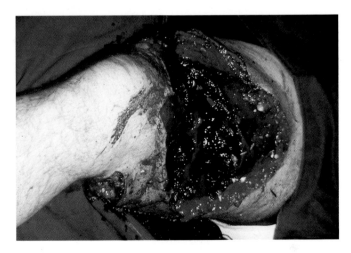

Fig. 8.9 Massive exit wound that can be created by a high velocity bullet.

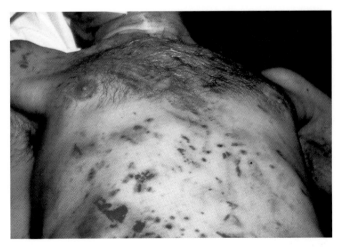

Fig. 8.12 Peppering due to secondary missiles from a bomb blast.

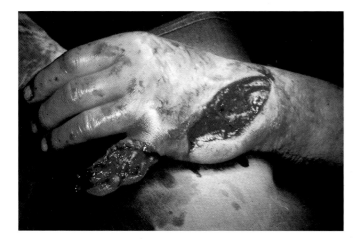

Fig. 8.13 Blast injury to the hand.

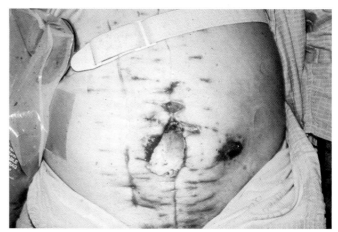

Fig. 9.2 Necrosis of skin bridge between two vertical incisions.

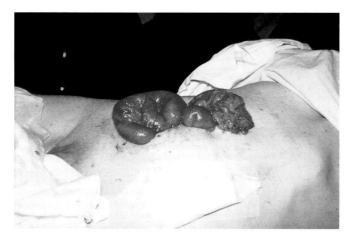

Fig. 9.3 Burst abdomen.

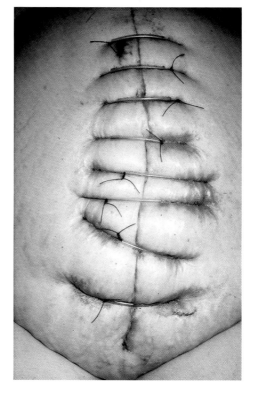

Fig. 9.5 Resutured burst abdomen.

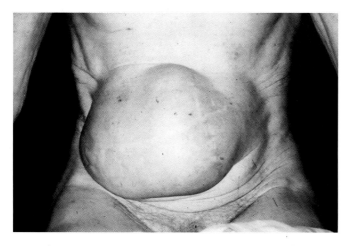

Fig. 9.4 Incisional hernia.

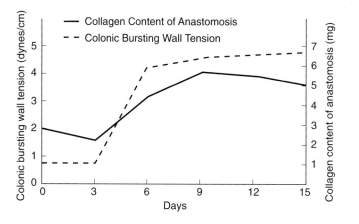

Fig. 9.7 Changes in the collagen content (solid line) and mechanical strength (point line) of the colonic anastomosis. A slight reduction in tensile strength during the first few days of healing is due to lysis of collagen in the edges of the wound.

a latent period following anastomosis of the intestine which lasts several days when there is no active wound healing, there is lysis of collagen in the wound edges, and the integrity of the intestinal suture line is entirely dependent on the support of the wound sutures. This brief period is followed by a proliferative phase of healing during which collagen and the other constituents of connective tissue repair are synthesized in large quantities and this is accompanied by a rapid decrease in the tensile strength of the anastomosis. Within ten days, the strength of the anastomosis is largely independent of the presence of suture materials. It follows, therefore, that there is no particular logic in using suture materials which retain their tensile strength for long or indefinite periods. The handling characteristics and ease of knotting are probably more important considerations in the choice of suture material.

In recent years surgeons have had the option of using stapling instruments rather than sutures for end-to-end anastomosis of the intestine. Modern stapling 'guns' enable secure anastomoses to be created with speed and relative simplicity. However, there is no evidence that such anastomoses have greater security or safety than hand-sewn anastomosis of the intestine in areas where surgical access may be difficult, such as anastomoses of the oesophagus or in low colorectal anastomoses. Stapling techniques for anastomosis may have a wider application as laparoscopic resections of the intestine are increasingly undertaken.

Sutureless techniques of intestinal anastomosis have rarely progressed beyond experimental studies. An exception is the Valtrac™ biofragmentable anastomosis ring (138). This device is composed of polyglycolic acid polymer and barium sulphate and it disintegrates in 16–23 days. The ring is secured by purse-string sutures of PDS placed in the cut edges of the bowel and it creates a secure inverted 'anastomosis' with serosal apposition. In a multicentre study of 101 anastomoses of the large bowel created with this technique there were only two cases of anastomotic dehiscence (139). A disadvantage

of the method at present is that it is unsuitable for low colorectal anastomosis.

Recent experimental studies have suggested that secure anastomoses of the intestine may be created by laser welding (140, 141), and this method may find a place in clinical practice with new advances in laser technology (142).

Problems of healing in oesophagus and colon

Anastomoses in the oesophagus and large intestine are associated with a particularly high incidence of failure and surgical mortality, and there are cogent arguments that the surgery of the oesophagus or large intestine should be undertaken only by surgeons who have specialist expertise in these areas.

In the UK large bowel cancer project, Fielding and his colleagues (128) studied the outcome of 1466 large bowel anastomoses performed by 84 surgeons in 23 hospitals and the incidence of anastomotic dehiscence in the hands of different surgeons ranged from 0.5 per cent to more than 30 per cent. Again, in a study of 1119 oesophageal resections in the West Midlands, Matthews and his colleagues (129) suggested that the experience of the surgeon was an important determinant of operative mortality. Surgeons performing three or less than three resections per year had an average operative mortality of 39 per cent whereas those who performed more than six resections per year had a mortality rate of 21 per cent.

What makes anastomoses of these organs so difficult or dangerous and how can the risks be minimized?

Oesophageal anastomoses

The factors which may be significant in anastomosis of the oesophagus are surgical access, the anatomy of the oesophagus, and the local and systemic effects of anastomotic dehiscence.

Surgical access

It is usually necessary to perform the anastomosis within the chest cavity and this is clearly a less satisfactory state of affairs than, for example, an anastomosis of the small intestine in which the ends of the intestine can be delivered to the skin surface.

Surgical anatomy

The wall of the oesophagus comprises an outer layer of longitudinal muscle, a submucosal layer, and an inner layer of oesophageal mucosa, which are not an optimal arrangement for suturing or stapling. The submucosal layer is thinner and has a much lower suture-holding capacity than the equivalent layer in the stomach, small intestine, or colon, and the mucosal layer of the oesophagus thus has greater significance in the suture of oesophageal anastomoses. Moreover, the longitudinal muscle of the oesophagus has a relatively poor capacity to hold sutures or staples.

The longitudinal orientation of the blood supply along the wall of the oesophagus is also a significant consideration in anastomoses. Care must be taken to avoid over-zealous mobilization of the oesophagus lest the blood supply to the anastomosis is compromised.

Anastomotic dehiscence

A major leak from an oesophageal anastomosis within the chest will result in a spreading mediastinitis, septicaemia, and death. A small proportion of patients may be salvaged by prompt surgical intervention. In cases of gross leakage this will involve drainage of the mediastinum, further oesophageal resection, and some arrangement which prevents further contamination of the chest cavity, such as a cervical oesophagectomy and abdominal gastrostomy. The mortality risk associated with the disruption of intrathoracic oesophageal anastomoses has been a significant factor in the development of the technique of transhiatal oesophagectomy (143). In this method the whole of the intrathoracic oesophagus is removed blindly by blunt dissection through the abdominal hiatus and an anastomosis is created in the neck between the cervical oesophagus and the stomach. Although anastomotic leaks are not uncommon, the consequences are generally less serious than leakage from an intrathoracic anastomosis. However, there are other risks attached to the transhiatal method (144) and it may give less effective clearance for oesophageal cancer (145).

There is a large variation in the mortality of oesophageal resection reported from different centres. The average mortality rates in published series from the USA and UK are 12 per cent and 16 per cent respectively (146) but mortality rates are undoubtedly influenced by the proportion of palliative operations and international comparisons are probably inappropriate. It would appear that the 'gold standard' for oesophageal resection is a mortality rate of around 4 per cent (147). The results suggest that there is probably little to choose between hand-sewn or stapled anastomoses (148–151) although postoperative stricture formation may be more common with the latter (152).

Large bowel anastomoses

The factors which have been implicated in the dehiscence of large-bowel anastomoses are emergency operations for acute complications of colonic disease (153, 154), faecal loading of the colon (155), and the operation of low anterior resection of the rectum (156).

Emergency operations

Operations performed for obstruction or perforation of the intestine are associated with an increased mortality by comparison with elective surgery. Elective operations are associated with mortality rates of 1–3 per cent whereas the mortality after emergency operations may exceed 20 per cent (157, 158). Much of this mortality is related to factors unassociated with the colonic anastomosis (154) but there is an increased incidence of dehiscence of anastomoses in emergency operations, particularly when primary anastomosis is performed after emergency resection of the left colon.

Faecal loading of the colon

It has been suggested that the problems of colonic anastomosis in emergency operations are largely due to the unprepared state of the bowel, although coexisting peritoneal sepsis is undoubtedly an important adverse factor in cases of colonic perforation (159). The risks of colonic anastomosis in the presence of faecal loading prompted Dudley and colleagues (160), to introduce a method of on-table lavage of the intestine, and clinical trials have suggested that the technique does remove much of the risk associated with primary anastomosis of the unprepared colon in emergency operations (161). Ravo (162) has approached the problem of the unprepared intestine in a different way with the development of an intracolonic bypass tube. Using absorbable sutures, this device is sewn into the bowel proximal to the left-sided anastomosis and it effectively prevents contact between the suture line and the colonic contents until it separates and is expelled spontaneously after two weeks. Despite these innovations, primary anastomosis of the left colon is a suitable procedure in only a minority of patients undergoing emergency operations for obstruction and probably not at all in cases of established colonic perforation. Many of these patients are elderly and already suffering from serious coexisting medical disorders. The appropriate treatment in most cases is a primary resection and end colostomy.

Low anterior resection

Most of the problems with elective anastomoses in the large intestine occur after the operation of low anterior resection in which the colon is joined to a short stump of rectum deep in the pelvis. In many respects the problems bear a similarity to those encountered in oesophageal anastomosis: access may be difficult; and, like the oesophagus, the rectum is a muscular tube devoid of a serosal coat. There is the added problem in low colorectal anastomoses of an infective bowel content, and faecal loading of the colon had been regarded as an adverse factor in the healing of these anastomoses (155). However, recent reports of this operation suggest that it can be performed with considerable safety and associated mortality rates of around 3 per cent (163, 164).

It is not easy to define the factors which have made anterior resection a safer procedure. The experience of the St Mary's large bowel cancer project (128) would suggest that the expertise of the surgeon may be the most significant factor but various aspects of surgical practice may be involved, including the preparation of the intestine, antimicrobial therapy, the methods of anastomosis, prevention of pelvic haematoma, and diversion of the faecal stream.

1. Preparation of the intestine. Preoperative mechanical preparation of the large intestine is standard practice before elective colorectal resections. Recently, the wisdom of this policy has been challenged (165) and there may be a case for a prospective study of the value of bowel preparation in low anterior resection (166). Meanwhile, most surgeons will continue to believe that effective mechanical preparation of the intestine is a significant safety factor in colorectal surgery.

2. Antimicrobial therapy. Recognition of the importance of *Bacteroides* species in the pathogenesis of septic complications after colorectal surgery has led to the introduction of more effective regimens of preoperative oral antimicrobial therapy and a reduction in wound sepsis after large-bowel resection (167). It has also been shown that the short term

use of intravenous broad-spectrum antibiotics during the perioperative period leads to a reduction in the septic complications of colonic surgery (168). A combination of metronidazole and a cephalosporin or aminoglycoside is generally preferred, and it has been suggested that such therapy is more effective than the use of oral antimicrobial agents before surgery (169). However, other studies have suggested that the perioperative use of intravenous antibiotics does not replace the requirement for traditional methods of intestinal preparation (170). Whilst there is convincing evidence that such therapy results in a reduction in the incidence of wound sepsis after colorectal surgery, it is less clear that it makes any difference to anastomotic healing or the incidence of anastomotic disruption.

3. Methods of anastomosis. The options are a single-layer sutured anastomosis or stapled anastomosis and, in practice, the choice is frequently determined by the personal preference and experience of the surgeon. There is no evidence that the stapled anastomosis is inherently safer, and the incidence of disruption in sutured and stapled anastomoses is very similar (171, 172). The attractions of the stapled anastomosis are that it is quicker and easier to perform than a hand-sewn anastomosis provided that the surgeon is familiar with the mechanical aspects of the stapling gun and the safety rules. The standard method of end-to-end stapled anastomosis involves the insertion of purse-string sutures in the cut ends of

the colon and rectum, and the 'anvil' and cartridge of staples are enclosed within the colon and rectum before the instrument is fired and the anastomosis completed. An easier method of stapled anastomosis involves the use of two stapling instruments and avoids the need for a purse-string suture in the rectum (Fig. 9.8) (173, 174). The rectum is divided and closed at the selected level with a transverse stapling instrument. Next, an end-to-end stapling gun with a detachable anvil is used to create an anastomosis between the stapled rectum and the end of the colon. The advantage of the technique is that it avoids the requirement to introduce a purse-string suture in a short and relatively inaccessible rectal stump. A potential disadvantage is the concern that the T-junction between the stapled rectum and the colorectal anastomosis may be potentially weak and some surgeons insert an outer layer of seromuscular sutures to cover the stapled closure. However, studies have shown that this double stapling technique is at least as safe as single stapled end-to-end anastomoses and it is simpler and quicker to perform (175). It is probably wise, but not critical, to test the integrity of the stapled closure by air insufflation of the rectal stump. Such tests may detect small leaks which can be repaired by simple suture without adverse clinical sequelae (166).

4. Prevention of pelvic haematoma. The operation of low anterior resection creates a considerable dead space in the pelvis with a potential for the accumulation of blood or serum. Such collections are regarded as a potent cause of anastomotic dehiscence and have led to the routine use of postoperative drains in the presacral space (176). An alternative or complementary method is to obliterate the presacral dead space by placing the mobilized greater omentum in the pelvis, and it is claimed that peritoneal drains may be unnecessary when this method is used (177).

5. Faecal diversion. The need to divert the faecal stream after low anterior resection remains the subject of considerable controversy with arguments for and against the use of a proximal stoma. However, the evidence suggests that there is an 8 per cent incidence of major anastomotic leaks and faecal peritonitis if the anastomosis is not defunctioned (178, 179). It has been suggested that a temporary loop ileostomy may be preferable to a transverse colostomy (180, 181). An ileostomy may be more acceptable to the patient and it is alleged that closure of this stoma is associated with fewer complications than closure of a colostomy (181). However, colostomy closure should be a safe uncomplicated operation (182) whereas closure of an ileostomy is the more hazardous procedure.

Anastomotic strictures

Stricture formation is uncommon after conventional sutured anastomoses in the gastrointestinal tract. Experimental studies have shown that two-layer inverting anastomoses cause more narrowing of the bowel lumen than single-layer anastomoses, at least during the early phase of healing (183), but this appears to have little significance in clinical practice. The factors which appear to be significant in stricture formation are anastomotic disruption, eversion of the suture line, stapled methods of anastomosis, and irradiation injuries of the bowel.

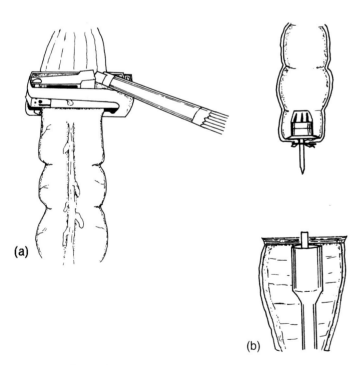

(a)

(b)

Fig. 9.8 Colorectal anastomosis by the double stapling method. (a) Transverse stapling: the rectum is divided flush with the edge of the stapler after the application of a proximal occlusion clamp. (b) An end-to-end stapler is used to create an end-to-end anastomosis between the colon and rectal stump.

Anastomotic disruption

Most colorectal surgeons have encountered anastomotic strictures as one of the sequelae of leakage from colorectal anastomoses and, in general, the severity of the stricture is proportional to the extent of the anastomotic disruption. The pathogenesis of the stricture would appear to be the excessive fibrous tissue which occurs as a result of granulation tissue formation and healing of the anastomosis by secondary intention.

Eversion of the suture line

The protagonists of everting anastomoses claimed that such techniques were bound to cause less narrowing of the bowel lumen than the standard inverting methods of suture (184, 185) but in clinical practice the everting anastomosis is associated with an unacceptable incidence of stricture formation (186). Again, the mechanism would appear to be excessive fibrosis resulting from the sequelae of anastomotic disruption. Everting anastomoses are associated with a high incidence of anastomotic leakage and perianastomotic sepsis (132, 133).

Stapled anastomoses

It is now recognized that stapled anastomoses are associated with a higher incidence of stricture formation than hand-sutured anastomoses although the mechanism of the stricture formation is obscure. Significant stenoses occur in about 10 per cent of stapled colorectal anastomoses (187, 188). The incidence of stricture formation in stapled oesophageal anastomoses seems to be higher in oesophagogastric anastomoses than in oesophagojejunal anastomoses (154).

Experimental studies have suggested that stapled anastomoses are associated with more necrosis and inflammation than hand-sewn anastomoses, and these observations may explain why strictures are more common in the former (189). However, some surgeons believe that strictures in stapled anastomoses are simply due to the use of too small a stapler (154, 187).

Irradiation

Experienced surgeons are familiar with the fact that irradiated tissues heal poorly, and anastomoses in irradiated bowel are associated with an increased incidence of leakage and stricture formation. In general, the problems are encountered in bowel which has been deliberately or inadvertently exposed to therapeutic doses of irradiation. Problems are rarely encountered with the radiation doses used in adjuvant therapy for rectal cancer. The basic injury in bowel affected by irradiation is an endarteritis obliterans of the blood vessels but strictures may result from disruption of the suture line and healing by secondary intention.

Biliary tract and liver

The specialty of hepatobiliary surgery has emerged in recent years with a new generation of surgeons specializing in liver resection and the surgery of the bile ducts. The apparent safety and the low mortality associated with these complex procedures are testimony to the skills of the surgeons but it must be emphasized that such skills are acquired only in

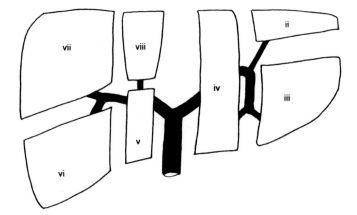

Fig. 9.9 The segmental anatomy of the liver, showing the eight segments of the two lobes.

specialist units. Hepatobiliary surgery is a regional or supraregional specialty and it is not a field which should be entered occasionally by inexperienced surgeons. The areas of interest in wound healing are liver injuries, liver resections, and the surgery of the bile ducts. The major advances in liver surgery and the surgery of the intra- and extrahepatic bile ducts are largely due to the recognition of the segmental anatomy of the liver and its significance in hepatobiliary surgery (Fig. 9.9).

Liver injury

Injuries of the liver are caused by stab wounds, high-velocity missiles, and blunt trauma. Blunt trauma, mostly road traffic accidents, is by far the most common cause of liver injury in the UK.

Blunt trauma to the liver may result in simple or stellate lacerations of the liver parenchyma and variable damage to the intrahepatic blood vessels and bile ducts. Haemorrhage is the major problem in all significant injuries of the liver and is proportional to the complexity and depth of the injury in the liver substance. Lacerations of the major blood vessels within the liver may result in rapid exsanguination, particularly when the major hepatic veins are involved.

Fortunately, the majority of liver injuries which result from blunt trauma can be managed without the need for liver resection. Simple lacerations with little continuing blood loss may be left alone or repaired with atraumatic mattress sutures of catgut mounted on a blunt-nosed needle. More complex or deeper lacerations of the liver substance, associated with significant blood loss, are often associated with a coagulopathy and should be treated by packing in the first instance. It is a mistake to pack the actual defect in the liver: this simply creates further separation of the liver parenchyma and encourages continuing bleeding. Packs should be placed around the liver in a fashion which supports the organ and brings the edges of the laceration together.

Nearly all blunt injuries of the liver can be managed by primary packing and, if necessary, the patient can be transferred to a specialist hepatobiliary unit with the packs *in situ* (190). All patients should receive broad-spectrum parenteral antibiotics because of the risk of infection. The packs are removed after 48 h at a second operation and further management depends on the presence or absence of re-bleeding. Haemorrhage from the liver substance may require further packing, hepatic artery ligation, or liver resection depending on the circumstances.

Liver resections are required when blood loss cannot be controlled by packing or by arterial ligation or embolization. When possible, segmental liver resections are performed rather than formal hepatectomy (191), the latter being associated with a formidable mortality (192, 193).

Liver resection

Various types of liver resection are now common practice in the management of malignancies and these range from resections of small segments to the removal of all of the right lobe and parts of the left lobe of the liver (trisegmentectomy). The liver has a considerable capacity for regeneration and major resections are remarkably well tolerated. Experimental studies have shown that mitosis occurs in parenchymal cells 24 h following liver resection and after 48 h in nonparenchymatous sinusoidal cells, the epithelium of bile ductules, connective tissue, and blood vessels (194). The rate of regeneration is partly related to the amount of functioning tissue lost but the process appears to be under hormonal control (195, 196) and insulin appears to be of particular importance (197).

The safety of liver resection is dependent on the expertise of the staff caring for the patient and the use of specialist equipment in the surgical operation. Proper case selection and preoperative evaluation are essential in the assessment of potential candidates. Greater surgical precision and reduced blood loss are achieved with the intraoperative use of ultrasound scanners (198) and the ultrasonic liver dissector (199).

Surgery of the bile ducts

In the western hemisphere, operations on the bile ducts are mostly required for cholelithiasis, primary or secondary malignancies, and iatrogenic injuries. Injuries to the bile ducts most frequently occur during the operation of cholecystectomy, the incidence being of the order of 1 in 300–500 open procedures (200). The incidence of ductal injury is higher after laparoscopic cholecystectomy (201). It is rarely possible to restore continuity of the bile ducts by direct anastomosis after deliberate or inadvertent resection of a segment and the usual practice is to create an anastomosis between the proximal cut end and the upper intestine, usually a Roux loop of jejunum. Problems of wound healing chiefly arise in the treatment of bile duct injuries and in resections of the bile duct for primary malignancies. These problems are largely due to the difficulties in access experienced in lesions or injuries in the liver hilum, and the remarkable propensity for stricture formation in anastomoses of the bile duct (202, 203).

Surgical access

Problems of access to the ducts in the porta hepatis and the difficulties of mucosal suture resulted in the development of the ingenious 'mucosal graft' technique of biliary–enteric anastomosis, a method which has enjoyed considerable success in the treatment of high bile duct strictures (204). However, this method has been largely superseded by other methods of intrahepatic cholangio-enteric anastomosis. Access to the intrahepatic ducts may be achieved by splitting the liver in the relatively avascular plane between the right lobe and medial segment of the left lobe (205) and this approach is used in the management of difficult benign strictures of the bile duct and in the resection of cholangiocarcinomas arising in the liver hilum (Klatskin tumour). Alternatively, obstruction of the extrahepatic bile ducts by benign or malignant lesions may be relieved by anastomosis of the intestine to the left hepatic duct either in the umbilical fissure (206) or in liver segment iii (Fig. 9.9) (207).

Stricture formation

Anastomoses of the bile ducts have a notorious reputation for stricture formation (204) but the factors involved in the pathogenesis of biliary strictures are somewhat obscure. Experimental studies have shown that transection and resuture of the bile duct is followed by the formation of excessive quantities of granulation tissue and a high rate of stricture formation (206), and it has been suggested that ischaemia and the noxious effects of bile may be responsible for these strictures. It has been shown that the biliary epithelium is highly susceptible to anoxic damage (207) and the anatomy of the blood supply to the extrahepatic ducts is such that it may be rather vulnerable to surgical damage (208). Evidence that bile may be involved in the pathogenesis of strictures stems from experimental observations that proximal biliary diversion prevents stricture formation in biliary anastomoses in dogs (209), and that bile simulates collagen synthesis and the formation of fibrous tissue (210, 211). Moreover, experimental studies have suggested that infected bile is particularly prone to cause stricture formation (212). The messages which emerge from these studies are that care should be taken to ensure that there is an adequate blood supply to the biliary anastomosis, that there is careful mucosal apposition of the suture line, and that steps are taken to limit any leakage of bile. It has been customary to splint or stent biliary anastomoses with indwelling tubes, largely because of the fear of stricture formation. Some surgeons retain their transhepatic splinting tubes for many months after surgery. In modern surgical practice, however, most surgeons retain splinting tubes for only a few weeks and the functions of the tube are to provide decompression of the biliary system in the early postoperative period and access for postoperative cholangiography.

All patients undergoing surgical operations on the bile ducts should be given broad-spectrum antibiotics, and nutritional support should be provided after surgery. It is recognized that some jaundiced patients are at an increased risk of complications of wound healing (213) and it appears that this is related to their poor nutritional status (214).

Pancreas

Ligation of the pancreatic duct in experimental animals is followed by destruction and atrophy of the acinar tissue, but the islet cells remain intact. Partial resection of the pancreas is followed by some degree of hypertrophy and hyperplasia of the acinar tissue and islet cells (215, 216) but the recovery is very modest by comparison with the changes which follow hepatic resection. The complications of pancreatic wound healing are mainly related to leakage from the pancreatic ducts or a secondary pancreatitis. The release of pancreatic secretions may have serious consequences: abscess formation and Gram-negative septicaemia are probable complications; and the proteolytic activity of the pancreatic secretion may result in the disruption of gastrointestinal anastomoses.

Pancreatic trauma

Isolated injuries of the pancreas are uncommon, with a mortality rate of 3–10 per cent. More often, the injury is associated with injuries to other organs and a higher overall mortality: 22 per cent with penetrating injuries; and 19 per cent with blunt injury (217). Injuries range from simple contusions with minimal parenchymal damage to complex combined pancreatico-duodenal injuries, which can be ranked into four grades of severity (218). The recommended methods of management (219–21) of these different categories are shown in Table 9.1.

Elective pancreatic resection

Elective resections of the pancreas are mainly performed for malignancies or chronic pancreatitis.

Table 9.1 Grades of pancreatic injury and methods of management

Grade	Definition	Surgical management
I	Simple contusion with minimal parenchymal damage	Simple drainage; possibly sump drains for 10 days
II	Deep lacerations with transection of body or tail of gland	Sump drainage if duct is intact. Resection for ductal damage. Suture of gland or repair of duct is impracticable
III	Severe crush, perforation, or transection of head and ductal damage	Sump drainage. On-lay Roux loop of jejunum if duct damaged
IV	Combined pancreatico-duodenal injuries	Pancreaticoduodenectomy has unacceptable mortality. Options are: (a) on-lay Roux loop of jejunum (b) duodenal diversion either by pyloric exclusion[1] or duodenal diverticulization[2]

[1] Suture of pylorus with polyglactin (Vicryl) and gastrojejunostomy.
[2] Duodenal repair, vagotomy, antrectomy, gastrojejunostomy and tube duodenostomy.

Distal resection

Resections of the tail or body and tail of the pancreas are generally associated with fewer complications than resections of the head of the pancreas although there is still some debate concerning the optimal method of management of the pancreatic stump. The reported incidence of pancreatic fistula ranges from 6 to 30 per cent (218, 222). The standard management of the pancreatic stump involves ligature of the pancreatic duct and closure of the stump with non-absorbable mattress sutures. More recently, lateral stapling instruments have been used to close the pancreatic stump, with or without ligation of the duct, and it appears that such techniques are associated with a low morbidity (218, 219, 223, 224). Drainage of the pancreatic stump into a defunctioned loop of jejunum appears to offer no significant advantage (225, 226) but mass ligature of the pancreatic stump with stout non-absorbable ligatures may be as safe as any method (227).

Proximal resection

Between 15 and 20 per cent of malignant tumours of the head of pancreas are resectable (228), and the mortality rate of such surgery worldwide is probably around 20 per cent (229). Much of this mortality is related to complications associated with the pancreatico-enteric anastomosis, and has prompted some surgeons to perform total pancreatectomy for tumours of the pancreatic head, thereby avoiding the problems of pancreatic anastomosis. However, total pancreatectomy has other disadvantages and it is apparent that specialists in pancreatic surgery can achieve remarkably low mortality rates following pancreaticoduodenectomy (230, 231).

Most surgeons anastomose the pancreatic remnant to the proximal jejunum either proximal or distal to the choledochojejunal anastomosis and this may be achieved either by infolding the pancreatic stump into the end of the jejunum or by lateral anastomosis to the jejunum. Whichever method is used, it is advisable to divert the pancreatic secretions away from the anastomosis with a splinting tube in the pancreatic duct.

Spleen

The spleen is an organ which is frequently damaged by blunt trauma to the abdomen and, occasionally, it is inadvertently damaged in the course of elective surgical operations in the upper abdomen. The extent of the injury ranges from a minor laceration of the splenic pulp or a capsular tear to a complete disruption of the organ or avulsion from its vascular pedicle. The splenic tissue and capsule of the spleen are not readily amenable to suture or repair and the standard surgical treatment for most splenic injuries has been total splenectomy. However, the spleen has a major role in humoral and cell-mediated immunity and splenectomy is followed by an increased risk of serious or fatal infection, particularly in young children (232, 233). Post-splenectomy infection usually occurs within two years of surgery but may occur up to 25 years after operation (234). The overall risk is 2.5 per cent (235) but it rises to 20–50 per cent in infants (233, 236). Once established, the mortality rate of post-splenectomy infection is 50–70 per cent (235, 237). The consensus view is that splenectomy

Table 9.2 Alternatives to splenectomy for trauma (after Cooper and Williamson, ref. 238)

Treatment	Examples
Conservative management	No laparotomy
Pressure plus topical agents	Microfibrillar collagen
	Thrombin
	Gelatin foam
	Cyanoacrylate adhesive
Splenorrhaphy	Mattress suture
	Omental wrap
	Suture ladders
	Polyglycolic acid mesh
Arterial ligation	Main trunk
	Primary divisions
Partial splenectomy	Upper pole
	Lower pole
Autotransplantation	Splenosis
	Deliberate implantation

should be avoided if possible in young children, particularly those under the age of two years (238), and this has led to the development of new techniques of splenic conservation. Some surgeons practise splenic conservation whenever possible in all patients, irrespective of their age. The techniques that have been used in splenic trauma (238) are listed in Table 9.2. Splenic suture or splenorrhaphy is easier in children than in adults because the splenic capsule is relatively thicker in children (239). Arterial ligation alone may be effective in the control of bleeding from the spleen and it permits splenic conservation but it may not protect patients from the risk of post-splenectomy sepsis. Likewise, autotransplantation of splenic cells within the peritoneal cavity may not reduce the risk of septic complications (238, 240).

Fifty per cent of infections following splenectomy are caused by *Streptococcus pneumoniae* but *Neisseria meningitidis*, *Escherichia coli*, *Haemophilus influenzae*, and *Staphylococcus aureus* have also been implicated (232, 235–237). Patients undergoing splenectomy should receive immunization with polyvalent pneumococcal vaccine and children under the age of two years should receive antibiotics for 3–5 years (238).

Orthopaedic surgery

The aim of the orthopaedic surgeon is to preserve and restore the skeletal system – the bones and joints, together with their associated muscles, tendons, and ligaments.

This section reviews the specialized techniques that have been developed in orthopaedic surgery to allow optimal healing of musculoskeletal tissues. Restoration of function is the prime objective.

Muscles

There are approximately 600 muscles in the body which together form 45 per cent of the body mass. There are surpris-ingly few pathological processes that affect skeletal muscle despite its large amount; however, it is susceptible to trauma. Most orthopaedic surgical procedures involve a degree of damage or disruption to muscle. Knowledge of the development of muscle provides a better understanding of its healing and repair. In the embryo, mesoderm gives rise to all the connective tissues of the body, which at first is a loose, space-filling, three-dimensional mesh of cells. These cells, known as mesenchyme, later differentiate into bone, cartilage, muscle, and fibrous tissue.

There are three major functions of muscles:

(1) motion – via the integrated function of bones, joints, and tendons

(2) maintenance of body position

(3) heat generation – 85 per cent of heat produced in the body is from muscular activity.

The main characteristics of muscle that enable these functions are listed below.

1. *Excitability*. Muscles produce electrical signals in response to chemicals released from nerves.
2. *Contractility*. Muscles shorten, thus exerting a force on the bones to which they are attached.
3. *Extensibility*. Muscles can be stretched without damage to the tissue.
4. *Elasticity*. Muscles return spontaneously to their original shape.

Structure (241, 242)

Muscles may be characterized by the arrangements of fibres within the tissue, which are essentially of three types.

1. In parallel muscles, the fibres run parallel to one another along the long axis of the muscle, e.g. sartorius.
2. In fusiform muscles, the fibres are nearly parallel but the 'belly' of the muscles is thicker than the ends, e.g. biceps brachii.
3. In pennate muscles, the fibres may attach obliquely to a tendon, e.g. deltoid.

Skeletal muscle is made of long, cylindrical cells called fibres which contain contractile proteins. The main contractile proteins, actin and myosin, are arranged into thin filaments and thick filaments. These overlap each other to a greater or lesser extent, depending on whether the muscle is contracting (maximum overlap) or relaxed (minimum overlap). These overlaps are regular and form the cross-striations that make the muscle appear striped under magnification. The cells contain large numbers of mitochondria, the 'power-houses', which provide the energy needed for contraction. Muscle cells are polynucleate, the nuclei lying along the edges of the cylinders, out of the way of the contractile tissue. The cells have a wall or plasma membrane, called the sarcolemma, and measure 10–100 μm in diameter and 30–100 μm in length.

Muscle fibres may have a high myoglobin content and a rich

blood supply, in which case they appear red and are relatively fatigue-resistant. These muscle fibres contract relatively slowly and are found in areas responsible for body posture, such as in the neck muscles. Alternatively the myoglobin content may be low; these muscles appear paler (often called white) and contain large amounts of glycogen. They are able to contract strongly and relatively rapidly and are composed of 'fast-twitch' fibres.

Dense, irregular connective tissue called endomysium surrounds each muscle cell (fibre). Bundles of 10–100 such fibres are in turn surrounded by perimysium. Most skeletal muscle is a mixture of red and white muscle fibres, the proportion being determined by the function of the muscle. Bundles of fibres in perimysium are grouped together and wrapped in a secondary layer of epimysium to form a whole muscle. This in turn is wrapped in the dense connective tissue, called deep fascia, that holds muscle together and divides if into separate groups. In the forearm, for example, there are three fascial compartments of muscle: superficial flexor, deep flexor, and extensor. The fascia allows free movement of muscles and carries nerves and blood vessels.

This deep fascia is itself surrounded by superficial fascia, adipose tissue, and areolar tissue. The superficial fascia stores water and fat, and insulates against heat loss. It also provides a pathway for nerves and blood vessels, which serve to protect the underlying tissues from trauma. This whole 'unit' is wrapped in skin.

The specialized development of the contractile apparatus in skeletal muscle and the syncytial nature of the fibre results in a modified pathological response.

1. *Fibre size.* Muscle fibres vary in diameter, and hypertrophy (increase in size but not number) occurs with increased workload. They atrophy (decrease in size) when this workload is removed (so-called 'disuse' atrophy) which is a normal, physiological response. Loss of nerve supply to a fibre also results in a decrease in cell size (neurogenic atrophy). Six months to two years after loss of innervation, muscle is one quarter of its original size and the fibres become replaced by fibrous tissue. The change to fibrous tissue is irreversible.

2. *Fibre distribution.* When a muscle loses its nerve supply and new nerves grow back to supply it, the fibres adopt new fibre types which are arranged in groups supplied by the same nerve type.

Pathological processes that affect muscle are rare but the muscular dystrophies are a group of inherited conditions in which progressive degeneration and destruction of muscle fibres occur. Primary neoplasms (rhabdomyosarcomas) are malignant, but rare tumours and secondary (metastatic) cancer deposits are also uncommon in muscle despite its bulk and rich blood supply.

Regeneration

Skeletal muscle fibres have little potential to divide after the first year of life – growth is due to an enlargement of existing cells rather than an increase in the number of fibres. In adults there is a low turnover of muscle tissue compared to other organs such as the intestine or skin. When voluntary muscle fibres are damaged they can be replaced on an individual basis depending on whether the cell membrane (sarcolemma) is still intact. If the sarcolemma does remain intact then considerable regeneration may occur.

In an area of muscle damage a haematoma forms, followed by a typical acute inflammatory response. Stem cells (satellite cells), which are usually dormant, begin to proliferate. In a young adult, these stem cells form 4–5 per cent of the cell population whereas in the elderly they represent 1 per cent. They can develop into myoblasts with one central nucleus per cell. Myoblasts can fuse together to form a new fibre with many nuclei (a syncytium) which initially has a row of central nuclei and is known as a myotube. These mature, increasing in girth, and the contractile protein that is packed into the nuclei displaces the nuclei to the edges of the fibres.

Muscle repair (243, 244)

Whatever the original cause of injury, muscle repair is a uniform response. After a mild insult by physical trauma or temporary ischaemia there is a rapid physical and electrical recovery. Intracellular oedema occurs with the loss of some myofibrils, but after only a few hours mechanical contractility and electrical activity reappear. Twenty four hours after injury, fibres are indistinguishable from normal.

After more severe damage, muscle fibre necrosis occurs with a typical acute inflammatory reaction. This is followed by phagocytosis – macrophages invade and clear the necrotic debris before regeneration begins. After six weeks, most of the damaged muscle appears normal, although there is a slight excess of collagen between fibres. Active muscle contraction assists regeneration after injury.

Widespread vascular insufficiency, for example from arterial occlusion, causes death of a large mass of muscle, which is slowly replaced by fibrous tissue that may contract tightly when it matures, causing a deformity. This is known as Volkman's ischaemic contracture and no muscle regeneration can occur in these circumstances.

Clinical aspects of muscle damage and repair

When planning an operation an approach should be planned between muscle planes or at the border of a muscle (e.g. a postero-lateral approach to the femur). This is not always possible, and an approach should then be made which splits the muscle along the line of the fibres rather than cutting across the muscle. Excessive diathermy should be avoided for the control of bleeding as this causes muscle necrosis. When closing a wound the fascia, made of mostly inert collagenous tissue, can be sutured together, but sutures should be avoided or tied loosely to avoid trauma and ischaemia.

Compartment syndrome

Muscles lie within relatively inelastic compartments of fibrous tissue which can deform to allow muscle contraction but do not allow much distension. If there is rapid expansion in a compartment, for example due to haemorrhage or post-traumatic oedema, the volume cannot increase and the compartment pressure increases. The pressure may become so high that the blood flow to the muscle is compromised, eventually resulting in ischaemic necrosis of the muscle. These fibres cannot regenerate and undergo fibrosis. A compartment syndrome should be decompressed as an emergency as soon as it is suspected. Early clinical signs include inappropriate pain following trauma to a limb, and pressure or stretching of the muscles in the affected compartment. The pressure in the compartment may be measured and should be less than 40 mmHg (5 kPa). Symptoms suggesstive of excessive pressure should be treated initially by removing any dressings around the limb; if this does not relieve the pain, progress to fasciotomy is required to split the fascia, open up the compartment, and relieve pressure.

Tendons

The word tendon comes from the Latin *tendere* (to stretch out). Tendons connect muscle to bone and their function is to transmit the pulling force of the muscle to the bone levers for movement or to maintain position. Injuries to tendons may be caused not only by direct trauma (e.g. knife wounds), but also by undue stresses, such as high impact sporting activities. It has been estimated that the economic loss following finger and hand injuries involving tendon damage is twice that due to long bone fractures. Successful surgery for repair, transposition, transplantation, or grafting requires a knowledge of normal tendon anatomy, physiology, function, and healing. The overall results depend upon careful surgical technique and postoperative management.

Function of tendons

Tendons contain no contractile units and cannot therefore generate force; instead they are designed to transmit force from muscles to bones. The mechanical advantages of having tendons are that

(1) they are made from a viscoelastic material and are able to store and release energy and thereby reduce the amount of work done by muscles;

(2) they reduce the bulk of a limb distally by allowing a muscle to be based proximally to the area upon which it works;

(3) they enable precise movements to be achieved by allowing long tendon excursions to be transmitted to small joints.

Anatomy (245, 246)

Tendons vary with the function and shape of muscle to which they are attached. They may be flattened as in muscle aponeuroses (abdominal oblique muscles), rounded, as in finger flexors, or somewhere in between, as in Achilles tendon. The tensile strength of the whole of a tendon is considerable and equivalent to that of bone. For example, a tendon of 1 cm diameter will support 600–1000 kg when under tension.

Tendons appear white because they do not contain an internal vascular network. They consist of 30 per cent collagen and 2 per cent elastin embedded in an extracellular matrix of which 68 per cent is water. All of these elements are made by fibroblasts. Collagen makes up 70 per cent of the dry mass of tendons, with type I being the most common. Collagen has a breaking point equivalent to that of steel but will only elongate to 104 per cent of its length. In contrast to globular proteins, fibrous proteins such as collagen and keratin in the skin, as well as elastin and fibrin, have a characteristically high percentage of glycine and regularly repeating amino acid sequences, which predisposes them to form helical structures. Mature collagen is composed of a triple helix of three tropocollagen strands that are extensively cross-linked by covalent bonds to form fibrils of great tensile strength. In tendons, the collagen fibrils are organized into parallel bundles aligned longitudinally with the major axis of stress on the tendon.

Elastin contributes greatly to the elasticity of tendons. This protein exists in several random coil conformations and can fluctuate from one to another. As in collagen, every third amino acid residue is glycine and it possesses a highly regular sequence, the other amino acids being mainly proline and valine. It can extend to up to 170 per cent of its resting length; it is highly cross-linked and it is these cross-links that enable elastin to return to its original shape after stretching. The fibrils are usually less than 1 μm long but can be stained and visualized in tissue sections by light microscopy.

The extracellular matrix is a highly viscous gel which provides structural support and a medium for nutrient materials. It is composed of proteoglycans and water.

An adequate supply of protein in the diet is necessary to provide the amino acids for the synthesis of collagen, and carbohydrate is needed to form the extracellular matrix. Collagen synthesis also requires iron and vitamin C (ascorbic acid). Collagen stability is influenced by the conversion of proline residues to hydroxyproline. The enzyme effecting this conversion requires oxygen, iron, and a reducing agent such as ascorbic acid. Collagen synthesized in the absence of these factors is insufficiently hydroxylated and the chains are readily degraded within the cell, giving rise to the fragile skin and blood vessels symptomatic of scurvy. Regular exercise increases collagen production; the number and size of fibrils increases, with the tensile and maximum static strength of the tendon.

Tendon structure

The collagen microfibrils are arranged with the elastin fibres around columns of modified fibroblasts called tenocytes, to form fascicles. The fascicles are surrounded by loose areolar tissue (endotendon) and clumped together to form tendons. The loose areolar tissue condenses to form an epitendon around the tendon. Where tendons pass under ligamentous bands, such as retinacula, they may be surrounded by another layer, the synovial sheath. The sheaths consist of two concentric cylinders (visceral and parietal) separated by a very thin film of synovial fluid. Their function is to allow the tendons to slide back and forth easily.

Blood supply

The preservation of blood supply is probably the most important factor in tendon healing. Although it can be very variable it is usually divided into three regions.

1. In the region close to the musculotendinous junction, small arterioles branch to supply both the muscle and tendon, although capillaries do not overlap.
2. The middle length of the tendon is supplied by vessels in the tissue around the tendon (paratenon), which then enter the endotenon. The paratenon is often clearly visible; for example, around the Achilles tendon.
3. In the region close to the bone–tendon junction, small arterioles branch to supply both bone and tendon but there is no supply across the junction.

The areas where two regions meet may be an area of relatively poor blood supply, which is particularly prone to tendinitis or rupture. A classic example is the area 2–6 cm above the insertion of the Achilles tendon to the heel. Inflammation of the tendons and tendon sheaths is termed tenosynovitis. Tendons commonly affected are in the wrists (De Quervain's tenosynovitis), shoulders (rotator cuff syndrome), elbow (tennis elbow), and fingers (trigger finger). The areas may become red and swollen with pain on movement at the joint. It often follows excessive repetitive exercise.

Tendon healing (247)

Interest in tendon healing dates back to at least the second century AD. Galen warned against surgical procedures involving tendon as they were thought to contain nervous tissue, and repair would result in gangrene and convulsions. Apart from Avicenna in the tenth century, this warning was largely heeded in Europe, and tendons largely ignored until 1767 when Hunter began his first experimental studies. Since then there has been continued disagreement regarding the precise healing mechanism of tendon, with three schools of thought:

(1) tendon repairs itself by reparative cellular growth from the cut ends of the tendon; or
(2) tendon is repaired by cellular activities of surrounding tissues which proliferate, invade the gap, and repair it; or
(3) tendons repair through a combination of the above two mechanisms.

A typical acute inflammatory response follows tendon injury which is followed by proliferation of fibroblasts at the tendon ends, which lay down collagen that is not in line with the long axis of the tendon. There are no cross-links between tropocollagen chains during this early phase when the collagen is still immature.

Collagen fibres become orientated within the line of major stress on the tendon as cells take on a mature appearance and reduce to normal numbers. The tensile strength of the tendon is restored to normal over months to years after the original injury.

Clinical aspects of tendon healing (248, 249)

The concept of 'one wound – one scar' summarizes the clinical challenge in tendon healing, in which satisfactory healing of the tendon is achieved without the repair being bound by adhesions to surrounding tissues. A good functional result requires a trade-off between the need to avoid tendon rupture and prevent the formation of adhesions during early mobilization. This is a particularly important consideration in tendons with the greatest amplitude of movement – the finger flexor tendons.

Surgical considerations in tendon repair

Factors that make adhesion more likely are dependent in part on the severity of the associated tissue damage at the time of the injury. Scarring and adhesive fibrosis are more likely after an injury in which the tendon is crushed or torn, or when infection has occurred. Associated injuries to nearby blood vessels, which compromise blood supply, and injury to juxtaposed joints, will also contribute to stiffness. Although these factors may be out of the surgeon's control, good surgical technique and postoperative rehabilitation will optimize the final outcome.

The following considerations of surgical technique help to achieve restoration of normal structure and function of the musculotendinous–skeletal unit (a secure tendon repair which glides without restriction):

(1) use of an atraumatic technique;
(2) the gliding surfaces should not be grasped with toothed forceps but handled as little as possible using thumb and finger or a sharp hook;
(3) the tendon should not be allowed to dry out and should be handled with moistened gloves;
(4) gauze should not be used around a tendon because this may damage its smooth surface;
(5) the operation should be planned so that the tendon is exposed for the minimum time;
(6) to preserve gliding and blood supply and to prevent adhesions, damage to the paratenon and synovial sheath should be avoided;
(7) tendon repair should be performed in an aseptic theatre area, within 6 h of injury, with good light, assistance, and magnification;
(8) the periosteum of nearby bone should not be traumatized otherwise it will need repair;
(9) the suture materials used for repair must be strong and cause little tissue reaction. Stainless steel and monofilament Nylon, Prolene, or Mersilene are suture materials of choice, mounted on an atraumatic needle.

Suturing techniques

The aim of the anastomosis is to approximate the two ends with as little damage as possible. In most techniques the ends are spliced together. Techniques commonly used in flexor tendon repair are outlined in Fig. 9.10. Kessler's suture may be modified by burying the knot within the repair to lessen adhesions using one suture or two sutures. Kleinert modified Bunnell's suture technique in the same way. These techniques may then also be augmented by a running epitendinous stitch (which can also be locked at each stitch) and thereby 'tidy' the repair and add to the reparative strength. The Pulvertaft end

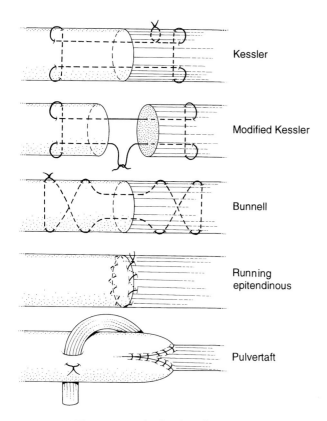

Kessler

Modified Kessler

Bunnell

Running
epitendinous

Pulvertaft

Fig. 9.10 Methods of tendon repair.

weave suture is the strongest repair, but is too bulky to use in the flexor tendons of the hand.

Grafts

Tendon grafting may be used to lessen the likelihood of adhesions when a gap exists between tendon ends, to avoid a direct repair in an area of scar tissue, or to avoid repairing a flexor tendon within a fibrous flexor sheath. The tendons of palmaris longus or plantaris are commonly used and may be harvested through a small incision using a tendon harvester. The important principle is to ensure correct tension so that contraction of the muscle produces the desired effect. This can be judged by comparing the tension with neighbouring tendons.

Tendon transfers

Tendons are transferred to restore function to dysfunctional musculotendinous units. A tendon may be disconnected from its distal end and reconnected to the proximal end of another tendon to 'motor' that unit. Active movement which has been lost owing to muscle or tendon damage or neurological disease may be restored. A synergistic muscle with a similar range of movement, which can be spared from its original function, is chosen for the transfer.

Mobilization

The postoperative management of tendon injuries is as important as the operative technique. Controlled mobilization is required to prevent adhesions. The biological basis for immo-

bilization is to allow revascularization to occur, rather than to prevent tension across the anastomosis from causing dehiscence. Studies suggest that active motion should not be attempted before three weeks. Active motion may be prevented with passive splints. However, dynamic splints can be used to enable passive motion but exclude active motion. Examples of dynamic splints are outriggers or Capner splints. Treatment regimens, such as the Belfast regimen, for flexor tendon physiotherapy have been developed to encourage early active movement.

Involvement of specialist physiotherapists and occupational therapists who are competent to deal with splintage techniques is essential. The importance of the ability and willingness of the patient to participate during the recovery phase cannot be overstated.

Bone and joint

The articulated framework of rigid struts upon which skeletal muscles act is made of bone. If this tissue is injured, it heals, in optimal conditions, by reconstituting tissue almost identical to its original form without scar formation. These conditions can be optimized by specialized techniques of surgery and splintage that have been developed for this unique tissue type.

Structure

Bone is a calcified connective tissue made up of cells embedded in a firm matrix. Despite its rigidity the structure is not permanent and is constantly being turned over. Thirty per cent of the matrix is made up of organic material consisting mainly of collagen fibrils. The remainder is inorganic bone salt, the main being hydroxyapatite ($Ca_{10}(PO_4)_6(OH)_2$). Other inorganic constituents include sodium, magnesium, chloride, fluoride, bicarbonate, and citrate ions, which make up crystals sized 2.5–5.0 nm by 40 nm.

In the embryo, bone is derived from mesenchyme and then ossified in one of two ways.

1. Most of the skeleton, in particular the long bones of the limbs and vertebrae, is first developed as 'models' or anlages made of cartilage. These grow slowly and are eventually replaced by bone.
2. Membranous bones, for example those in the face, develop directly from the mesenchyme and do not go through the intermediate cartilage model stage.

Bone structure is described as being of two types – cortical, which forms the bone tube of long bones, or cancellous, which can be found in the metaphyses of long bones; in the iliac crest for example.

Cortical bone comprises concentric layers (lamellae) of matrix around a central (Haversian) canal which contains blood vessels. Within this matrix are channels and spaces which contain cells. There are two main types of active cells: osteoblasts, which lay down the inorganic part of the matrix, and osteoclasts, which resorb the mineralized bone. Eventually osteoblasts which start on the surface get buried in the matrix where they become dormant osteocytes. Tiny channels (canaliculi), which transport nutrients, run between the main canal and these cells and between each level of lamellae. Cancellous bone (spongy/trabecular bone) is made up of large (trabeculae) and smaller (spiculae) units of bone. Osteoblasts on the side of these units deposit inorganic matrix. Trabeculae are most prominent along lines of mechanical stress. Around the outside is a dense layer of connective tissue (periosteum). Bundles of fibres from the periosteum pierce the bone and act as a firm insertion for tendons.

Bone healing (250)

The aim of bone healing is not only to restore continuity but also stability. This requires that broken bone is repaired with bone. For this to occur, there must be an adequate supply of osteoblasts, fibroblasts, osteoclasts, and cartilage cells (chondroblasts). These cells are activated by chemical mediators and mechanical stimuli.

When a bone is exposed to a form that exceeds its modulus of elasticity, it fractures along the line of least resistance. This disrupts bony and soft tissue and releases chemical and electrical stimuli which trigger the healing process. Bones are said to heal by first or second intention, as described below.

1. Primary (or direct) healing, with no callus, occurs in fractures that are well apposed, with minimal movement and a good blood supply. This is the mode of healing of fractures which have been fixed with plates.

2. Secondary bone healing is the more common type of healing in which a supporting callus helps to splint and immobilize the fracture ends. The more common secondary bone healing occurs in several stages after the fracture (or osteotomy):

    (a) Inflammatory stage: an acute inflammatory reaction is initiated in the area of injury.

    (b) Granulation stage: resting cells are stimulated, granulation tissue develops, and haematoma is removed by phagocytosis. The bone ends are essentially avascular and do not play a part in the healing process. However, fibroblasts from the endosteum, periosteum, and surrounding soft tissues become active within 8–16h and begin to deposit collagen, which splints the fracture site. Osteoclasts remove the necrotic, traumatized bone at the fracture ends.

    (c) Formation of primary callus: callus formation depends on the specialized cells which form bone cartilage and fibrous tissue. Cells and blood vessels come from the periosteum, medullary endosteum, trabecular marrow, and from the soft tissues. After 4 days, progenitor resting cells differentiate to become the extracellular matrix that will become bone and cartilage. This mineralizes after 4–16 weeks, becoming increasingly rigid and helping to further immobilize the fracture ends. The more motion at the fracture site, the more callus that is formed.

    (d) Proliferative phase: the bone ends are gradually repaired by osteoclasts and progressively replaced by trabecular bone derived from the callus. Eventually all of the damaged bone and haematoma is replaced.

    (e) Remodelling phase: the excess callus is removed and the mineralized cartilage gradually changes to woven bone and then to lamellar bone. This phase may take from 1 to 4 years. Eventually this remodelled bone looks virtually normal, even under the microscope. Deformity associated with the fracture is sculpted to a smooth contour with time. This remodelling is occurs in response to the mechanical stress applied to the bone.

Primary healing of bone

Primary healing of bone occurs when there is virtually no motion at the fracture site. This can be achieved by using internal fixation, with screws and plates across the fracture. No callus is formed but the gap between the fracture ends is filled with trabecular bone from the periosteum and endosteum. The Haversian systems can join across the fracture and reform. Eventually the two ends are welded together.

Factors affecting bone healing

Fracture healing is a biomechanical process and the factors that affect fracture healing may be considered as principally biological or mechanical.

There are many biological factors that play a role. A satisfactory blood supply is essential to healing. Soft-tissue injuries, which are not obvious by X-ray examination, may influence the final outcome, and the blood supply to the region may be disturbed to a variable extent by the original injury. The general nutrition of a patient, particularly in the elderly, may be inadequate to enable satisfactory healing. Important deficiencies may include proteins, vitamin D, and calcium but these are rare in the UK from a practical point of view. As in other tissues, healing can be adversely affected by steroids and diabetes mellitus. Infection of the fracture site is a serious potential problem which may result in osteomyelitis, bone necrosis, collagenolysis, and failure of matrix formation.

Mechanical factors also affect healing. Any soft tissue that is interposed between the bone ends may act as a mechanical barrier to fracture union. Inadequate immobilization of the fracture ends may also result in delayed healing and result either in abundant callus formation, which is produced to splint the ends, or in a failure of union. The bone ends must also be close enough for callus to bridge the gap, otherwise callus involutes.

Clinical aspects of fracture treatment

The aim of treatment is to achieve restoration of a stable continuity of bones in satisfactory alignment and adequate length, retaining as good a range of movement as possible at the associated joints. Immobilization at the fracture site is required to achieve pain relief and sound union. Conversely, joint mobilization is important in preserving functional movement. The methods of treatment described in Table 9.3 may be used alone or in combination. These methods of treating

Table 9.3 Methods of fracture treatment

Immobilization method	Advantages	Disadvantages
External splinting with plaster casts (or similar), splints, strappings, and slings	Closed technique Less invasive	Joints are immobilized (cast-bracing may help) Difficult to obtain and maintain perfect reduction Some bones are not amenable to treatment by this method
Internal fixation with screws or plates, wires, intramedullary nails or pins. These devices share the load until bone has sufficient independent strength	Secure and accurate reduction may be achieved and maintained Early joint movement is possible	Stripping of the soft tissues may compromise the blood supply and predispose to delayed union or non-union Risk of infection is higher after surgery
External skeletal fixation, transfixing the bones with pins on either side of the fracture. The fracture is stabilized by the clamps and rods which connect the pins	Adjustable Less invasive Allows access to soft tissues at trauma site Useful in open fractures May allow mobilization of nearby joints	Risk of pin site infection May be bulky

broken bones have been used widely over many years. Orthopaedic techniques and instruments have been developed to promote the optimal healing of bone. These techniques have enabled the majority of patients to recover after a fracture with normal function and anatomy.

Mal-union, delayed union, and non-union

A fracture which heals in a non-anatomical and unsatisfactory position is said to be mal-united. The mal-union may involve angular or rotational deformity or shortening. While it has been suggested that deformity in any plane causes asymmetrical loading of the juxtaposed joint (and the development of osteoarthritis) correction should mainly be reserved to improve function.

Delayed union and non-union are quite different complications. In delayed union, fracture healing fails to keep pace with a predicted time scale for a given fracture site, whereas in non-union, the fracture fails to be completed and the healing process stops, despite the fracture still being present. Unfortunately there is no one measure of fracture healing, but delayed or non-union may be diagnosed on combinations of clinical features, such as persistent pain, fracture site mobility, and radiographic features. Specialized tests such as bone scans are also useful. Problems with union are encountered more commonly in open, comminuted, high energy fractures, pathological fractures, and in areas with an impaired blood supply.

Non-union may be either hypertrophic, when there is abundant callus formation about the fracture site, or atrophic, where there is paucity of bone. Essentially, hypertrophic non-union requires stabilization while atrophic non-union requires vitalization; infection should be eradicated, bone stock renewed and stabilized, and a healthy soft tissue envelope provided. New bone may be taken as a graft from elsewhere in the body. A cancellous bone graft is best, and these are commonly taken from the iliac crest. A vascularized bone graft may be taken as a segment of a long bone, for example, a fibula or a rib, and the blood supply joined to the local blood vessels by microvascular surgical techniques.

Articular cartilage (251)

This is a hard but flexible tissue which can resist tensile and compressive forces. It is a connective tissue in which cells are embedded in a resilient matrix of chondroitin, with collagen fibrils woven in, which resist tensile forces. The matrix is deposited by chondrocytes which lie in spaces (lacunae) in the matrix. There is a denser layer of cells with types I and II collagen at the edge of the cartilage – the perichondrium. New chondroblasts are found here and add to the matrix.

Unlike bone matrix, cartilage matrix is deformable and therefore cartilage can grow by swelling, as more cells embed in the matrix and secrete more matrix. Chondrocytes (dormant chondroblasts) may also divide in their lacunae to form two sister cells which then develop a layer of matrix between them and separate.

There are three types of cartilage.

1. Hyaline cartilage has a matrix of a semi-transparent material made of chondroitin, sulphate and collagen. There are no connections between lacunae, unlike bone, and no blood vessels in the matrix. All exchange of nutrient material depends on the slow process of diffusion. This type of cartilage is found in articulating bone ends, in the nose, and in the embryonic skeleton. It is hydrophilic and its ultrastructure can resist impact loading.

2. White fibrous cartilage is densely packed with collagen fibres to produce greater tensile strength but less flexibility. This is found in intervertebral discs, the symphysis pubis, and ligamentous capsules of joints.

3. Yellow elastic cartilage has a semi-opaque network of yellow elastic fibres that make the tissue more elastic. This is found in the ear and epiglottis.

Articular cartilage healing

William Hunter (1743) first observed that articular cartilage did not heal and this limited repair response to injury has since been confirmed. The avascularity of cartilage inhibits normal repair mechanisms; diffusion is the main mode of transport of nutrients within cartilage.

Thus in contrast to other tissues, the normal response to injury does not occur in cartilage. Cartilage cells in the area of injury may die but necrosis is minimal. As there are no blood vessels, acute inflammation does not occur and there are few cells present to mount a repair response.

Superficial cartilage injury is relatively unimportant and has no consequences. Damage becomes neither larger nor smaller, and osteoarthritic change is uncommon. If the injury extends deeper, down to the level where bone and cartilage meet, the situation is different. An example of this is the intra-articular fracture where there is minimal displacement. The healing response derived from the vascular subarticular injured bone fills the defect in the cartilage inorganising haematoma, which becomes granulation tissue, and eventually matures into fibrocartilage. If, following an intra-articular fracture the alignment is not perfect and there is irregularity of the weight-bearing surface, osteoarthritis is likely to develop in time. Severe blunt trauma to articular cartilage which exceeds the capacity of cartilage to resist deformation results in injuries that may progress rapidly to osteoarthritis.

Following injury to a limb it is important to mobilize joints as soon as possible. This has two advantages: first, mobilization helps to distribute synovial fluid, which contains nutrients, and enhances the diffusion process. Second, after only three weeks of immobilization, fibrous tissues which surround the joint (the capsule) can contract and form adhesions. These contractures can limit the range of movement of the joint and limit the function of the limb following its recovery.

Vascular surgery

Healing following surgery to blood vessels requires not only consideration of the normal physiological processes, but is tempered by the need for immediate haemodynamic and functional success. This is not required in bowel or orthopaedic surgery where the strength of an anastomosis or repair can be allowed to increase over a period of days or weeks before full function is restored. Additionally patients with peripheral vascular disease are usually elderly, with diseased tissue from atheroma or dilatation leading to weakness and the inability to hold sutures. Paradoxically, tissue growth and collagen deposition at the site of an anastomosis may be reduced by the compromised circulation that the surgery is intended to improve. Although inadequacies of surgical technique may present immediately with vessel thrombosis, restenosis from progression of atherosclerosis or intimal hyperplasia often do not manifest until years after surgery.

Vessel trauma and repair

Blood vessels are composed of three layers (Fig. 9.11) with the media providing strength, elasticity, and compliance; the endothelium has antithrombogenic properties; whilst the adventitia blends with the surrounding connective tissue. In veins the muscular media and adventitia are less prominent. On simple division and suture of an artery there is initial loss of endothelium at the site of trauma. The endothelium is

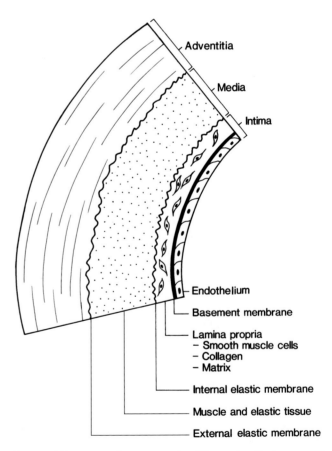

Fig. 9.11 Diagrammatic cross-section illustrating the layers of the arterial wall.

antithrombogenic, locally releasing active prostaglandins and fibrinolytic factors which prevent thrombotic vessel occlusion. Conversely, the collagenous stroma of the exposed media is intensely thrombogenic, attracting platelet adhesion and clot formation. The endothelial defect is replaced by ingrowth of cells from the viable edges and this is normally rapid and complete (252). Whilst platelet adhesion to any suture line is required for haemostasis, overactivation of the clotting cascade may lead to vessel occlusion in the early postoperative period. Repair of blood vessels is similar to other tissues, with an acute inflammatory response, and neovascularization within the adventitia and media. Collagen formation occurs over the following weeks and full strength of an anastomosis may take months to develop and may permanently be compromised in atherosclerotic vessels. The compliance and elasticity of a vessel may never return because of surrounding fibrosis. Many vascular procedures, such as application of arterial clamps, balloon embolectomy, transluminal dilatation, and vessel flushing may cause significant loss of endothelium, increasing the risk of thrombosis (253, 254).

Endothelialization of extensive areas of injury, such as endarterectomy sites with a plane of cleavage through the media, are inadequately covered by endothelial ingrowth. Multipotent cells from the blood may cover the defect but it is likely that endothelialization occurs from migration of cells from the vasa vasorum or by transformation of medial smooth muscle cells (255–258). Deeper endarterectomy accelerates endothelial coverage as exposure of vasa vasorum facilitates cellular migration over shorter distances (257). In response to injury, smooth muscle cells within the media proliferate and migrate to the subintimal layers. This migration may be initiated by the release of platelet derived growth factor from repeated platelet–vessel wall interaction. After migration, smooth muscle proliferation continues and extracellular matrix is laid down within the neointima. This proliferation reaches a peak at two weeks (in a rat model) but then stabilizes at a rate equal to cell death (259). Although this process is reparative, if injury is repetitive or the initial proliferation is florid, a hyperplastic intima may develop, leading to vessel stenosis and occlusion. Following carotid endarterectomy 10–20 per cent of patients will develop restenosis from intimal hyperplasia (260–262). This, however, does not normally produce thromboembolic symptoms, possibly due to the non-ulcerative nature of the intima. Restenosis following the trauma of transluminal ballon angioplasty is likely to be due to intimal hyperplasia or fibrosis. Platelet inhibitory therapy reduces this incidence of restenosis, and the role of expandable mesh stents to maintain patency is gaining popularity (263, 264). Femoro-popliteal vein grafts are prone to develop stenoses, particularly within the first two years after implantation. At the anastomotic sites these stenoses may represent intimal hyperplasia secondary to turbulent flow whilst mid-graft stenoses are fibrotic and relate to rough operative graft handling (Fig. 9.12). Turbulent anastomotic flow is accentuated by vessel diameter mismatch, intimal irregularity, an inappropriate angle between graft and host vessel, and compliance mismatch. The latter assumes importance in anastomoses involving calcified atherosclerotic vessels or prosthetic grafts. Although platelet inhibitory drugs reduce

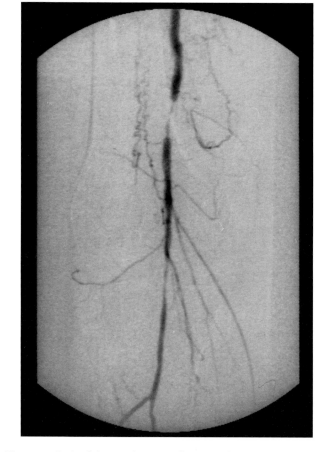

Fig. 9.12 Intimal hyperplasia producing a long stenosis at the lower end of a femoro-popliteal reversed vein graft.

graft occlusion rats (265), their influence on intimal hyperplasia is unclear and management is directed to identifying graft stenoses before occlusion occurs (266, 267).

Prosthetic grafts

Prosthetic implants are inferior to natural vascular autologous grafts but are expedient in areas where large diameters are required such as aorta or iliac vessels, and when lower limb veins are inadequate. The major disadvantages of man-made prosthetic grafts are lack of compliance and secretory endothelium. In the human, prosthetic grafts do not ususaly endothelialize apart from one centimetre next to the anastomosis where migration of cells occurs from the host artery (268, 269). The remaining graft luminal surface becomes covered with a pannus of thrombus and connective tissue known as neointima, which remains intensely thrombogenic indefinitely (268). Patchy islands of endothelium have been demonstrated away from the anastomosis but only limited areas are covered (270). Experimentally, both polytetrafluoroethylene and Dacron grafts have been seeded successfully with autologous endothelial cells producing a confluent covering (271–273). Endothelial adhesion to grafts is increased following precoating with fibronectin, collagen, or laminin (274–276). Improved patency and reduction in luminal thrombus formation has been demonstrated in animal endothelial seeded grafts (272, 273). Clinical use in humans has been restricted by inadequate endothelialization and the risk of infection from the cultures necessary to seed the grafts. The graft itself becomes incorporated in a fibrous capsule of connective tissue. Infiltration of connective tissue into the graft, which may prevent graft infection, is dependent upon the closeness of the fabric weave (277). Loosely knit Dacron grafts are well incorporated and the ease of connective tissue infiltration allows ingrowth of a plexus of capillaries, which helps to maintain and organize the fibrous intima but may reduce any compliance (277). A loose weave has the disadvantage that the graft will be porous and leak blood when initially implanted. This has been overcome by preclotting the graft at the time of surgery or impregnating the graft with collagen or gelatin during manufacture. The nature of healing in grafts placed transfemorally without a formal arteriotomy is subject to study. The vascular trauma is reduced, although intimal damage occurs, and the prosthesis is held in place by expandable metallic mesh stents. These may endothelialize with time but can dislodge or produce stenoses (278, 279).

Surgical technique

Exposure of blood vessels should involve the minimum dissection necessary to apply clamps and obtain sufficient mobilization. Over-extensive mobilization of an artery may damage vasa vasorum which supply the adventitial capillary network and oxygen to the outer two thirds of the wall. The majority of surgery is performed for ischaemia and this will reduce healing in local connective tissue and skin leading to necrosis of skin edges. Lymphatic channels should be retracted, especially in the groin, in order to prevent postoperative lymphoedema. If it is necessary to divide a lymphatic, the vessel should be tied to avoid the development of a lymphatic fistula which may lead to wound infection.

Clamps should be applied gently as stenosis at the clamp site is well recognized. Silicone cushions within the jaws may reduce vessel damage. Vein grafts should never be clamped. The theoretical advantages of a transverse arteriotomy with avoidance of stenosis on closure may not be applicable to atherosclerotic vessels. A longitudinal arteriotomy may easily be extended to visualize major arterial branches or endarterectomy end points. Too deep an endarterectomy can lead to subsequent arterial dilatation or rupture, whereas a superficial endarterectomy may not remove all disease. An intimal flap at the distal endarterectomy site should be sutured firmly to the vessel wall using a Kunlin suture to avoid it occluding the vessel when flow is restored (Fig. 9.13).

Although silk sutures have been used in the past for closing arteriotomies and anastomosing vessels, the knots formed foci of infection and the material itself slowly degenerated and was phagocytosed. Almost universally, monofilament non-absorbable polymeric sutures are now used (such as nylon or polypropylene). They maintain the strength and integrity of an anastomosis over a period of months. Whilst non-diseased vessels and those of children exhibit a normal

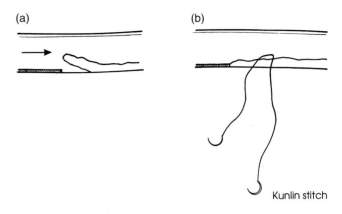

Fig. 9.13 Avoidance of atheromatous flap: (a) an atheromatous flap at the distal limit of the endarterectomy which may occlude flow. (b) Use of a double ended polypropylene stitch to anchor the atheroma to the vessel wall.

collagenous healing process this is delayed in atherosclerotic arteries, particularly where a prosthetic graft is involved and permanent anastomotic strengthening by sutures may be required. Indeed the strength of an arterial closure may be dependent upon a periadventitial fibrous reaction. Intimal apposition is required, unlike the inverting anastomoses within bowel, to prevent turbulence and maintain secretory endothelial confluence. A patch is applied to close an arteriotomy if primary closure stenoses the vessel. The width of the patch must be sufficient to maintain host vessel diameter without producing dilatation. Traditionally, the needle travels from the luminal to the adventitial surface in order to avoid lifting an atheromatous flap which may lead to early thrombosis or late intimal hyperplasia. The depth and distance between stitches is dependent upon the size and strength of the vessels but 2 mm respectively is suitable for femoral vessels. Sutures that are loose or too spaced apart may predispose to false aneurysm formation, particularly if a patient is given anticoagulant therapy postoperatively. Excessive tension on the suture line when the vessel has been weakened by an endarterectomy may tear the vessel, again leading to false aneurysm formation. Continuous sutures are used for speed but, in children and venous surgery, interrupted sutures may be more appropriate to prevent anastomotic narrowing.

Complications associated with healing

Thrombosis, intimal hyperplasia, and false aneurysm formation form the majority of undesirable outcomes and have been discussed. Subcutaneous infection following vascular surgery, especially in the groin, is not uncommon. Fortunately, infection within native blood vessels or grafts is rare, but is disastrous. Predisposing factors to wound infection include ischaemic tissues, debility, lengthy surgical procedures, gangrene, or infection distal to an anastomosis. It is unusual for autologous vessels to become infected, particularly if monofilament sutures are used. The incidence of prosthetic graft infection is reported to be between 1 and 6 per cent

(280). Organisms involved include *Staphylococcus aureus* and *S. epidermidis* with other skin commensals and coliforms. Haematogenous spread may occur and infect a graft months or years after implantation. Infection occurs insidiously and may present clinically only months after contamination with sinus formation, septicaemia, or disruption of an anastomosis. Prosthetic graft infection tracks throughout the length of the prosthesis with the development of a perigraft collection of fluid. Involvement of the anastomoses, particularly when immediately after surgery, causes necrosis and weakening of native vessels in apposition to the graft, with the development of a false aneurysm and torrential bleeding. Classical treatment involves complete removal of the infected prosthesis with replacement by autologous grafts of extra-anatomic bypass together with systemic antibiotics (281, 282). Due to the high mortality of these procedures and the difficulty in identifying suitably sized autologous grafts to replace aortic prostheses, some centres have reported encouraging results using local graft excision and replacement together with antibiotic irrigation (283–285).

Prevention of graft infection involves careful aseptic technique and administration of prophylactic antibiotics over the perioperative period. Bathing the patient in an antiseptic solution prior to surgery is practised but all methods of prevention are difficult to compare scientifically due to the low rate and late presentation of graft infection. Antibiotic impregnation of grafts is being attemped but this is applicable to only a minority of antibiotics (286, 287). Polytetrafluoroethylene may be more resistant to infection than Dacron and improved tissue incorporation with knitted loose weave Dacron grafts may be beneficial.

Rarely patients may exhibit an autoimmune reaction to compounds within a Dacron graft but not by Dacron itself (288). If recognized and life threatening, treatment is by immediate graft excision.

The urinary tract

Healing follows injury, which can take a variety of forms in the urinary tract. The result depends on the cause of the injury, the viability of the tissues, and their response to local factors and to treatment. Trauma from high-speed deceleration accidents and iatrogenic causes account for the majority of injuries; tissue viability may be compromised by previous surgery or radiotherapy, and urine presents a unique environmental factor influencing treatment. In normal circumstances the urothelium provides a lining, from the calyces to the external urethral meatus, which is impermeable to urine but if this is damaged, urinary extravasation occurs which stimulates an inflammatory response. The extravasated urine may be absorbed or it may become localized into a collection or 'urinoma', with the potential risk of infection, septicaemia, abscess, or fistula formation.

Establishing haemostasis, a water-tight closure, and unobstructed urinary drainage are important principles in the management of injuries, but often involve the use of sutures, catheters, or stents. Any foreign material introduced within the urinary tract may act as a nidus for crystals to deposit and

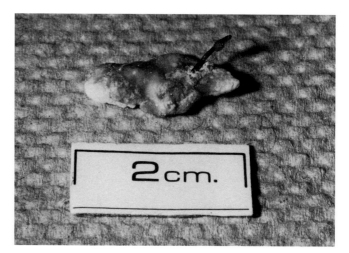

Fig. 9.14 Stone formation on a Nylon suture inadvertently passed through the bladder wall.

to form stones (Fig. 9.14). A knowledge of the interaction between the tissues, urine, and the foreign materials used in repair forms an important basis to the management of these injuries. The clinical objective is to preserve renal function by controlling haemorrhage and restoring urinary drainage; 30 per cent function of one kidney is sufficient to maintain adequate renal function and to avoid the need for dialysis.

Kidney

The renal parenchyma consists of soft friable tissue contained within a strong fibrous capsule. The kidneys are well protected, lying in the paravertebral gutters, in front of the lower ribs and the quadratus lumborum muscles, and behind the peritoneal cavity with the upper abdominal viscera. The kidneys are surrounded and cushioned by dense perinephric fat which is enclosed by Gerota's fascia. Their blood supply follows a relatively constant pattern (289) which is of particular relevence to the surgeon exploring a renal injury. The renal artery approaches the sinus of the kidney between the vein anteriorly and the pelvis posteriorly before dividing into an anterior and posterior trunk. The anterior trunk subdivides into four segmental arteries namely the apical, upper, middle, and lower branches which are end-arteries supplying corresponding segments of the kidney; the posterior trunk becomes the posterior segmental artery crossing the back of the renal pelvis at its junction with the superior calyx.

The majority of renal injuries arise from blunt trauma and heal without operative intervention. They have been classified broadly into three groups in order of their severity, namely contusions, lacerations, and pedicle injuries. Accurate staging of these by computed tomography (CT) has contributed to their management, but the condition of a severely injured patient may not permit time for this. Intravenous urography with a 20 min film may be sufficient to demonstrate a functioning kidney. Ultrasonography and selective renal arteriography may provide additional imaging techniques for assessment.

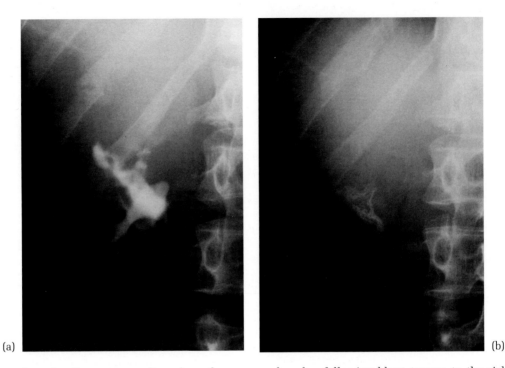

(a)   (b)

Fig. 9.15 (a) Extravasation of radio-opaque medium from the upper pole calyx following blunt trauma to the right kidney. (b) Dystrophic calcification occurring after the injury.

Renal contusion is associated with renal or perirenal haematoma; minor capsular lacerations may be present but there is no extravasation of urine. Healing is normally uneventful but may result in atrophic scarring of the cortex if arterial damage arises. Antibiotic cover has been advocated as a prophylactic measure (290) because of the risk of infection, although opinions differ on this policy (291). Extracorporeal shock wave lithotripsy can induce perirenal haematomas. Knapp and colleagues (292) reported an incidence of 0.66 per cent (24 haematomas following 3620 treatments) on the Dornier HM3 machine; the incidence was 2.5 per cent for patients with preexisting hypertension and 3.8 pen cent for those whose hypertension was not under satisfactory control.

Renal lacerations may pass through the cortico-medullary junction into the collecting system or involve the renal pelvis (293), causing varying degrees of urinary extravasation. This does not appear to be associated with serious complications unless infection supervenes. The pathological kidney (affected by disease) is more vulnerable to relatively minor trauma; in the series of 151 patients reviewed by Slade (290), nine patients had a moderate or severe hydronephrosis and six of these required interval nephrectomy. Dystrophic calcification can arise in the region of the damaged renal parenchyma (Fig. 9.15) during the healing process and later reabsorb spontaneously.

Small urinomas do not require drainage but leakage may persist and, if signs of infection become evident, the collection should be drained percutaneously or by open operation. A persistent urinoma can form a renal pseudocyst which may

not be recognized for months or years after injury (294). Crabtree (295) reported 23 cases of pararenal cysts occurring within the fatty tissue around the kidney following a traumatic breach of the renal calyx, pelvis, or ureter. The characteristic feature of the cyst is its fibrous tissue lining which has no epithelium. Alternative names for these collections include pseudohydronephrosis, perirenal or perinephric cyst, and hydrocoele renalis.

Pawlowski (296) described a peculiar type of inflammation that arises in the fatty tissue adjacent to the renal pelvis which contains numerous eosinophilic nodules. Mitchinson and Bradley-Watson (297) coined the term peripelvic urine granuloma for this condition, which was considered to be due to extravasation of urine. However, it is still controversial whether urinary extravasation produces any serious sequelae. Small amounts of urinary extravasation through the fornix of a calyx have been shown to occur on sudden increase in intrapelvic pressure during excretion urography when external compression is applied over the ureters (298), during acute renal colic, or on retrograde pyelography (299).

Pedicle injuries are usually associated with multiple organ injuries but they present varying degrees of severity. Intimal tears of the segmental or renal arteries cause atrophic scarring of the renal parenchyma whilst avulsion or tearing of the arterial or venous walls can produce massive haemorrhage, demanding early exploration.

In a series of 1363 patients reported by McAninch and colleagues (300), renal exploration was required in 127; 2.4 per cent of blunt injuries, 45 per cent of stab wounds, and 96 per cent of gunshot wounds required surgery and the majority were associated with multiple organ injuries. The kidney has a remarkable capacity to heal if bleeding and urinary leakage can be controlled. The absolute indications for renal exploration include a pulsatile haematoma in the loin or continued bleeding in a haemodynamically unstable patient.

The success of renal surgery for trauma is based on early vascular control. The nephrectomy rate rises sharply, up to 60 per cent, with the more aggressive approach to renal trauma (301, 302). Sagalowsky and colleagues (303) reported an overall total nephrectomy rate of 26.5 per cent in 185 patients undergoing renal surgery and rates of 36 per cent and 30 per cent for blunt and gunshot trauma respectively. Bleeding can be difficult to control on opening Gerota's fascia, which releases the perirenal tamponade, and an arterior abdominal approach to the hilar vessels is therefore advocated. The small bowel is lifted up and an incision made at the base of its mesentery through the haematoma to expose the aorta which is then traced up to the renal veins. Slings are placed around the renal arteries and veins on both sides and the retroperitoneal space is opened lateral to the colon to expose the kidney. Control of the bleeding and closure of the renal lacerations are the essential aims of the operative procedure (304). Non-viable renal parenchyma should be removed, bleeding vessels and the collecting system should be sutured with 4/0 chromic catgut, and a partial nephrectomy performed for severe damage to an upper or lower pole of the kidney. Various techniques of 'renorrhaphy' have been described to close the parenchyma. Primary closure of the strong renal capsule is performed, when intact, with or without a haemostatic bolster such as Oxycel or free fat. If the capsule has been damaged, cover may be obtained with a pedicle of omentum, a peritoneal graft, or synthetic mesh. Albarran (305) encapsulated the kidney with catgut sutures but various synthetic biodegradable materials are now available. In an experimental study (306), polyglycolic acid mesh stimulated a thick fibroblastic proliferation at one month with the formation of a neocapsule at three months and complete resorption of the mesh. The mesh stopped the bleeding immediately during lower pole partial nephrectomy. Schoenberger and colleagues (307) used Vicryl mesh in another experimental study and Scott and colleagues (308) have investigated the properties of a collagen membrane reinforced with Vicryl mesh in renal, ureteric, and bladder surgery.

Page (309) produced hypertension in dogs by wrapping one or both kidneys in cellophane and it has been considered that subcapsular or perirenal haematomas might cause a similar result. The incidence of hypertension following renal injury has been variously quoted at between 0.7 and 33 per cent, but recent studies suggest it to be little more than an incidental finding. McAninch and colleagues (300) reported three patients with hypertension in their series of 1363, of whom two resolved spontaneously. Furthermore, non-disturbance of the infarcted kidney appears to cause no significant risk of hypertension or any other morbid sequelae (290, 293, 300).

Ureter

The mobility and muscular pliability of the ureters safeguards them from blunt injury but they can be damaged by penetrating or iatrogenic injuries. The blood supply is derived from a variable number of sources that feed into a plexus of vessels between the adventitia and muscular layers. At the upper end the major contribution comes from the lower segmental branch of the renal artery and at the lower end from the superior and inferior vesical arteries. Additional branches arise from the gonadal, the abdominal aorta, and the iliac arteries entering the ureteric vascular plexus from the medial side above the pelvic brim and the lateral side below this level.

There are three intrinsic narrow segments in the ureter: at the pelviureteric junction, the pelvic brim, and the ureterovesical junction (which is the most significant). Any injury above the intramural part of the ureter can lead to the development of a urinoma, infection, fistula, or stricture. Intubation of the damaged ureter with a fine catheter such as an 8FG infant-feeding tube brought out through the bladder, or the passage of a pig-tail stent, can avoid such a sequence of complications.

The ureter is particularly vulnerable during pelvic surgery, with reports of 0.3–3 per cent of routine gynaecological procedures resulting in injury to a ureter. In recent years the advent of the ureteroscope for diagnostic and stone surgery has introduced a further hazard, with an incidence of complications between 10 and 17 per cent, particularly in those ureters damaged by previous surgery or radiotherapy (310, 311).

Many penetrating and intraoperative injuries to the ureter are not recognized at operation and are associated with delayed diagnosis, which presents with persistent loin or abdominal pain, fever, ileus, abscess, urinary ascites, or increased discharge from a drain or the vagina. If the concentration of urea in the 'discharge' exceeds that in the blood, a fistula is certain. An IVU has been the essential investigation followed by bilateral ureterograms but CT is also of value in these cases. Percutaneous nephrostomy is rarely necessary but may be indicated if a pyonephrosis is suspected (312). Following gynaecological surgery the diagnosis may not be made until urinary incontinence is obvious and that raises the question of the timing of the repair. Badenoch and colleagues (313) strongly advocate early intervention for inadvertent injuries to the bladder or ureter following gynaecological surgery; delay increases fibrosis and may reduce the patient's morale. The choice of repair includes the spatulated uretero-ureterostomy, the transuretero-ureterostomy, and the ureteroneocystostomy. Successful treatment of gynaecological injuries to the ureter by means of ureteric stenting has been reported and should certainly be attempted if a guide wire can be passed through the damaged segment. If a long length of ureter is deficient, ureteric replacement with ileum and renal autotransplantation also need to be considered.

Injuries to the upper or middle third of the ureter may be treated by uretero-ureterostomy if the ends of the ureters are healthy after adequate debridement and can be approximated without tension. The ureters should be cut obliquely to spatulate their ends and anastomosed with a 3/0 catgut or polyglactin-910 suture to give a water-tight closure. A drain should be placed adjacent to the anastomosis.

The role of ureteric stenting is controversial. Various types of stents are available which can provide internal or external drainage. In the upper ureter it can be difficult to be confident that an internal pig-tail stent is lying within the bladder and problems can arise if it migrates up or down in the early postoperative period. Nephrostomy catheters of the rat-tail type or a silicone T-tube with a long distal limb can be passed down the ureter from the kidney or the renal pelvis across the anastomosis, thereby providing access for a ureterogram 7–10 days postoperatively to check the anastomosis before the removal of the catheter.

If there is loss of, or damage, to the distal ureter 5 cm or more above the bladder, transuretero-ureterostomy provides a satisfactory method of establishing urinary drainage by anastomosing the damaged ureter to the healthy one on the contralateral side. Irvine Smith (314) described the operation as simple and safe. The upper ureter is mobilized and brought across the abdominal aorta and inferior vena cava either above or below the inferior mesenteric artery. The ureter is cut obliquely to spatulate the end to a diameter of about 1 cm and an incision of similar length is made in the healthy ureter. A drain placed down to the site of the anastomosis is essential (315) but the question of ureteric stenting is best left to the discretion of the surgeon.

The common sites of injury to the distal ureter are at the level of the pelvic brim, the infundibulopelvic ligament, and the ureterovesical junction (316). The ureter may be inadvertently clamped, divided, or partially ligated. If it is possible to pass a guide wire through the damaged section of the ureter, ureteric stenting alone may be sufficient to allow healing of the ureter to occur (317). When the ureter is obstructed or a fistulous track has been established, direct reimplantation of the ureter into the bladder is the treatment of choice, but tension must be avoided. The psoas-hitch procedure and the Boari flap are popular methods of treatment, avoiding tension on the anastomosis by mobilizing the bladder.

For the psoas-hitch procedure the bladder is first mobilized from the contralateral wall by division of the superior vesical vessels. Turner-Warwick (318) described a method of elongating the bladder by making an accurately placed transverse incision across the anterior wall and closing this vertically so that it reaches a point 3 cm above the iliac vessels. Large bites of psoas minor, avoiding the nerve trunks (or of the tendon of psoas minor when present), are taken with chromic catgut to fix the bladder securely to the pelvic wall. A 3 cm suburothelial tunnel is then constructed for the ureter which is intubated with an 8FG catheter.

The construction of the Boari flap may require division of the superior vesical artery on the contralateral side to the injured ureter. Blandy advises filling the bladder with saline so that a broad-cased U-shaped flap of bladder can be marked out before it is cut and shaped to meet the ureter without tension (Fig. 9.16) (319). A submucosal tunnel is formed for the ureteric anastomosis and the ureter is catheterized with an 8FG Gibbon catheter which is brought out through the abdominal wall as a splint.

The commonest ureteroscopic injury is perforation of the ureter and the upper ureter is particularly at risk – the use of ultrasonic or electrohydraulic lithotripsy can cause thermal damage and traction on an impacted stone basket can avulse the ureter. The use of the miniscopes with a fibre-optic system

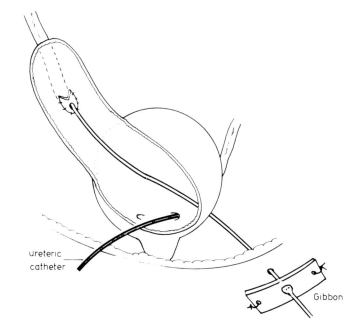

ureteric catheter

Gibbon

Fig. 9.16 The Boari flap: a broad-based bladder flap has been developed and the ureter implanted without tension.

and an external diameter of 6FG–7.5FG has facilitated the introduction of the instrument without the need for ureteric dilatation. Guidelines have been suggested: if dilatation of the lower ureter is required, hydrostatic balloon dilatation is less likely to damage the ureter than the graduated bougies. A guide wire should be passed to the renal pelvis under radiological control and it should remain in place throughout the procedure. If difficulty is encountered passing the instrument, or if damage to the ureter is suspected, a ureteric stent can be left *in situ* and the examination postponed for a few days. Whenever possible, screening facilities should be available during ureterosopic procedures.

Ureteric dilatation in response to intubation was noted by Wiseman (320) and this facilitates the introduction of a ureteroscope at a later session.

Bladder

The bladder is the most resilient part of the urinary tract. The wall consists of an adventitial outer layer of connective tissue, a well developed muscular layer and an inner urothelial lining. The smooth muscle bundles form a meshwork and are not arranged in layers. The blood supply comes from branches of the internal iliac artery; the superior vesical and inferior vesical arteries are the two named branches, but additional vessels arise from the obturator and inferior gluteal arteries.

The bladder and the urothelial lining heal rapidly. Hastings and colleagues (321) showed that bladder wounds gained rapid strength, attaining 100 per cent of the strength of the unwounded tissue in 14–21 days, and that the urothelium covered both the wound and the exposed sutures five days after the injury. If the bladder is totally denuded of mucosa it will be completely re-epithelialized in 16 weeks.

Injuries to the bladder may cause severe bruising that may be associated with gross haematuria or rupture of the bladder which may be associated with either extraperitoneal or intraperitoneal extravasation of urine. Prior to the antibiotic era, rupture of the bladder had a high mortality rate with reports of over 40 per cent mortality (322).

Extraperitoneal rupture is usually associated witih fractures of the pelvis or occur as a result of inadvertent injury during pelvic or transurethral surgery. Urethral drainage alone is sufficient in most cases and drainage of the retroperitoneal space should be performed if there is a large collection of urine.

Intraperitoneal rupture can arise from a severe blow to the distended bladder which ruptures at its weakest point in the dome. Trauma sufficent to rupture the bladder is liable to be associated with other visceral injuries demanding exploration. Exploration and closure of the rupture with suprapubic drainage is advocated for these injuries. A cystogram is performed 14 days later and, if no leakage is demonstrated, the suprapubic catheter is removed. The suprapubic tract closes rapidly in the absence of urethral obstruction.

Vesicovaginal fistula is a complication of abdominal hysterectomy and is usually closed through an abdominal approach. The fistulous track should be opened and the vaginal and bladder walls closed separately with interposition of omentum. Suprapubic drainage of the bladder is normally advocated after bladder repair or reconstruction. The use of omentum has been strongly advocated in reconstructive urological procedures and its use as a pedicle graft has been promoted by Turner-Warwick (323). The pedicle graft is based on the right gastro-epiploic artery and in this manner it can be brought well down into the perineum. The omentum naturally becomes adherent to healing structures but once that process has resolved the omentum regains its suppleness and is relatively easy to separate if re-exposure of the structures is necessary. The use of omentum in urological surgery has gained wide application and it is now frequently employed to reinforce renal, ureteric, bladder, and even urethral closures.

Urethra

Urethral injuries invariably present with blood at the external urethral meatus and they can lead to serious debilitating complications resulting in incontinence, stricture, periurethral abscess, fistula, and impotence (324). In an animal model, the post-traumatic inflammatory response was shown to be much more severe when extravasation of urine had occurred (325). Injuries to the urethra are rare and the late complications of stricture are the domain of the specialist in a tertiary referral centre. They are divided into anterior and posterior urethral injuries.

Anterior urethral injuries are mainly related to 'fall astride' injuries when the urethra is crushed against the inferior margin of the pubic arch. If the bruising is severe and associated with retention of urine, suprapubic catheterization should be performed. Urethrography may reveal extravasation at the the site of the injury but urethral catheterization should be avoided. Before the suprapubic catheter is removed two

weeks after the injury a micturating cystogram is performed to exclude extravasation at the site of the injury.

Iatrogenic injuries of the anterior urethra are normally recognized at the time of instrumentation. Again, suprapubic catheter drainage of the bladder allows the urethral laceration to heal and radiological assessment to be undertaken.

Posterior urethral injuries are associated with fractures of the pelvis usually arising in the region of the apex of the prostate at the junction of the prostatic and membanous parts of the urethra. The acute problem should be investigated by urethrography to identify the site of the urethral disruption and urethral catheterization should be avoided. The bladder can be drained by suprapubic catheterization during the initial management of the patient. If surgery is indicated and external fixation of the pelvic fracture planned, realignment of the urethra over a urethral catheter should be considered at the same time. These are rare and complex problems demanding an experienced urological opinion.

Sutures

Any foreign material in the urinary tract can form a nidus for stone formation and hence only absorbable sutures can be used. The ideal suture should be as strong as the structures it approximates and it should maintain its strength until healing is complete before undergoing complete absorption without stone formation. There are two groups of absorbable sutures, namely collagen and the synthetic polymers. The problem with the collagen sutures, plain and chromic catgut, is their variable strength and unpredictable absorption, which was shown to be longer in traumatized tissues (326). The manufacture of the synthetic sutures polyglycolic acid and polyglactin-910, which are absorbed by hydrolysis, allows their quality to be standardized. Edlich and colleagues (327) considered the braided polyglycolic acid and polyglactin-910 sutures to be ideally suited for the urinary tract, maintaining their strength for approximately 21 days yet being totally reabsorbed by 80 days. Holbrook (328) showed that polyglycolic acid sutures appeared to lose tensile strength rapidly when incubated in urine infected with *Proteus mirabilis* and suggested that they should not be used in the presence of proven proteus infections. Polydioxanone (PDS) was introduced in 1981 as a monofilament absorbable suture but it retains its strength longer than chromic catgut and it was suggested that its slower absorption by hydrolysis could possible give rise to stone formation if used within the urinary tract.

Catheters, stents, and encrustation

Catheters provoke an inflammatory reaction from the urothelium. An outbreak of reports of urethral stricture following cardiac surgery in the early 1980s drew attention to the severe reaction that can occur; patients experienced a severe burning sensation in the penis within two days of insertion of a latex catheter. This was considered to be related to the composition of the catheter because the problem resolved when the brand of catheter was changed (329, 330). Ohkawa and colleagues (331) showed that urethral catheters develop a fine fibrillar material on their surface, within three days of

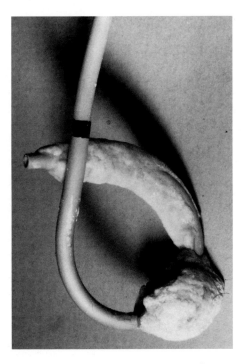

Fig. 9.17 Stone formation on a pig-tail stent.

insertion, containing fibrin and cellular debris from the urothelium. Microorganisms adhere to this layer and produce a mass of fibres consisting of polysaccharides which form the glycocalyx. Costerton and Marrie (332) drew attention to the concept of the planktonic microorganisms in the urine and the adherent sessile bacteria, with a glycocalyx, which are relatively resistant to antibiotics. In one study biofilms were demonstrated on about 50 per cent of urethral catheters but their formation was not related to the length of time that the catheter remained in place (333). Crystals become attached to the glycocalyx and these form the basis for encrustation and stones. Catheter encrustation is usually associated with urea-splitting organisms such as *Proteus*, *Klebsiella*, *Pseudomonas*, and *Providentia* which cause the urine to become alkaline with a high ammonia content. Struvite ($MgNH_4PO_4{\cdot}6H_2O$) and carbonate–apatite ($Ca_{10}(PO_4,CO_3)_6{\cdot}(OH,CO_3)_2$) form the main constituents of these deposits (334). Bruce and colleagues and Kunin *et al.* (335, 336) have noted the individual variation amongst patients in blocking catheters. The relationship between the surface morphology of catheters and their susceptibility to bacterial colonization and encrustation has not received sufficient attention (337). Encrustation of ureteric stents develops rapidly in stone-forming patients (Fig. 9.17) and has been observed within two weeks of insertion of the catheter (338). Pocock and colleagues (339) advised that the stent should be left *in situ* for a period of less than six weeks in this group. Less encrustation occurred on silicone material, which may be related to the smoothness of the surface (340).

References

1. Odland, G. R. (1983). Structure of the skin. In *Biochemistry and physiology of skin*, (ed. L. A. Goldsmith), Ch. 1, pp. 3–63. Oxford University Press, New York.
2. Robson, M. C., Krizek, T. J., and Wray, R. C. Jr (1979). Care of the thermally injured patient. In *The management of trauma*, (ed. Ballinger, Rutherford, and Zuidema), Ch. 23, pp. 666–730. W. B. Saunders, Philadelphia.
3. Robson, M. C. and Smith, D. J. (1990). Care of the thermally injured victim. In *Plastic surgery: principles and practice*, Ch. 50, pp. 1355–410. C. V. Mosby, St Louis.
4. Briggaman, R. A. (1983). The epidermal–dermal junction and genetic disorders of this area. In *Biochemistry and physiology of skin*, (ed. L. A. Goldsmith), Ch. 42, pp. 1001–24. Oxford University Press, New York.
5. Shilbert, J. E. (1983). Proteoglycans and glycosaminoglycans. In *Biochemistry and physiology of skin*, (ed. L. A. Goldsmith), Ch. 20, pp. 448–61. Oxford University Press, New York.
6. Horstmann, E. (1966). The lymph vessels of skin. *Die Ernahrangsindustrie*, **68**, 379–83.
7. Robson, M. C. and Parsons, R. W. (1988). Reconstructive and plastic surgery. In *Essenital surgical practice*, (ed. A. Cushieri, G. R. Giles, and A. R. Moossa), (2nd edn), Ch. 22, pp. 328–42. John Wright, London.
8. Gillies, H. and Millard, D. R. (1957). Reducation and aesthetic surgery. In *The principles and art of plastic surgery*, (ed. Gillies and Millard), Ch. 20, pp. 391–429. Little, Brown & Co, Boston.
9. Phillips, L. G. and Heggers, J. P. (1988). Better laceration repair with layered closure. *Postgrad. Med.*, **83**, 142–52.
10. Robson, M. C. and Zachary, L. S. (1992). Repair of traumatic cutaneous injuries involving the skin and soft tissues. In *Textbook of plastic, maxillofacial, and reconstructive surgery*, (ed. Georgiade, Georgiade, Riefkohl, and Barwick), (2nd edn), Ch. 5, pp. 129–33. Williams and Wilkins, Baltimore.
11. Hamer, M. L., Robson, M. C., Krizek, T. J., and Wouthwisk, W. O. (1975). Quantitative bacterial analysis of comparative wound irrigations. *Ann. Surg.*, **181**, 819–22.
12. Robson, M. C. (1991). Wound healing and wound closure. In *Quantitative bacteriology: its role in the armamentarium of the surgeon*, (ed. J. P. Heggers and M. C. Robson), Ch. 6, pp. 55–66. CRC Press, Boca Raton.
13. Robson, M. C. (1991). Plastic surgery. In *Quantitative bacteriology: its role in the armamentarium of the surgeon*, (ed. J. P. Heggers and M. C. Robson), Ch. 8, pp. 71–84. CRC Press, Boca Raton.
14. Robson, M. C., Duke, W. F., and Krizek, T. J. (1973). Rapid bacterial screening in the treatment of civilian wounds. *J. Surg. Res.*, **14**, 426–30.
15. Halsted, W. S. (1890). The treatment of wounds with especial reference to the value of blood clot in the management of dead space. *Johns Hopkins Hospital Reports*, **2**, 255–314.
16. Ricketts, C. R., Squire, J. R., Topley, E., and Lilly, H. A. (1951). Human skin lipids with particular reference to the self-sterilizing power of the skin. *Clin. Sci.*, **10**, 89–111.
17. Krizek, T. J., Robson, M. C., and Kho, E. (1967). Bacterial growth and skin graft survival. *Surg. Forum*, **18**, 518–19.
18. Littlewood, A. H. M. (1960). Seroma: an unrecognized cause of failure of split-thickness skin grafts. *Brit. J. Plast. Surg.*, **13**, 42–6.
19. Robson, M. C. (1988). Disturbances of wound healing. *Ann. Emerg. Med.*, **54**, 559–663.
20. Kraissl, J. (1951). The selection of appropriate lines for elective surgical incisions. *Plast. Reconstr. Surg.*, **8**, 1–28.

21. Koss, N. (1976). The mathematics of flap design. In *Symposium on basic science in plastic surgery*, (ed. T. J. Krizek and J. E., Hoopes), Ch. 31, pp. 274–83. C. V. Mosby, St Louis.

22. Larson, D. L., Abston, A., Evans, E. B., Dobrkovsky, M., and Linares, H. A. (1971). Techniques for decreasing scar formation and contractures in the burn patient. *J. Trauma*, **11**, 807–23.

23. Linares, H. A. and Larson, D. L. (1978). Proteoglycans and collagenase in hypertrophic scar formation. *Plast. Reconstr. Surg.*, **62**, 589–93.

24. Berman, B. and Duncan, M. R. (1989). Short-term keloid treatment *in vivo* with interferon alpha-2B results in a selective and persistent normalization of keloidal fibroblast collagen, glycosaminoglycans, and collagenase production *in vitro*. *J. Am. Acad. Dermatol.*, **21**, 694–702.

25. Duncan, M. R. and Berman, B. (1985). Gamma interferon is the lymphokine and beta interferon the monokine responsible for inhibition of fibroblast collagen production and late but not early fibroblast proliferation. *J. Exp. Med.*, **162**, 516–27.

26. Zacarian, S. A. (1985). Cryogenics: the cryolesion and the pathogenesis of cryonecrosis. In *Cryosurgery for skin and cutaneous disorder*, (ed. S. Zacarian), Ch. 11, pp. 1–30. C. V., Mosby, St Louis.

27. Mohs, F. E. (1980). Chemosurgery. *Clin. Plast. Surg.*, **65**, 656–64.

28. Tromovitch, T. and Stegman, S. (1978). Microscopic-controlled excision of cutaneous tumours: chemosurgery, fresh-tissue technique. *Cancer*, **41**, 653–8.

29. Mohs, F. E. (1978). *Chemosurgery, microscopically controlled surgery for skin cancer*. Charles C Thomas, Springfield, IL.

30. Robson, M. C. (1988). Burn sepsis. *Critical Care Clinics of North America*, **4**, 281–98.

31. Moritz, A. R. and Henrique, F. C., Jr (1947). Studies of thermal injury: the relative importance of time and surface temperature in the causation of cutaneous burns. *Am. J. Pathol.*, **23**, 695–720.

32. Raine, T. J., Heggers, J. P., Robson, M. C., London, M. D., and Johns, L. (1981). Cooling the burn wound to maintain microcirculation. *J. Trauma*, **221**, 394–7.

33. Heggers, J. P., Robson, M. C., London, M. D., Raine, T. J., and Becker, B. (1982). Cooling and the prostaglandin effect in thermal injury. *J. Burn. Care. Rehab.*, **3**, 350–4.

34. Heggers, J. P., Ko, F., Robson, M. C., Heggers, R., and Craft, K. E. (1980). Evaluation of burn blister fluid. *Plast. Reconstr. Surg.*, **65**, 798–804.

35. Zawacki, B. E. (1974). Reversal of capillary stasis and prevention of necrosis in burns. *Ann. Surg.*, **186**, 99–102.

36. McHugh, T. P., Robson, M. C., Heggers, J. P., Phillips, L. G., Smith, D. J., and McCollum, M. C. (1986). Therapeutic efficacy of Biobrane® in partial thickness and full thickness thermal injury. *Surgery*, **100**, 661–4.

37. Robson, M. C., Smith, D. J., and Heggers, J. P. (1988). Innovations in burn wound management. *Adv. Plast. Reconstr. Surg.*, **4**, 149–76.

38. Jackson, D. McG. (1953). The diagnosis of the depth of burning. *Brit. J. Surg.*, **40**, 388.

39. Robson, M. C. (1983). Reconstruction and rehabilitation from admission: a surgeon's role at each phase. In *Comprehensive approaches to the burned person*, (ed. N. T. Bernstein and M. C. Robson), Ch. 4, pp. 35–48. Medical Exam Publ., New Hyde Park, NY.

40. Robson, M. C., Samburg, J. L., and Krizek, T. J. (1973). Quantitative comparison of biological dressings. *J. Surg. Res.*, **14**, 431–4.

41. Roberts, L. W., McManus, W. F., Shirani, K. Z., Mason, A. D., and Pruitt, B. A. (1985). Biobrane and porcine: a comparative study. *Proc. Am. Burn Assoc.*, **18**, 168.

42. Purdue, G. F., Hunt, J. L., Gillespie, R. W., Hansbrough, J. F., Dominic, W. J., Robson, M. C., *et al.* (1987). Biosynthetic skin substitute versus frozen human cadaver allograft for temporary coverage of excised burn wounds. *J. Trauma*, **27**, 155–7.

43. Robson, M. C., Barnett, R. A., Leitch, I. O. W., and Hayward, P. G. (1992). Prevention and treatment of post-burn scars and contracture. *World J. Surg.*, **16**, 87–96.

44. Rees, R. S., Nanney, L. B., Fleming, P., and Cary, A. (1986). Tissue expansion: its role in traumatic below-knee amputation. *Plast. Reconstr. Surg.*, **77**, 133–7.

45. Paul, M. E., Wall, W. J., and Duff, J. H. (1976). Delayed primary closure in colon operations. *Canadian J. Surg.*, **19**, 33–6.

46. McLachlin, A. D. and Wall, W. (1976). Delayed primary closure of the skin and subcutaneous tissue in abdominal surgery. *Canadian J. Surg.*, **19**, 37–40.

47. Stuart, M. (1976). The role of delayed primary wound closure in the prevention of wound sepsis after appendectomy. *Med. J. Aust.*, **2**, 421–2.

48. Ellis, H., Coleridge-Smith, P. D., and Joyce, A. D. (1984). Abdominal incisions – vertical or transverse? *Postgrad. Med. J.*, **60**, 407–10.

49. Bucknall, T. E., Cox, P. J., and Ellis, H. (1984). Burst abdomen and incisional hernia: a prospective study of 1129 major laparotomies. *Br. Med. J.*, **284**, 931–3.

50. Guillou, P. J., Hall, T. J., and Donaldson, D. R. (1980). Vertical abdominal incisions – a choice? *Br. J. Surg.*, **67**, 395–9.

51. Capperauld, I. (1989). Suture materials: A review. *Clinical Materials*, **4**, 3–12.

52. MacKenzie, D. A. C. (1971). A short history of sutures. Based on a paper presented to the Royal College of Surgeons of Edinburgh.

53. Moynihan, B. G. A. (1914). *Abdominal operations*. W. B. Saunders, Philadelphia.

54. Moynihan, B. G. A. (1920). The ritual of a surgical operation. *Br. J. Surg.*, **8**, 27–35.

55. Dudley, H. A. F. (1970). Layered and mass closure of the abdominal wall. A theoretical and experimental analysis. *Br. J. Surg.*, **57**, 664–7.

56. Kennedy, J. W. (1934). Tragedies of the abdominal incision. *Am. J. Surg.*, **25**, 512–20.

57. Nayman, J. (1976). Mass single layer closure of abdominal wounds. *Med. J. Aust.*, **1**, 183–6.

58. Bucknall, T. E. (1983). Factors influencing wound complications: a clinical and experimental study. *Ann. Roy. Coll. Surg. Engl.*, **65**, 71–7.

59. Pollock, A. V., Greenall, M. J., and Evans, M. (1979). Single-layer mass closure of major laparotomies by continuous suturing. *J. Roy. Soc. Med.*, **72**, 889–93.

60. Wadstrom, J. and Gerdin, B. (1990). Closure of the abdominal wall: how and why? Clinical review. *Acta Chirurgica Scandinavica*, **156**, 75–82.

61. Karakousis, C. P. (1980). One layer closure of the abdominal wall. *Surgery, Gynecology and Obstetrics*, **150**, 243–4.

62. Jones, T. E., Newell, E. T., and Brubaker, R. E. (1941). *Surgery, Gynecology and Obstetrics*, **72**, 1056.

63. Irvin, T. T. (1985). Simple skin closure. *Br. J. Hosp. Med.*, **33**, 325–30.

64. Milewski, P. J. and Thomson, H. (1980). Is a fat stitch necessary? *Br. J. Surg.*, **67**, 393–4.

65. Sapala, J. A., Brown, T. E., and Sapala, M. A. (1986). Anatomic staple closure of midline incision of the upper part of the abdomen. *Surgery, Gynecology and Obstetrics*, **163**, 282–4.

66. Wissing, J., van Vroonhoven, T. J., Schattenkerk, M. E., Veen, H. F., Ponsen, R. J., and Jeekel, J. (1987). Fascia closure after

midline laparotomy: results of a randomised trial. *Br. J. Surg.*, **74**, 738–41.

67. Read, R. C. and Yoder, G. (1989). Recent trends in the management of incisional herniation. *Arch. Surg.*, **124**, 485–8.

68. Bucknall, T. E., Teare, L., and Ellis, H. (1983). The choice of a suture to close abdominal incisions. *Euro. Surg. Res.*, **15**, 59–66.

69. Bucknall, T. E. (1981). Abdominal wound closure: choice of suture. *J. Roy. Soc. Med.*, **74**, 580–5.

70. Bucknall, T. E. and Ellis, H. (1981). Abdominal wound closure – a comparison of monofilament nylon and polyglycolic acid. *Surgery*, **89**, 672–7.

71. Howes, E. L. and Harvey, S. C. (1929). The strength of healing wounds in relation to the holding strength of catgut suture. *New Eng. J. Med.*, **200**, 1285–90.

72. Grace, D. M. (1976). Dexon: an excellent suture for midline incisions. *Can. J. Surg.*, **19**, 54–8.

73. Jenkins, T. P. (1976). The burst abdominal wound: a mechanical approach. *Br. J. Surg.*, **63**, 873–6.

74. Campbell, J. A., Temple, W. J., Frank, C. B., and Huchcroft, S. A. (1989). A biomechanical study of suture pullout in linea alba. *Surgery*, **106**, 888–92.

75. Gallup, D. G., Nolan, T. E., and Smith, R. P. (1990). Primary mass closure of midline incisions with a continuous polyglyconate monofilament absorbable suture. *Obstetrics and Gynaecology*, **76**, 872–5.

76. Krukowski, Z. H., Cusick, E. L., Engeset, J., and Matheson, N. A. (1989). Polydioxanone or polypropylene for closure of midline abdominal incisions: a prospective comparative clinical trial. *Br. J. Surg.*, **74**, 828–30.

77. Fisher, G. T., Fisher, J. B., and Stark, R. B. (1980). Origin of the use of subcuticular sutures. *Ann. Plast. Surg.*, **4**, 144–8.

78. Onwuanyi, O. N. and Evbuomwan, I. (1990). Skin closure during appendectomy: a controlled clinical trial of subcuticular and interrupted transdermal suture techniques. *J. Roy. Coll. Surg. Edin.*, **35**, 353–5.

79. Ftahi, Z. and Snow, W. N. (1989). The buried running dermal subcutaneous suture technique. *J. Dermat. Surg. Onc.*, **15**, 264–6.

80. Gatt, D., Quick, C. R., and Owen-Smith, M. S. (1985). Staples for wound closure: a controlled trial. *Ann. Roy. Coll. Surg. Engl.*, **67**, 318–20.

81. Doody, D. P., Albert, D. L., and Laberge, J. M. (1986). Zipper closure of the abdominal wall in the treatment of recurrent intra-abdominal abscesses. *J. Paed. Surg.*, **21**, 1195–7.

82. Aprahamian, C., Wittman, D. H., Bergstein, J. M., *et al.* (1990). Temporary abdominal closure (TAC) for planned relaparotomy (etappen-lavage) in trauma. *J. Trauma*, **30**, 719–23.

83. Irvin, T. (1981). *Wound healing – principles and practice.* Chapman and Hall, London.

84. Ellis, H. (1962). The aetiology of post-operative abdominal adhesions. *Br. J. Surg.*, **50**, 10–16.

85. Karipineni, R. C., Wilk, P. J., and Danese, C. A. (1976). The role of the peritoneum in the healing of abdominal incisions. *Surgery, Gynaecology and Obstetrics*, **142**, 729–30.

86. Ellis, H. and Heddle, R. (1977). Does the peritoneum need to be closed at laparotomy? *Br. J. Surg.*, **64**, 733–6.

87. McGinn, F. P. and Hamilton, J. C. (1976). Ascorbic acid levels in stored blood and in patients undergoing surgery after blood transfusion. *Br. J. Surg.*, **63**, 505–7.

88. Taube, M., Elliott, P., and Ellis, H. (1981). Jaundice and wound healing: a tissue culture study. *Br. J. Exp. Path.*, **62**, 227–31.

89. Bayer, I. and Ellis, H. (1976). Jaundice and wound healing: an experimental study. *Br. J. Surg.*, **63**, 392–6.

90. Colin, J. F., Elliott, P., and Ellis, H. (1979). The effects of uraemia upon wound healing: an experimental study. *Br. J. Surg.*, **66**, 793–97.

91. Goodson, W. H. 3d and Hunt, T. K. (1979). Wound healing and aging. *J. Invest. Derm.*, **73**, 88–91.

92. Bucknall, T. E. (1980). The effect of local infection upon wound healing – an experimental study. *Br. J. Surg.*, **67**, 851–5.

93. Leaper, D. J. and Simpson, R. A. (1986). Antiseptics and healing. *J. Antimicr. Chemot.*, **17**, 135–7.

94. Bannister, G. C. (1995). Personal communication.

95. Saxe, J. M., Ledgerwood, A. M., and Lucas, C. E. (1991). Management of the difficult abdominal closure. *Surg. Cl. N. Am.*, **73**, 243–51.

96. Bucknall, T. E., Cox, P. J., and Ellis, H. (1982). Burst abdomen and incisional hernia: a prospective study of 1129 major laparotomies. *Br. Med. J.*, **284**, 931–3.

97. Leaper, D. J., Pollock, A. V., and Evans, M. (1977). Abdominal wound closure: a trial of nylon, polyglycolic acid and steel sutures. *Br. J. Surg.*, **64**, 603–6.

98. Pollock, A. V., Greenall, M. J., and Evans, M. (1979). Single-layer mass closure of laparotomies by continuous suturing. *Proceedings of the Royal Society of Medicine*, **72**, 889–93.

99. Poole, G. V., Meredith, J. W., Kon, N. D., Martin, M. B., *et al.* (1984). Suture technique and wound bursting strength. *American Surgeon*, **50**, 569–72.

100. Adamson, R. J., Musco, F., and Enquist, I. F. (1964). The relationship of collagen content to wound strength in normal and scorbutic animals. *Surgery, Gynaecology and Obstetrics*, **119**, 323–9.

101. Högström, H. and Haglund, U. (1986). Postoperative decrease in suture holding capacity in laparotomy wounds and anastomoses. *Acta. Chirurgica Scandinavica*, **151**, 533–5.

102. Högström, H., Haglund, U., and Zederfeldt, B. (1985). Suture technique and early breaking strength of intestinal anastomoses and laparotomy wounds. *Acta. Chirurgica Scandinavica*, **151**, 441–3.

103. Senapati, A. (1982). Spontaneous dehiscence of an incisional hernia. *Br. J. Surg.*, **69**, 313.

104. Bettman, R. B. and Kobak, M. W. (1960). Relative frequency of evisceration after laparotomy in recent years. *J. Am. Med. Assoc.*, **172**, 1764.

105. Keill, R. H., Keitzer W. F., Nichols W. K., Henzel, J., and DeWeese, M. S. (1973). Abdominal wound dehiscence. *Ann. Surg.*, **106**, 573–7.

106. Miles, R. M., Moore, M., Fitzgerald., and Gillespie, H. (1964). The aetiology and prevention of abdominal wound disruption. *American Surgeon*, **30**, 566–73.

107. Reitamo, J. and Möller, C. (1972). Abdominal wound dehiscence. *Acta. Chirurgica Scandinavica*, **138**, 170–5.

108. Reid, M. R., Zinninger, M. M., and Merrell, P. (1933). Closure of abdomen with through and through silver wire sutures in cases of acute abdominal emergencies. *Am. J. Surg.*, **98**, 890–4.

109. Dayton, M. T., Buchele, B. A., Shirazi, S. S., *et al.* (1986). Use of an absorbable mesh to repair contaminated abdominal wall defects. *Arch. Surg.*, **121**, 954–60.

110. Stone, H. H., Fabian, T. C., Turkles, M. L., *et al.* (1981). Management of acute full-thickness losses of the abdominal wall. *Ann. Surg.*, **193**, 612–16.

111. Voyles, C. R., Richardson, J. D., Bland, K. I., *et al.* (1981). Emergency abdominal wall reconstruction with polypropylene mesh. *Ann. Surg.*, **194**, 219–23.

112. Tejani, F. H. and Zamora, B. O. (1977). Placement of retention sutures. *Surgery, Gynecology and Obstetrics*, **144**, 572–3.

113. Faxen, A., Meurling, S., and Borkowski, A. (1976). A new kind of 'deep retention suture'. *Acta. Chirurgica Scandinavica*, **142**, 13–14.

114. Chávez-Cartaya, R., Jirón-Vargas, A., Pinto, A., *et al.* (1992). Adjustable nylon ties for abdominal wall closure. *Am. J. Surg.*, **163**, 609–12.

115. Mayer, A. D., Ausobsky, J. R., Evans, M., and Pollock, A. V. (1981). Compression suture of the abdominal wall: a controlled trial in 302 major laparotomies. *Br. J. Surg.*, **68**, 632–4.

116. Mudge, M. and Hughes, L. E. (1985). Incisional hernia: a 10 year prospective study of incidence and attitudes. *Br. J. Surg.*, **72**, 70–1.

117. Shepherd, J. H., Cavanagh, D., Riggs, D., Praphat, H., and Wisniewski, B. J. (1983). Abdominal wound closure using a non-absorbable single-layer technique. *Obstetrics and Gynaecology*, **61**, 248–52.

118. Bentley, P. G., Owen W. J., Girolami, P. L., and Dawson, J. L. (1978). Wound closure with Dexon (polyglycolic acid) mass suture. *Ann. Roy. Coll. Surg. Engl.*, **60**, 215–17.

119. Ellis, H., Gajraj, H., and George, C. D. (1983). Incisional hernias: when do they occur? *Br. J. Surg.*, **70**, 290–1.

120. Pollock, A. V. and Evans, M. (1989). Early prediction of late incisional hernias. *Br. J. Surg.*, **76**, 953–4.

121. Cleveland, R. D., Zitsch, R. P. 3d, and Laws, H. L. (1989). Incisional closure in morbidly obese patients. *American Surgeon*, **55**, 61–3.

122. Lamont, P. M. and Ellis, H. (1988). Incisional hernia in re-opened abdominal incisions: an overlooked risk factor. *Br. J. Surg.*, **75**, 374–6.

123. Urschel, J. D., Scott, P. G., and Williams, H. T. (1988). Aetiology of late developing incisional hernias – the possible role of mechanical stress. *Medical Hypotheses*, **25**, 31–4.

124. Jenkins, T. P. (1980). Incisional hernia repair: a mechanical approach. *Br. J. Surg.*, **67**, 335–6.

125. Walker, P. M. and Langer, B. (1976). Marlex mesh for repair of abdominal wall defects. *Can. J. Surg.*, **19**, 211–13.

126. van der Linden, F. T. and van Vroonhoven, T. J. (1988). Long-term results after surgical correction of incisional hernia. *Netherlands J. Surg.*, **40**, 127–9.

127. Plaus W. J. (1993). Laparoscopic trocar site hernias. *J. Laparoend. Surg.*, **3**, 567–70.

128. Fielding, L. P., Stewart-Brown, S., Blesovsky, L., and Kearney, G. (1980). Anastomotic integrity after operations for large-bowel cancer: a multicentre study. *Br. Med. J.*, **281**, 411–14.

129. Matthews, H. R., Powell, D. J., and McConkey, C. C. (1986). Effects of surgical experience on the results of resection for oesophageal carcinoma. *Br. J. Surg.*, **73**, 621–3.

130. Devlin, H. B. (1992). Findings of the NCEPOD report for 1990. *Br. J. Hosp. Med.*, **47**, 723–4.

131. Campling, E. A., Devlin, H. B., Hoile, R. W., and Lunn, J. N. (eds) (1992). *Report of the National Confidential Enquiry into Perioperative Deaths 1990*. National Confidential Enquiry into Perioperative Deaths, London.

132. Irvin, T. T. and Edwards, J. P. (1973). Comparison of single-layer inverting, two-layer inverting and everting anastomoses in the rabbit colon. *Br. J. Surg.*, **60**, 453–7.

133. Goligher, J. C., Morris, C., McAdam, W. A. F., DeDombal, F. T., and Johnston, D. (1970). A controlled clinical trial of inverting versus everting intestinal suture in clinical large bowel surgery. *Br. J. Surg.*, **57**, 817–22.

134. Matheson, N. A. and Irving, A. D. (1975). Single layer anastomosis after recto-sigmoid resection. *Br. J. Surg.*, **62**, 239–42.

135. Carly, N. J., Keating, J., Campbell, J., Karanjia, N., and Heald, R. J. (1991). Prospective audit of an extramucosal technique for intestinal anastomosis. *Br. J. Surg.*, **78**, 1291–6.

136. Leverment, J. N. and Mearns Milne, D. (1974). Oesophagogastrectomy in the management of malignancy of the thoracic oesophagus and cardia. *Br. J. Surg.*, **61**, 683–8.

137. Kratzer, G. L. and Onsanit, T. (1974). Single layer steel wire anastomosis of the intestine. *Surg. Gynecol. Obstet.*, **139**, 93–5.

138. Hardy, T. G., Pace W. G., Maney, J. W., Katz, A. R., and Kaganov, K. L. (1985). A biofragmentable ring for sutureless bowel anastomosis. *Dis. Colon Rectum*, **28**, 484–90.

139. Cahill, C. J., Betzler, M., Gruwez, J. A., Jeekel, J., Patel, J. C., and Zederfeldt, B. (1989). Sutureless large bowel anastomosis: European experience with the biofragmentable anastomosis ring. *Br. J. Surg.*, **76**, 344–7.

140. Costello, A. J., Johnson, D. E., Cromeens, D. M., Wishnow, K. I., von Eschenbach, A. C., and Ro, J. Y. (1990). Sutureless end-to-end bowel anastomosis using Nd:YAG and water-soluble intraluminal stent. *Lasers Surg. Med.*, **9**, 70–3.

141. Sauer, J. S., Hinshaw, J. R., and McGuire, K. P. (1989). The first sutureless, laser-welded, end-to-end bowel anastomosis. *Lasers Surg. Med.*, **9**, 70–3.

142. McCue, J. L. and Phillips, R. K. S. (1991). Sutureless intestinal anastomoses. *Br. J. Surg.*, **78**, 1291–6.

143. Orringer, M. B. (1983). Transhiatal oesophagectomy. In *Operative surgery*, (ed. H. Dudley, W. Pories, and D. Carter), p. 192. Alimentary Tract and Abdominal Wall. Butterworths, London.

144. Hankins, J. R., Miller, J. E., Allar, S., and McLaughlin, J. S. (1987). Transhiatal esophagectomy for carcinoma of the esophagus: experience with 26 cases. *Ann. Thorac. Surg.*, **44**, 123–7.

145. Barber, P. A., Luder, P. J., Schupfer, G., Becker, C. D., and Wagner, H. E. (1988). Quality of life and patterns of recurrence following transhiatal esophagectomy for cancer: results of a prospective follow-up in 50 patients. *World J. Surg.*, **12**, 270–6.

146. Muller, J. M., Erasmi, H., Stelzner, M., Zieren, U., and Pichlmaier, H. (1990). Surgical therapy of oesophageal carcinoma. *Br. J. Surg.*, **77**, 845–57.

147. Paterson, I. M. and Wong, J. (1989). Anastomotic leakage: an avoidable complication of Lewis–Turner oesophagectomy. *Br. J. Surg.*, **76**, 127–9.

148. Akiyama, H., Tsurumaru, M., Kawamura, T., and Ono, Y. (1981). Principles of surgical treatment of carcinoma of the esophagus. *Ann. Surg.*, **194**, 438–46.

149. Fabri, B. and Donnelly, R. J. (1982). Oesophagogastrectomy using the end-to-end anastomosing stapler. *Thorax*, **37**, 296–9.

150. West, P. N., Marbarger, J. P., Martz, M. N., and Roper, C. L. (1981). Esophagogastrectomy with the EEA stapler. *Ann. Surg.*, **193**, 825–30.

151. Fekete, F., Breil, P. H., Ronsse, H., Tossen, J. C., and Langonnet, F. (1981). EEA stapler and omental graft in esophagogastrectomy. *Ann. Surg.*, **193**, 825–30.

152. Ingake, M., Yamane, T., Kitao, Y., Okuzumi, J., Kutata, K., Yamaguchi, T., *et al.* (1992). Balloon dilatation for anastomotic stricture after upper gastrointestinal surgery. *World J. Surg.*, **16**, 541–4.

153. Waldron, R. P., Donovan, I. A., Drumm, J., Mottram, S. N., Tedman, S. (1986). Emergency presentation and mortality from colorectal cancer in the elderly. *Br. J. Surg.*, **73**, 214–16.

154. Irvin, T. T. (1988). Prognosis of colorectal cancer in the elderly. *Br. J. Surg.*, **75**, 419–21.

155. Irvin, T. T. and Goligher, J. C. (1973). Aetiology of disruption of intestinal anastomoses. *Br. J. Surg.*, **60**, 461–4.

156. Goligher, J. C., Graham, N. G., and DeDombal, F. T. (1970). Anastomotic dehiscence after anterior resection of rectum and sigmoid. *Br. J. Surg.*, **57**, 109–18.

157. Irvin, T. T. and Greaney, M. G. (1977). The treatment of colonic cancer presenting with intestinal obstruction. *Br. J. Surg.*, **64**, 741–4.

158. Runkel, N. S., Schlag, P., Schwarz, V., and Herfarth, C. (1991). Outcome after emergency surgery for cancer of the large intestine. *Br. J. Surg.*, **78**, 183–8.

159. Irvin, T. T. (1976). Collagen metabolism in infected colonic anastomoses. *Surg. Gynecol. Obstet.*, **143**, 220–4.

160. Dudley, H. A. F., Radcliffe, A. G., and McGeehan, D. (1980). Intraoperative irrigation of the colon to permit primary anastomosis. *Br. J. Surg.*, **67**, 80–1.

161. Koruth, N. M., Krukowski, Z. H., Youngson, G. G., Hendry, W. S., Logie, J. R. C., Jones, P. F., and Munro, A. (1985). Intraoperative colonic irrigation in the management of left-sided large bowel emergencies. *Br. J. Surg.*, **72**, 708–11.

162. Ravo, B. (1988). Colorectal anastomotic healing and intracolonic bypass procedure. *Surg Clin. North. Am.*, **68**, 1267–94.

163. Jones, P. F. and Thompson, H. J. (1982). Long-term results of a consistent policy of sphincter preservation in the treatment of carcinoma of the rectum. *Br. J. Surg.*, **69**, 564–8.

164. Dixon, A. R., Maxwell, W. A., and Thorton Holmes, J. (1991). Carcinoma of the rectum: a 10 year experience. *Br. J. Surg.*, **78**, 308–11.

165. Irving, A. D. and Scrimgeour, D. (1987). Mechanical bowel resection for colonic resection and anastomosis. *Br. J. Surg.*, **74**, 580–1.

166. Johnston, D. (1987). Bowel preparation for colorectal surgery. *Br. J. Surg.*, **74**, 553–4.

167. Goldring, J., McNaught, W., Scott, A., and Gillespie, G. (1975). Prophylactic oral anti-microbial agents in elective colonic surgery: a controlled clinical trial. *Lancet*, **ii**, 997–9.

168. Willis, A. T., Ferguson, I. R., Jones, P. H., Phillips, K. D., Tearle, P. V., *et al.* (1977). Metronidazole in prevention and treatment of *Bacteroides* infections in elective colonic surgery. *Br. Med. J.*, **i**, 607–10.

169. Galland, R. B., Saunders, J. H., Moseley, J. G., and Darrell, J. H. (1977). Prevention of wound infection in abdominal operations by preoperative antibiotics of povidone–iodine. *Lancet*, **ii**, 1043–5.

170. Condon, R. E., Bartlett, J. G., and Nicholls, R. L. (1979). Preoperative prophylactic cephalothin fails to control septic complications of colorectal operations: results of a controlled clinical trial. *Am. J. Surg.*, **137**, 68–71.

171. Brennan, S. S., Pickford, I. R., Evans Mary, and Pollock, A. V. (1982). Staples or sutures for colonic anastomoses: a controlled clinical trial. *Br. J. Surg.*, **69**, 722–4.

172. Beart, R. W. and Kelly, K. A. (1981). Randomized prospective evaluation of the EEA stapler for colorectal anastomoses. *Am. J. Surg.*, **141**, 143–7.

173. Knight, C. D. and Griffen, F. D. (1980). An improved technique for low anterior resection of the rectum using the EEA stapler. *Surgery*, **88**, 710–14.

174. Cohen, Z., Myers, E., Langer, B., Taylor, B., Railton, R. H., and Jamieson, C. (1982). Double stapling technique for low anterior resection. *Dis. Colon Rectum.*, **26**, 231–5.

175. Moritz, E., Achleitner, D., Holbling, N., Miller, K., Speil, T., and Weber, F. (1991). Single vs. double stapling technique in colorectal surgery, a prospective randomized trial. *Dis. Colon Rectum.*, **34**, 495–7.

176. Fazio, V. F. (1978). Symposium: factors that make low colorectal anastomoses safe. *Dis. Colon Rectum*, **21**, 401–5.

177. Smith, S. R. G., Swift, I., Gompertz, H., and Baker, W. N. W. (1988). Abdominoperineal and anterior resection of the rectum with retrocolic omentoplasty and no drainage. *Br. J. Surg.*, **75**, 1012–15.

178. Karanjia, N., Corder, A., Holdsworth, P., and Heald, R. (1991). Risk of peritonitis and fatal septicaemia and the need to defunction the low anastomosis. *Br. J. Surg.*, **78**, 196–8.

179. Mealy, K., Burke, P., and Hyland, J. (1992). Anterior resection without a defunctioning colostomy: questions of safety. *Br. J. Surg.*, **79**, 305–7.

180. Fasth, S., Hulten, L., and Palselius, I. (1980). Loop ileostomy – an attractive alternative to a temporary transverse colostomy. *Acta Chir. Scand.*, **146**, 203–7.

181. Williams, N. S., Nasmyth, D. G., Jones, D., and Smith, A. H. (1986). De-functioning stomas: a prospective controlled trial comparing loop ileostomy with loop transverse colostomy. *Br. J. Surg.*, **73**, 566–70.

182. Irvin, T. T. (1987). Recent results of colostomy closure: a prospective study of 98 operations. *J. R. Coll. Surg. Edinb.*, **32**, 352–4.

183. Hamilton, J. E. (1967). Reappraisal of open intestinal anastomoses. *Ann. Surg.*, **165**, 917–24.

184. Getzen, L. C., Roe, R. D., and Holloway, C. K. (1966). Comparative study of intestinal anastomotic healing in inverted and everted closures. *Surg. Gynecol. Obstet.*, **123**, 1219–27.

185. Ravitch, M. M., Canalis, F., Weinshelbaum, A., and McCormick, J. (1967). Studies in intestinal healing, III. Observations on everting intestinal anastomoses. *Ann. Surg.*, **166**, 670–80.

186. Irvin, T. T. (1975). Factors affecting the healing of colonic anastomoses. ChM Thesis, University of Aberdeen.

187. Smith, L. E. (1981). Anastomosis with EEA stapler after anterior colonic resection. *Dis. Colon Rectum*, **24**, 236–42.

188. Kissin, M. W., Cox, A. G., Wilkins, R. A., and Kark, A. E. (1985). The fate of the EEA stapled anastomosis: a clinicoradiological study of 38 patients. *Ann. R. Coll. Surg. Engl.*, **67**, 20–2.

189. Dziki, A. J., Duncan, M. D., Harmon, J. W., Saini, N., Malthaner, R. A., Trad, K. S., *et al.* (1991). Advantages of handsewn over stapled bowel anastomosis. *Dis. Colon Rectum*, **34**, 442–8.

190. Watson, C. J. E., Caine, R. Y., Padhani, A. R., and Dixon, A. K. (1991). Surgical restraint in the management of liver trauma. *Br. J. Surg.*, **78**, 1071–5.

191. Sherlock, D. J. and Bismuth, H. (1991). Secondary surgery for liver trauma. *Br. J. Surg.*, **78**, 1313–17.

192. Bismuth, H., Castaing, D., and Houssin, D. (1985). Die leberresektion, indikabionen und ergiebnisse. *Chirurgie*, **56**, 203–10.

193. Moore, F. A., Moore, E. E., and Seagroves, A. (1985). Non-resectional management of major hepatic trauma. *Am. J. Surg.*, **150**, 725–32.

194. Abercrombie, M. and Harkness, R. D. (1951). The growth of cell populations and the properties in tissue culture of regenerating liver of the rat. *Proc. R. Soc. Med.*, **B138**, 544–61.

195. Bucher, N. L. R., Scott, J. F., and Aub, J. C. (1951). Regeneration of the liver in parabiotic rats. *Cancer Res.*, **11**, 457–65.

196. Sigel, B., Baldia, L. B., Dunn, M. R., and Menduke, H. (1967). Humoral control of liver regeneration. *Surg. Gynecol. Obstet.*, **123**, 1023–31.

197. Starzl, T. E., Porter, K. A., and Kashiwagi, N. (1975). Portal hepatotrophic factors, diabetes mellitus and acute lever atrophy, hypertrophy and regeneration. *Surg. Gynecol. Obster.*, **141**, 843–58.

198. Bismuth, H., Castaing, D., and Garden, J. (1987). The use of operative ultrasound in surgery of primary liver tumours. *World J. Surg.*, **11**, 610–14.

199. Hodgson, W. J. B. and Del Quercio, L. R. M. (1984). Preliminary experience in liver surgery using the ultrasonic scalpel. *Surgery*, **95**, 230–4.

200. Garden, O. J. (1991). Iatrogenic injury to the bile duct. *Br. J. Surg.*, **78**, 1412–13.

201. Cameron, J. L. and Gadacz, T. R. (1991). Laparoscopic surgery. *Ann. Surg.*, **213**, 1–2.

202. Smith, R. (1979). Obstructions of the bile duct. *Br. J. Surg.*, **66**, 69–79.

203. Blumgart, L. H. (1983). Hepatic resection. In *Operative surgery: alimentary tract and abdominal wall*, 2, (ed. H. Dudley, W. J. Pories, and D. C. Carter), pp. 477–99. Butterworths, London.

204. Blumgart, L. H. and Kelley, C. J. (1984). Hepaticojejunostomy in benign and malignant high bile duct stricture: approaches to the left hepatic ducts. *Br. J. Surg.*, **71**, 257–61.

205. Traynor, O., Castaing, D., and Bismuth H. (1987). Left intrahepatic cholangioenteric anastomosis (round ligament approach): an effective palliative treatment for hilar cancers. *Br. J. Surg.*, **74**, 952–4.

206. McWhorter, G. L. (1929). New methods of anastomosis of common bile duct; experimental study. *Arch. Surg.*, **18**, 117–28.

207. Myers, R. T., Meredith, J. H., Rhodes, J., and Gilbert, J. W. (1960). The fate of free grafts in the common bile duct. *Ann. Surg.*, **151**, 776–82.

208. Northover, J. M. A. and Terblanche, J. (1979). A new look at the arterial supply of the bile duct in man and its surgical implications. *Br. J. Surg.*, **66**, 379–84.

209. Douglass, T. C., Lounsbury, B. F., Cutter, W. W., and Wetzel, N. (1950). Study of healing in the common bile duct. *Surg. Gynecol. Obster.*, **91**, 301–5.

210. Carlson, E., Zukoski, C. F., Campbell, J., and Chvapil, M. (1977). Morphologic, biophysical and biochemical consequences of ligation of the common biliary duct in the dog. *Am. J. Path.*, **86**, 301–20.

211. Rains, A. J. H. (1959). Biliary obstruction in the region of the porta hepatis. *Ann. R. Coll. Surg. Engl.*, **24**, 69–100.

212. Rozga, J., Ahren, B., Andersson, R., Emody, L., Wadstrom, T., and Bengmark, S. (1991). Effect of biliary infection on common bile duct healing in the rat. *Br. J. Surg.*, **78**, 1329–31.

213. Irvin, T. T., Vassilakis, J. S., Chattopadhyay, D. K., and Greaney, M. G. (1978). Abdominal wound healing in jaundiced patients. *Br. J. Surg.*, **65**, 521–2.

214. Armstrong, C. P., Dixon, J. M., Duffy, S. W., Elton, R. A., and Davies, G. C. (1984). Wound healing in obstructive jaundice. *Br. J. Surg.*, **71**, 267–70.

215. Shaw, J. W. and Latimer, E. O. (1926). Regeneration of pancreatic tissue from the transplanted pancreatic duct in the dog. *Am. J. Physiol.*, **76**, 49–53.

216. Raitsina, S. S., Farutina, L. M., and Kashintseva, V. N. (1965). Regeneration hypertrophy of the pancreas in simians. *Ark. Anat. Histol. Embriol.*, **49**, 43–8.

217. Campbell, R. and Kennedy, T. (1980). The management of pancreatic and pancreaticoduodenal injuries. *Br. J. Surg.*, **67**, 845–50.

218. Patcher, H. L., Pennington, R., Chassin, J., and Spencer, F. C. (1979). Simplified distal pancreatectomy with the Auto Suture stapler: preliminary clinical observations. *Surgery*, **85**, 166–70.

219. Fitzgibbons, T. J., Yellin, A. E., Maruyama, M. M., and Donovan, A. J. (1982). Management of the transected pancreas following distal pancreatectomy. *Surg. Gynecol. Obstet.*, **154**, 225–31.

220. Bach, R. D. and Frey, C. F. (1971). Diagnosis and treatment of pancreatic trauma. *Am. J. Surg.*, **121**, 20–9.

221. Graham, J. M., Mattox, K. L., and Jordan, G. L. (1978). Traumatic injuries of the pancreas. *Am. J. Surg.*, **136**, 744–8.

222. Papachristou, D. N., D'Agostino, H., and Fortner, J. G. (1980). Ligation of the pancreatic duct in pancreatectomy. *Br. J. Surg.*, **67**, 260–2.

223. Lansing, P. B., Browder, I. W., Harkness, S. O., and Kitahama, A. (1983). Staple closure of the pancreas. *Am. Surg.*, **49**, 214–17.

224. Anderson, D. K., Bolman, R. M. III, and Moylan, J. A. Jr (1980). Management of penetrating pancreatic injuries: subtotal pancreatectomy using the Auto Suture stapler. *J. Trauma*, **20**, 347–9.

225. Leger, L. (1958). Technique de la pancreato-jejunostomie après pancreatectomie gauche pour pancreatite chronique. *J. Chir. Paris*, **76**, 93–115.

226. Shankar, S., Theis, B., and Russell, R. C. G. (1990). Management of the stump of the pancreas after distal pancreatic resection. *Br. J. Surg.*, **77**, 541–4.

227. Sadek, S., Holdsworth, R., and Cuschieri, A. (1988). Experience with pancreatic banding: results of a simple technique for dealing with the pancreatic remnant after distal partial pancreatectomy. *Br. J. Surg.*, **75**, 486–7.

228. Watanapa, P. and Williamson, R. C. N. (1992). Surgical palliation for pancreatic cancer: developments during the past two decades. *Br. J. Surg.*, **79**, 8–20.

229. Carter, D. C. (1987). Cancer of the pancreas. In *Surgery*, Vol. 1, (ed. J. S. P. Lumley and J. L. Craven), pp. 1002–7. Medical Education (International), Oxford.

230. Matsuno, S. and Sato, T. (1986). Surgical treatment for carcinoma of the pancreas, experience in 272 patients. *Am. Surg.*, **152**, 499–504.

231. Trede, M., Schwall, G., and Saeger, H. (1990). Survival after pancreato-duodenectomy: 118 consecutive resections without an operative mortality. *Ann. Surg.*, **211**, 447–58.

232. Francke, E. L. and New, H. C. (1981). Postsplenectomy infection. *Surg. Clin. North Am.*, **61**, 135–55.

233. Walker, W. (1976). Splenectomy in childhood: a review in England and Wales. *Br. J. Surg.*, **63**, 36–43.

234. Grinblat, J. and Gilboa, Y. (1975). Overwhelming pneumococcal sepsis 25 years after splenectomy. *Am. J. Med. Sci.*, **270**, 523–4.

235. Singer, D. B. (1973). Postsplenectomy sepsis. In *Perspectives in paediatric pathology*, (ed. H. S. Rosenberg), Vol. 1, pp. 285–311.

236. Heier, H. E. (1980). Splenectomy and serious infections. *Scand. J. Haematol.* **24**, 5–12.

237. Dickerman, J. D. (1979). Splenectomy and sepsis: a warning. *Paediatrics*, **64**, 938–40.

238. Cooper, M. J. and Williamson, R. C. N. (1984). Splenectomy: indications, hazards and alternatives. *Br. J. Surg.*, **71**, 173–80.

239. Gross, P. (1965). Zur kinklichen traumatischen Milzupteren. *Beitr. Klin. Chir.*, **208**, 396–402.

240. McIntyre, P. A. and Wagner, H. N. (1970). Current procedures for scanning of the spleen. *Ann. Intern. Med.*, **73**, 995–1001.

241. Harriman, D. G. F. (1990). Normal muscle. In *Systemic pathology*, Vol. 4: *Nervous system, muscles and eyes*, (ed. R. O. Weller). Churchill-Livingstone, Edinburgh.

242. (1989). Excitation and contraction of skeletal muscle. In *Physiological basis for medical practice*, (ed. C. H. Best, N. B. Taylor, and J. B. West), (11th edn), Ch. 4, pp. 58–106. Williams and Wilkins, London.

243. Allbrook, D. (1992). Muscle breakdown and repair. In *Scientific foundations of orthopaedics and traumatology*, (ed. R. Owen, J. Goodfellow, and P. Bullough), pp. 306–15. William Heinemann Medical, London.

244. Hurme, T., Kalino, H., Lehto, M., and Jarvinen, M. (1991). Healing of skeletal muscle injury: an intrastructural and immunobiochemical study. *Medicine and Science in Sports and Exercise*, **23**, 801–10.

245. O'Brien, M. (1992). Functional anatomy and physiology of tendons. *Clinics in Sports Medicine*, **11**, 509–20.

246. Dykyj, D. and Jules K. T. (1991). Clinical anatomy of tendons. *Journal of the American Pediatric Medical Association*, **81**, 358–65.

247. Potenza, A. P. (1992). Tendon and ligament healing. In *Scien-*

tific foundations of orthopaedics and traumatology. (ed. R. Owen, J. Goodfellow, and P. Bullough), pp. 300–5. William Heinemann Medical, London.

248. Scheider, L. H. and Bush, D. C. (1989). Primary care of flexor tendon injuries. *Hand Clinics*, **5**, 383–94.

249. Stewart, K. M. (1991). Review and comparison of the current trends in the post-operative management of tendon repairs. *Hand Clinics*, **7**, 447–60.

250. Sharrard, W. J. W. (1984). Bone and joint. In *Wound healing for surgeons*, (ed. T. E. Bucknall and H. Ellis), Ch. 14, pp. 261–85. Baillière Tindall, London.

251. Bentley, G. (1992). Repair of articular cartilage. In *Scientific foundations of orthopaedics and traumatology*, (ed. R. Owen, J. Goodfellow, and P. Bullough), pp. 297–9. William Heinemann Medical, London.

252. Isogai, N., Kamiishi, H., and Chichibu, S. (1988). Re-endothelialisation stages at the microvascular anastomosis. *Microsurgery*, **9**, 87–94.

253. Mansfield, P., Hall, D., Di Benedetto, G., *et al.* (1978). The care of the vascular endothelium in pediatric surgery. *Ann. Surg.*, **188**, 216–28.

254. Ramos, J., Berger, K., Mansfield, P., and Sauvage, L. (1976). Histologic fate and endothelial changes of distende and non-distende vein grafts. *Ann Surg.*, **183**, 205–28.

255. O Neal, R., Jordan, G., Rabin, R., De Bakey, M., and Lalpart, B. (1964). Cells grown on isolated intravascular Dacron hub: an electron microscopic study. *Exp. Mol. Pathol.*, **3**, 403–12.

256. Goff, S., Wu, H., Sauvage, L., Usui, Y., Wechezak, A., Coan, D., *et al.* (1988). Differences in reendothelialisation after balloon catheter removal of endothelial cells, superficial endarterectomy, and deep endarterectomy. *J. Vasc. Surg.*, **7**, 119–29.

257. Shi, Q., Wu, H., Sauvage, L., Durante, K., Patel, M., Wechezak, A., *et al.* (1990). Re-endothelialisation of isolated segments of canine carotid artery with reference to the possible role of the adventitial vasa vasorum. *J. Vasc. Surg.*, **12**, 476–85.

258. Spaet, T., Stemerman, M., Veith, F., and Lejnieks, I. (1975). Intimal injury and regrowth in the rabbit aorta. Medial smooth muscle cells as a source of neointima. *Circulation Research*, **36**, 58–70.

259. Clowes, A., Clowes, A., and Reidy, M. (1986). Kinetics of cellular proliferation after arterial injury. III. Endothelial and smooth muscle growth in chronically denuded vessels. *Lab. Invest.*, **54**, 295.

260. De Letter, J., Moll, F., Welten, R., Eikelboom, B., Ackerstaff, R., Vermeulen, F., and Algra, A. (1994). Benefits of carotid patching: a prospective randomized study with long-term follow-up. *Ann. Vasc. Surg.*, **8**, 54–8.

261. Kieny, R., Hirsch, D., Seiller, C., Thiranos, J., and Petit, H. (1993). Does carotid eversion endarterectomy and reimplantation reduce the risk of restenosis? *Ann. Vasc. Surg.*, **7**, 407–13.

262. Magee, T., Earnshaw, J., Cole, S., Hayward, J., Baird, R., and Horrocks, M. (1992). A 5-year review of carotid endarterectomy in a vascular unit using a computerised audit system. *Ann. Roy. Coll. Surg.*, **74**, 430–3.

263. Pomerantz, R., Kuntz, R., Carrozza, J., Fishman, R., Mansour, M., Schitt S., *et al.* (1992). Acute and long term outcome of narrowed saphenous venous grafts treated by endoluminal stenting and directional athrectomy. *Am. J. Cardiol.*, **70**, 161–7.

264. Davies, A., Magee, T., Thompson, J., Murphy, P., Jones, H., Horrocks, M., *et al.* (1993). Stenting for vein graft stenosis. *Eur. J. Vasc. Surg.*, **7**, 339–41.

265. Anonymous (1994). Collaborative overview of randomised trials of antiplatelet therapy – II: Maintenance of vascular graft or arterial patency by antiplatelet therapy. Antiplatelet Trialists' Collaboration. (Review.) *Br. Med. J.*, **308**, 159–68.

266. Davies, A., Magee, T., Tennant, S., Lamont, P., Baird, R., and Horrocks, M. (1994). Criteria for the identification of the 'at risk' infrainguinal bypass graft. *Eur. J. Vasc. Surg.*, **8**, 315–19.

267. Ida, M., Tryen, E., and Bata, J. (1992). Surveillance of lower extremity vein grafts. *Eur. J. Vasc. Surg.*, **6**, 456–62.

268. Berger, K., Sauvage, L., Rao, A., and Wood, S. (1972). Healing of arterial prostheses in man: its incompleteness. *Ann. Surg.*, **175**, 118–27.

269. Koegel, H., Vollmar, J., Cyba-Altunbay, S., Mohr, W., and Frosch, D. (1989). New observations on the healing process in prosthetic substitution of large veins by microporous grafts – animal experiments. *Thoracic and Cardiovascular Surgeon*, **37**, 119–24.

270. Sauvage, L., Berger, K., Beilin, L., Smith, J., Wood, S., and Mansfield, P. (1975). Presence of endothelium in an axillary-femoral graft of knitted Dacron with an external velour surface. *Ann. Surg.*, **182**, 749–53.

271. Herring, M., Dilley, R., Gardner A., and Glover, J. (1978). A single staged technique for seeding vascular grafts with autogenous endothelium. *Surgery*, **84**, 498–504.

272. Stanley, J., Burkel, W., Ford, J., Vinter, D., Kahn, R., Whitehouse, W., and Graham, L. (1982). Enhanced patency of small diameter, externally supported Dacron iliofemoral grafts seeded with endothelial cells. *Surgery*, **92**, 994–1005.

273. Douville, E., Kempczinsky, R., Birinyi, L., and Ramalanjna, G. (1987). Impact of endothelial cell seeding on long term patency and subendothelial proliferation in a small caliber highly porous polytetrafluoroethylene graft. *J. Vasc. Surg.*, **5**, 544–50.

274. Seeger, J. and Klingman, N. (1988). Improved in vivo endothelialisation of prosthetic grafts by surface modification with fibronectin. *J. Vasc., Surg.*, **8**, 476–82.

275. Kaehler, J., Zilla, P., Fasol, R., Deutsch, M., and Kadletz, M. (1989). Precoating substrate and surface configuration determine adherence and spreading of seeded endothelial cells on polytetrafluoroethylene grafts. *J. Vasc. Surg.*, **9**, 535–41.

276. Li, J., Menconi, M., Wheeler, B., Rohrer, M., Klassen, V., Ansell, J., and Appel, M. (1992). Precoating expanded polyterafluroethylene grafts alters production of endothelial cell-derived thrombomodulators. *J. Vasc. Surg.*, **15**, 1010–17.

277. Wesolowski, S., Fries, C., and Karlson, K. (1961). Porosity: primary determinant of ultimate fate of synthetic vascular grafts. *Surgery*, **50**, 91–6.

278. Bergeron, P., Rudondy, P., Poyer, V., Pinot, J., Alessandri, C., and Hartelet, J. (1991). Long term peripheral stent evaluation using angioscopy. *Int. Angiol.*, **10**, 182–6.

279. den Heijer, P., van Dijk, R., Twist, S., and Lie, K. (1933). Early stent occlusion is not always caused by thrombosis. *Catheter and Cardiovascular Diagnosis*, **29**, 136–40.

280. O'Brien, T. and Collin, J. (1992). Prosthetic vascular graft infection. *Br. J. Surg.*, **79**, 1262–7.

281. Bandyk, D. and Esses, G. (1994). Prosthetic graft infection. (Review.) *Surgical Clinics of North America*, **74**, 571–90.

282. Sharp, W., Hoballah, J., Mohan, C., Kresowik, T., Martinasevic, M., Chalmers, R., and Corson, J. (1994). The management of the infected aortic prosthesis: a current decade of experience. *J. Vasc. Surg.*, **19**, 844–50.

283. Miller, J. (1993). Partial replacement of an infected arterial graft by a new prosthetic polytetrafluoroethylene segment, a new therapeutic option. *J. Vasc. Surg.*, **17**, 546–58.

284. Lai, D., Huber, D., and Hogg, J. (1993). Obturator foramen bypass in the management of infected prosthetic vascular grafts. *Aus. NZ. J. Surg.*, **63**, 811–14.

285. Morris, G., Friend, P., Vassallo, D., Farrington, M., Leapman, S., and Quick, C. (1994). Antibiotic irrigation and conservative surgery for major aortic graft infection. *J. Vasc. Surg.*, **20**, 88–95.

286. Chervu, A., Moore, W., Chvapil, M., and Henderson, T. (1991). Efficacy and duration of antistaphylococcal activity comparing three antibiotics bonded to Dacron vascular grafts with a collagen release system. *J. Vasc. Surg.*, **13**, 897–901.

287. Strachan, C., Newsom, S., and Ashton, T. (1991). The clinical use of an antibiotic-bonded graft. *Eur. J. Vasc. Surg.*, **5**, 627–32.

288. De Clerck, L., Houthooft, D., Vermeylen, J., (1990). Delayed reaction to a Dacron velour bypass graft. *J. Cardiovasc. Surg.*, **31**, 124–6.

289. Graves, F. T. (1954). The anatomy of the intrarenal arteries and its application to segemental resection of the kidney. *Br. J. Surg.*, **42**, 132–8.

290. Slade, N. (1971). Management of closed renal injuries. *Br. J. Urol.*, **43**, 639–45.

291. Pryor, J. P. and Williams, J. P. (1975). A study of 137 cases of renal trauma. *Br. J. Urol.*, **47**, 45–9.

292. Knapp, P. M., Kulb, T. B., Lingeman, J. E., Newman, D. M., Mertz, J. H. O., Mosbaugh, P. G., *et al.* (1988). Extracorporeal shock wave lithotripsy-induced perirenal haematomas. *J. Urol.*, **25**, 892–5.

293. Cass, A., Bubrick, M., Luxenberg, M., Gleisch, P., and Smith, C. (1985). Renal pedicle injuries. *J. Trauma*, **25**, 892–5.

294. Arnold, E. P. (1972). Pararenal pseudocyst. *Br. J. Urol.*, **44**, 40–6.

295. Crabtree, E. G. (1935). Pararenal pseudo-hydronephrosis. *Trans. Am. Assoc. Genito-Urinary Surgery*, **28**, 9–40.

296. Pawlowski, J. M. (1960). Peripelvic urine granuloma. *Am. J. Clin. Pathol.*, **34**, 6–65.

297. Mitchinson, M. J. and Bradley-Watson, J. D. (1966). Peripelvic urine granuloma. *Br. J. Urol.*, **38**, 453–6.

298. Daughtridge, T. G. (1965). Ureteral compression device for excretory urography. *Am. J. Roentgenol.*, **95**, 431–6.

299. Landes, R. R. and Hooker, J. W. (1952). Sclerosing lipogranuloma and peri-ureteral fibrosis following extravasation of urographic contrast media. *J. Urol.* (Baltimore), **68**, 403–6.

300. McAninch, J. W., Carroll, P. R., Klosterman, P. W., Dixon, C. R., and Greenblatt, M. N. (1991). Renal reconstruction after injury. *J. Urol.*, **68**, 932–7.

301. del Villar, R. G., Ireland, G. W., and Cass, A. S. (1972). Management of renal injury in conjunction with the immediate surgical treatment of the acute severe trauma patient. *J. Urol.*, **107**, 208–12.

302. Cass, A. S., Luxenberg, M., Gleich, P., and Smith, C. (1987). Long term results of conservative and surgical management of blunt renal lacerations. *Br. J. Urol.*, **59**, 17–20.

303. Sagalowsky, A. I., McConnell, J. D., and Peters, P. C. (1983). Renal surgery requiring surgery, an analysis of 185 cases. *J. Trauma*, **23**, 128–31.

304. Scott, R. J. Jr and Selzman, H. M. (1966). Complications of nephrectomy: review of 450 patients and a description of a modification of the transperitoneal approach. *J. Urol.*, **95**, 307–11.

305. Albarran, J. (1909). *Médecine opératoire des voies urinaires; anatomie normale et anatomie pathologique chirurgicale*, 28–0286. Masson et Cie, Paris.

306. Mounzer, A. M., McAninch, J. W., and Schmidt, R. A. (1986). Polyglycolic acid mesh in repair of renal injury. *Urol.*, **28**, 127–30.

307. Schoenberger, A., Mettler, D., Roesler, H., Zimmerman, A., Bilweis, J., Schilt, W., *et al.* (1985). Surgical repair of the kidney after blunt lesions of intermediate degree using a vicryl mesh: an experimental study. *J. Urol.*, **134**, 804–8.

308. Scott, R., Gorman, S. D., Aitcheson, M., Bramwell, S. P., Speakman, M. J., and Medding, R. N. (1991). First clinical report of a biodegradable membrane for use in urological surgery. *Br. J. Urol.*, **68**, 421–4.

309. Page, I. H. (1939). Compression of renal parenchyma by a perirenal process as a cause of hypertension. *J. Am. Med. Assoc.*, **113**, 2046–8.

310. Stackl, W. and Marberge, M. (1986). Late complications of the management of ureteral calculi with the ureteroscope. *J. Urol.*, **49**, 401–4. .

311. Daniels, G. F., Garnett, J. E., and Carter, M. F. (1988). Ureteroscopic results and complications, experience with 130 cases. *J. Urol.*, **139**, 710–13.

312. Mann, W. J. (1991). Intentional and unintentional ureteral injuries: surgical treatment in gynaecological procedures. *Surg. Gynecol. Obstet.*, **172**, 453–6.

313. Badenoch, D. F., Tiptaft, R. C., Thakar, D. R., Fowler, C. G., and Blandy, J. P. (1987). Early repair of accidental injury to the ureter or bladder following gynaecological surgery. *Br. J. Urol.*, **59**, 516–18.

314. Smith, I. B. (1969). Trans-uretero-ureterostomy. *Br. J. Urol.*, **41**, 14–22.

315. Smith I. B. and Smith, J. C. (1975). Trans-uretero-ureterostomy, British experience. *Br. J. Urol.*, **47**, 519–23.

316. Tarkington, M. A., Dejter, S. W., and Presette, J. F. (1991). Early surgical management of extensive gynaecological/ureteral injuries. *Surg. Gynae. Obstet.*, **173**, 17–21.

317. Turner, W. H., Cranston, D. W., Davies, A. H., Fellows, G. J., and Smith, J. C. (1990). Double J stents in the treatment of gynaecological injury to the ureter. *J. R. Soc. Med.*, **83**, 623–4.

318. Turner-Warwick, R. T. (1988). The Turner-Warwick bladder-elongation psoas-hitch procedure for substitution ureteroplasty. In *Controversies and innovations in urological surgery*, (ed. J. C. Gingell and P. Abrams), pp. 109–14. Springer, London.

319. Blandy, J. P. (1988). Boari flap. In *Controversies and innovations in urological surgery*, (ed. J. C. Gingell and P. A. Abrams), pp. 101–8. Springer, London.

320. Wiseman, J. L. (1934). Observations of the stimulating influence of temporary rubber splinting on regeneration following ureteral resection. *Br. J. Urol.*, **6**, 11–16.

321. Hastings, J. C., Van Winkle, W., Barker, E., Hines, D., and Nochols, W. (1975). The effect of suture materials on healing wounds of the bladder, *Surg. Gynecol. Obstet.*, **156**, 933–7.

322. Bacon, S. K. (1943). Rupture of the urinary bladder; clinical analysis of 147 cases in the past 10 years. *J. Urol.*, **49**, 432–5.

323. Turner-Warwick, R. (1976). The use of the omental pedicle graft in urinary tract reconstruction. *J. Urol.*, **116**, 341–7.

324. McAninch, J. W. (1990). Urethral injuries. *World J. Urol.*, **7**, 184–8.

325. Singh, M. and Blandy, J. P. (1976). Pathology of urethral stricture. *J. Urol.*, **115**, 673–6.

326. Bartone, F. F. and Shires, T. K. (1969). The reaction of the urinary tract to catgut and reconstituted collagen sutures. *J. Urol.*, **101**, 411–15.

327. Edlich, R. F., Rodeheaver, G.T., and Thacker, J. G. (1987). Considerations in the choice of sutures for wound closure of the genito-urinary tract. *J. Urol.*, **137**, 373–9.

328. Holbrook, M. C. (1982). The resistance of polyglycolic acid sutures to attack by infected human urine. *Br. J. Urol.*, **54**, 313–5.

329. Ruutu, M., Alfthan, O., Heikkinen, L., Jarvinen, A., Lehtonen, T., Merikallio, L., *et al.* (1982). 'Epidemic' of acute urethral stricture after open heart surgery. *Lancet*, **i**, 218.

330. Sutherland, P. D., Maddern, J. P., Jose, J. S., and Marshall, V. R. (1983). Urethral stricture after cardiac surgery. *Br. J. Urol.*, **55**, 413–16.

331. Ohkawa, M., Sugata, T., Sawaki, M., Nakashima, T., Fuse, H., and Hisazumi, H. (1990). Bacterial and crystal adherence to the surfaces of indwelling urethral catheters. *J. Urol.*, **143**, 717–21.

332. Costerton, J. W. and Marrie, T. J. (1983). The role of the bacterial glycocalyx in resistance to antimicrobial agents. *Med. Microbiol.*, **3**, 63–6.

333. Ramsay, J. W. A., Garnham, A. J., Mulhall, A. B., Crow, R. A., Bryan, J. M., Eardley, I., *et al.* (1989). Biofilms, bacteria and bladder cathethers: a clinical study. *Br. J. Urol.*, **64**, 395–8.

334. Hukins, D. W. L., Hickey, D. S., and Kennedy, A. P. (1983). Catheter encrustation by struvite. *Br. J. Urol.*, **55**, 304–5.

335. Bruce, A. W., Sira, S. S., and Clark, A. F. (1974). The problem of catheter encrustation. *Can. Med. Assoc. J.*, **111**, 238–41.

336. Kunin, C. M., Chin, Q. F., and Chambers, S. (1987). Blockage of urinary catheters. *Am. J. Med.*, **82**, 405–11.

337. Cox, A. J. (1990). Comparison of catheter surface morphologies. *Br. J. Urol.*, **65**, 55–60.

338. Ramsay, J. W. A., Crocker, P. R., Ball, A. J., Jones, S., Payne, S. R., Levison, D. A., *et al.* (1987). Urothelial reaction to ureteric intubation: a clinical study. *Br. J. Urol.*, **60**, 504–5.

339. Pocock, R. D., Stower, M. J., Ferro, M. A., Smith, P. J. B., and Gingell, J. C. (1986). Double J stents: a review of 100 patients. *Br. J. Urol.*, **58**, 629–33.

340. Kohri, K., Yamate, T., Amasaki, N., Ishikawa, Y., Umekawa, T., Imanishi, M., *et al.* (1991). Characteristics and usage of different ureteral stent catheters. *Urol. Int.*, **47**, 131–7.

10

Clinical aspects of healing by secondary intention

G. D. MULDER, B. A. BRAZINSKY, D. FARIA, K. G. HARDING,
J. L. RODRIGUEZ, P. BARAGWANATH, R. SALAMAN,
and J. SALAMAN

Venous ulcers

Developments in pathophysiology and treatment

Despite their prevalence, venous ulcers remain a multidisciplinary problem and a clinical challenge. For example in the United States alone, between 500 000 and 1 000 000 people are afflicted with venous ulcers. As the elderly population increases, a rise in this number can be expected. This section addresses the pathogenesis, clinical features, and non-surgical options for venous ulcerations.

Non-invasive venous studies

A variety of techniques can be used to assess venous insufficiency. One of the simplest tests to perform is Doppler ultrasonography, but it is sometimes difficult to differentiate between superficial and deep venous insufficiency. The important factors in a venous Doppler examination are the presence and spontaneity of a signal. In addition, the frequency and pitch of the signal is important for diagnosing a venous disorder. For example, a high pitch signal with little fluctuation may be an indirect confirmation of venous stasis or occlusion (1).

Normal venous flow velocity fluctuates with respiratory excursions. Any deviation from this path may be indicative of venous insufficiency. Venous flow is also affected by external compression. Under normal conditions, proximal compression of a vessel leads to a brief sound followed by a zero velocity signal. Distal compression, however, produces an increase in signal frequency (augmentation) that is followed briefly by a zero velocity signal upon release and then by a rapid normalization of flow. Distal compression resulting in augmentation but then followed upon release by a backflow signal is indicative of the presence of valvular insufficiency (1).

Photoplethysmography (PPG) is a useful test to identify venous disease and to differentiate between superficial and deep vein incompetence. PPG works by assessing the variations in light absorption of the skin by haemoglobin in the dermal venous plexus. A full dermal venous plexus and high venous pressure will absorb light. The transmission of light increases as venous pressure decreases and the venous plexus empties (2). Additional tests used to determine venous insufficiency include strain-gauge plethysmography, light reflex rheography, foot volumetry, and phlebography. Of late, duplex Doppler ultrasound has been used in the assessment of venous reflux and venous thrombosis.

Anatomy

A review of venous anatomy is essential to a clear understanding of the development of venous stasis ulceration. Anatomically, the long and short saphenous veins communicate with the deep venous system.

The long, or great, saphenous vein is the longest vein in the body and the largest superficial vein of the lower extremity. It originates as a continuation of the medial marginal vein on the dorsum of the foot and courses anterior to the medial malleolus. The vein ascends the leg and remains medial and parallel to the tibia. It then passes behind the medial condyle of the tibia and femur and courses superiorly along the medial side of the thigh. It then penetrates through the fascia lata at the fossa ovalis and terminates at the femoral vein. The great saphenous vein has between 10 and 20 valves, with a greater number being located in the leg than the thigh. The number and position of communicating branches with the deep venous system may vary considerably (3, 4).

The long and small saphenous veins communicate with each other as well as the deep veins of the leg through perforating veins. The majority of perforating veins connect the long saphenous vein with the deep venous system in three sets; with one major communication located just proximal to the ankle joint. Related to this anatomy (and, of course, many other factors) any trauma to the long saphenous vein results in increased risk of ulceration occurring around the medial malleolar region.

Pathophysiology

The primary function of the venous system in the lower extremity is the return of venous blood from the capillary network to the heart. Three mechanisms account for this action; first, capillary pressure; second, intrinsic leg muscles with venous valvular competency; and third, of least importance in an erect position, intrathoracic pressure associated with respiration.

Venous stasis resulting from poor venous return may have numerous causes, including congestive heart failure, low serum protein level, pregnancy, obesity, postphlebitic syndrome, and incompetent valves leading to venous reflux. These conditions all tend to increase venous hydrostatic pressure, overcoming the osmotic pressure gradient and resulting in oedema.

Excessive venous pressure causes prolonged stasis leading to a rupture of venules. This causes extravasation of blood into the tissue, leading to red blood cell lysis which in turn causes increased haem production and a resulting haemosiderosis. Hyperpigmentation develops and skin breakdown occurs (3). Incompetent valves within the perforating veins connecting the superficial to the deep systems in the leg cause an increased venous tension and an inability to reduce venous tension on exercise. With sustained venous hypertension, blood is diverted from closed to open capillaries. There is a decrease in the number of capillary loops, which when damaged, allow leakage of fibrinogen and subsequent fibrin barrier formation. This relates to ulceration, with associated induration and hyperpigmentation (lipodermatosclerosis) (4).

Fibrinolysis

Theories were once held that venous stasis, with resulting anoxia, led to venous ulcers. It is now believed that venous ulcers occur when pericapillary fibrin layers are deposited from fibrinogen leakage in limbs with venous disease and unrelieved venous pressure (3, 4) (Fig. 10.1). The frequent presence of fibrin cuffs may prevent oxygen and nutrient diffusion and contribute to ulcer formation.

In patients with preulcerative changes, the accumulation of fibrin around capillaries may be due to a deficiency of fibrinolytic activity (tissue plasminogen activator) (3, 4). The presence of dermal pericapillary fibrin may be of diagnostic value in the evaluation of ulcers of uncertain aetiology (4).

White blood cells

Little or no apparent blood flow in some areas of skin may be present in patients with chronic venous insufficiency. A decrease in blood flow causes white blood cells to become trapped, causing capillary occlusion and the release of proteolytic enzymes and superoxide radicals (3). A study by Thomas and colleagues revealed a 30 per cent trapping of white blood cells in patients with venous disease compared with 7 per cent in control subjects (5). Lying down after standing may represent a form of ischaemia–reperfusion injury.

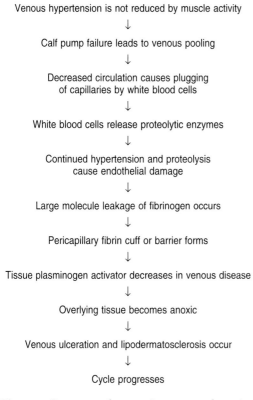

Venous hypertension is not reduced by muscle activity

↓

Calf pump failure leads to venous pooling

↓

Decreased circulation causes plugging
of capillaries by white blood cells

↓

White blood cells release proteolytic enzymes

↓

Continued hypertension and proteolysis
cause endothelial damage

↓

Large molecule leakage of fibrinogen occurs

↓

Pericapillary fibrin cuff or barrier forms

↓

Tissue plasminogen activator decreases in venous disease

↓

Overlying tissue becomes anoxic

↓

Venous ulceration and lipodermatosclerosis occur

↓

Cycle progresses

Fig. 10.1 Sequence of events in venous ulceration

Patients with chronic venous insufficiency have a decreased number of capillary loops in dependent legs (4). These capillary loops are visible only when containing red blood cells. This finding is explained by a reduced capillary flow rate in the trapping of white blood cells. White cells take 1000 times longer than red cells to deform on entering the capillary bed; because no red cells are present, the capillary loops are invisible (6). The white blood cells release toxic oxygen metabolites and enzymes that damage capillaries, causing leakage of large fibrinogen molecules and the formation of a fibrin cuff barrier. Therefore, the white blood cells are implicated as a responsive mediator for ischaemia during the capillary occlusion process.

This explanation does not conflict with data suggesting that patients with venous stasis have increased blood flow in subcutaneous tissue. It is believed that blood is diverted from closed to open capillaries in these patients. A diverted flow causes uneven oxygen perfusion, which may explain the uneven yet well defined borders of venous ulcers. Based on this explanation, white blood cells play a major role in the formation of venous ulcers.

Location and clinical features

The size and location of venous ulcers vary, yet they are most commonly found on the medial aspect of the leg. The long saphenous vein is the primary drainage of the medial site of the ankle and any damage to this vein may result in ulceration. Certainly, the medial side of the ankle is a more common site of ulceration than either the lateral ankle or upper leg (3).

Venous ulcers generally have irregular borders. A foul exudate is usually, but not always, associated with these ulcers. Induration and scaling of the skin are often found in association with the ulcers, as is peri-wound inflammation. Lipodermatosclerosis of surrounding tissue is also a common finding. Decreased tissue fibrinolytic activity has been observed in patients with lipodermatosclerosis (5). This decreased fibrinolytic activity can be determined through the measuring of tissue plasminogen activator as well as measurement of fibrin degradation products. Pain, when present, is often relieved by elevation of the involved extremity. Additionally, the presence of prominent subcutaneous venules over the medial malleolus when a patient stands (ankle flare sign) is often present with venous ulcers.

Venous ulcers must be differentiated from other lesions of the lower extremity including lesions of diabetic, arterial, neuropathic, bacterial, and malignant aetiology (Table 10.1). In addition, venous ulcers are often complicated by bacterial infection.

Treatment

Many clinicians believe that venous ulcers will resolve with complete bed rest and elevation of the affected extremity. This approach, however, does not address or reverse the physiologic damage already incurred. Furthermore, the ulcer will usually recur when the patient resumes a dependent position. Due to the inability to reverse the destruction of the involved venous system, treatment is often based on symptoms alone.

Three major issues must be addressed when dealing conservatively with venous ulcers: fibrinolysis, venous return, and wound repair. A variety of compressive wraps, stockings, pumps, ointments, drugs, and dressings are available for the treatment of venous ulcers (Table 10.2). The use of a single treatment modality often addresses only one of these issues. A multidisciplinary treatment directed toward the patient's specific needs, as well as requirements of wound therapy, should prove most effective.

Compressive modalities

The compressive modalities include the Unna's boot bandage wraps, elastic stockings, and external mechanical pumps. All of these modalities should be graduated in pressure in order to promote the most improvement in venous return.

Stockings

The benefit of compressive stockings as an aid to venous return is well supported in clinical studies (4, 6). Elastic stockings which provide graduated external compression help prevent fluid extravasation into subcutaneous tissue by aiding venous blood return and reducing oedema. External compression is also believed to decrease oedema through maintaining empty peri-ulceration venous channels, which reduces hyperstatic pressure (7). Ideally, all patients who can tolerate compression support stockings should wear them. Unfortunately, elderly, disabled, or arthritic patients may have

Table 10.1 Causes of leg ulceration

Vascular disorders	Venous stasis*
	Deep venous occlusion
	Deep superficial valvular incompetence
	Arterial insufficiency
	Atherosclerosis (peripheral vascular disease)
	Acute peripheral thrombosis/embolism
	Hypertension – Martorell's ulcer
	Vasculitis (primary acute-leucocytoelastic/ mononuclear; chronic granulomatous)
	Connective tissue disease
	Rheumatoid arthritis
	Systemic lupus erythematosus
	Scleroderma
	Cryofibrinogen
	Cryoglobulin
	Anticardiolipin
	Lymphatics
	Congential
	Acquired
	Congestive heart failure
	Dependency or immobility
Infections (local or systemic)	Fungal
	Syphilitic
	Bacterial
	Parasitic
Metabolic disorders	Diabetic ulcer (distal vascular disease, neuropathy, hyperglycaemia, and depressed leucocyte factor)
	Necrobiosis lipidica diabeticorum
	Hypothyroidism
	Liver disease
	Renal disease
Malignancy	Squamous cell carcinoma (and Marjolin's ulcer)
	Kaposi sarcoma
	Malignant melanoma
Haematological disease	Red blood cell disorders
	Sickle cell anaemia
	Thalassaemia
	Polycythemia vera
	White blood cell disorders
	Leukaemia
Miscellaneous	Neurotrophic ulcer (systemic disease – diabetes or multiple sclerosis; local disease – spina bifida, injury)
	Chemical burns
	Thermal injury
	Insect bites
	Radiation
	Frostbite
	Factitial (self-induced) injury
	Traumatic tissue loss
	Osteomyelitis

* 90% of lower extremity venous ulcers are a result of chronic venous insufficiency. Most also have an element of arterial insufficiency.

extreme difficulty, or be unable to put the stockings on their legs themselves.

The exact amount of calf and ankle pressure necessary to heal a venous ulcer has yet to be determined. The external pressure needed would be expected to be related to the amount of damage to the venous system. However, as little as 24 mmHg (3 kPa) of pressure at the ankle, and 16 mmHg (2 kPa) at the calf, have been found to assist the healing of venous ulcers (4). Although some patients may be unable to tolerate high compression (pressure of more than 24 mmHg or 3 kPa) stockings, even low compression (less than 18 mmHg or 2.4 kPa) stockings are thought to be of some benefit. Compression of 30–40 mmHg (4–5 kPa) is usually recommended in patients with venous ulcers. Maximum benefit from any pressure on compression is achieved when the stockings are applied upon first awakening in the morning before blood has a chance to pool in the lower extremities due to dependency.

Unna boot

The Unna boot is one of the most popular modalities in the USA for the treatment of venous ulcers. The boot generally consists of white cloth or cotton gauze impregnated with zinc oxide, gelatin, and, frequently, calamine paste. Many patients react to the calamine and therefore an Unna boot without calamine is preferential. Although the Unna boot has been the standard of conservative treatment for venous ulcers for many years, little evidence is available to support its advantage over other forms of treatment. In a study by Hendricks and Swallow, comparing the Unna boot and elastic support stockings, the success rate of healing with both modalities was found to be 78 per cent. The average healing time was somewhat faster with Unna boots, but the success rate in healing stasis leg ulcers was statistically equivalent between the two groups (7). Both therapies help decrease oedema and improve venous haemodynamics of the leg.

Unna boots are useful when applied to patients who may not be compliant with other compressive modalities, or who are unable to use elastic wraps or compressive stockings. The boots are often found to be uncomfortable by many patients and can interfere with daily hygiene. Geriatric and other patients with friable, sensitive tissue should not be treated with the Unna boot. However, when used judiciously, the Unna boot may expedite wound closure.

Elastic wraps

Elastic wraps are commonly used in the treatment of venous ulcers due to their availability and accessibility to patients and clinicians. Elastic wraps are most useful for patients who are unable to wear elastic stockings, cannot tolerate Unnas boots, or do not have access to mechanical pumps. Compressive wraps are more effective on small, fresh ulcers, than on large, chronic lesions.

Unfortunately, elastic wraps are often inappropriately applied. This may further impede venous return (8). Compressive wraps are contraindicated in patients with associated arterial occlusive disease, weeping stasis dermatitis, and infectious disease of the lower extremity.

Table 10.2 Medical therapy for venous ulcers

Treatment	Advantages
Compressive modalities	
Stockings	Maintain desired compression level; aid venous return; can be washed and reused
Elastic wraps	Aid venous return
Unna boot (paste bandages)	Possibly stimulates re-epithelialization; aids venous return
Pumps	Promote enhanced venous return; reduce oedema; have possible fibrinolytic effect; may promote wound closure
Dressings*	
Hydrocolloids	Easy to apply; good retention on low and moderately exuding wounds; water impermeable; self-adhesive; absorb exudate
Foams	Beneficial for high-exudate wounds
Polyurethanes	Very easy to apply; conform well to irregular surfaces; decrease periwound maceration; good on very superficial wounds; maintain moist environment
Topical medications[†]	
Fibrinolysin and desoxyribonuclease	Aids fibrinolysis and wound debridement, thus promotes granulation
Silver sulphadiazine	Promotes re-epithelialization
Povidone-iodine	Bactericidal at 1 in 10^3 dilution

* None of the dressings addresses the problem of venous stasis.
[†] Topical medications are of questionable benefit; they are directed at the wound, not the venous aetiology.

Sequential compression devices

The most recent advances in compression technology include the automated compression and sequential compression devices, which are mechanical means of aiding venous return. The use of sequential compression in preventing deep venous thrombosis is very well documented (9, 10). The benefits of sequential compression in expediting venous ulcer closure has recently been studied in Finland (5). More recent studies indicate that sequential compression stimulates fibrinolysis. Increased fibrinolysis with decreased amounts of fibrin around capillary walls has been postulated to reduce the probability of venous ulcer occurrence.

One study found that 100 per cent of patients with post-thrombotic leg ulcers healed with the use of sequential and graded pressure devices on the lower extremity, even after conservative measures failed (4). In all eight patients in this study skin oxygen tension increased and healing rates correlated with decreased leg swelling.

Through experience, pneumatic compression and ulcer resolution has been well achieved with a device that provides consistent, known levels of compression to the leg. This device consists of a controller and leg sleeves which are con-

nected by hoses. The sleeve is divided into six chambers, with a peak pressure of 45–60 mmHg (6–8 kPa) in the ankle. The two ankle chambers inflate first, followed 2.5 sec later by the inflation of the two calf chambers; 3.5 sec later the two thigh chambers inflate to a pressure of 25–30 mmHg (3–4 kPa). All chambers remain inflated for 5.5 sec then simultaneous deflation occurs. This cycle is repeated every 71 seconds. Good control of oedema has been established with the use of a foot pump. Sequential compression is found to be of greater benefit to patients unable to tolerate or use other compressive modalities.

Local wound care

Compression wraps and stockings play a role in wound repair by reducing stasis and oedema, but they do not directly address the wound environment. Topical wound dressings may be used to aid in tissue repair. During the past decade, numerous new products have been introduced, all with varying claims. In addition to gauze dressings, polyurethane, hydrocolloid, hydrogel, biological, occlusive, and semiocclusive dressings have been introduced. Protocols and algorithms may be devised locally which may aid the clinician in choosing an appropriate dressing based on wound appearance.

Occlusive and semiocclusive dressings

The benefits of occlusive modalities in wound repair has been supported in numerous studies (6, 10). Occlusive and semiocclusive dressings (see Chapter 11) promote repair primarily by maintaining an appropriate moist environment. They also protect the wound surface from outside contamination, provide a small amount of debridement, and reduce the need for frequent dressing changes.

Prior to initial application of an occlusive or semiocclusive dressing, wounds should be debrided of all excessive necrotic debris and cleansed with non-cytotoxic solution, such as sterile saline. The amount of time dressings can be worn varies with the amount of wound exudate and ranges from 2 to 7 days. Dressings should be changed when exudate begins to leak from the margins.

When the dressings are removed, a thick, often malodorous, pustular-appearing gel is often present. This gel is a by-product of wound exudate and dressing components, particularly hydrocolloids. The wound should be cleansed between dressing changes. It should always be examined for signs of infection such as increased necrosis, cellulitis, tissue breakdown, extensive erythema, and sinus tracts with purulent drainage.

The fear of bacterial infection is always a concern when physically occluding a wound. While culturing of chronic venous ulcers will most likely produce bacterial growth, distinction must be made between contamination and true infection (usually associated with a bacterial growth of more than 1×10^5 per cm^2). Although numerous organisms have been cultured from chronic wounds (4–7), the effect of bacteria on wound closure is both questionable and debatable. In most cases, cultures of chronic venous ulcers are not clinically useful. (See also later in this chapter, Chapter 7 and Chapter 9.)

Occlusive dressings may be disadvantageous when used on highly exuding wounds. Excessive maceration may occur, resulting in increased tissue damage. Certain dressings contain adhesives to which patients may develop a contact dermatitis. Dressing materials may adhere to patient's clothes and bed linen, making patients reluctant to use them. While hydrocolloid dressings tend to be easy to use, and are retained for longer periods, polyurethanes are difficult to handle and poorly contain or absorb wound fluids.

Hydrocolloid dressings are the most advantageous of the presently available materials. They are especially beneficial when used in conjunction with a compressive treatment modality. Caution must be taken when patients have an associated vasculitis, diabetes, or arterial disease. It is not recommended that an occlusive dressing be used on patients with unusually large ulcers, fragile skin, dermatological diseases, or sinus tracts.

Topical medications

Frequent use is made of sprays, ointments, and topical antibiotics in the treatment of venous ulcers. All are of questionable benefit. Systemic antibiotics should not be used unless cellulitis and other definite signs of infection, such as sepsis, are present.

Topical antibiotics may be of little or no benefit on wounds as they are unable to eradicate contaminants. The contaminants themselves have not been shown to present a high risk of becoming an infection in chronic wounds. Topical antimicrobial agents, such as hydrogen peroxide, povidone–iodine (Betadine), and sodium hypochlorite should be avoided in high concentrations because of their cytotoxicity and questionable benefits as wound cleansers (8). Ointments should be avoided on open wounds, particularly those containing petroleum, which has been shown to retard healing (9).

Debriding agents, including fibrinolytic, proteolytic, and collagenolytic agents may be useful for debridement of some dermal ulcers (4, 5, 10). Surgical debridement may be necessary in order to obtain the best dermal base for wound repair on those wounds with extensive eschar and necrotic tissue.

Cultured epidermal grafting

Autografts

New approaches in the treatment of venous stasis ulceration include the use of cultured epidermal cells (keratinocytes) as a skin graft (see also Chapter 11). Several burn centres in the US and Europe have found that application of these cultured cells can promote granulation tissue formation and wound healing (11–13). Angiogenic properties have been seen in association with a variety of growth factors. These include fibroblast growth factor, transforming growth factor alpha and beta, and epidermal growth factors (12, 13). In addition, platelet derived growth factor appears to increase the tensile strength of wounds (14).

In a study using human recombinant epidermal growth factor, the rate of re-epithelialization of venous ulcers was modestly improved over placebo, but the difference was not statistically significant (15). A similar study showed a 15 per cent acceleration in healing time with the use of epidermal growth factor in partial thickness grafts (16). The practical implications of these studies remain debatable. Other studies have demonstrated that less expensive treatment modalities such as occlusive hydrocolloid dressings produce similar or better results than growth factors (17). More research into the effects of growth factors must be performed before the actual beneficial effects on wound healing can be determined.

Adjuvant pharmacotherapy

The use of systemic medications for venous ulcerations should only be considered in addition to standard ulcer treatments. The use of drugs to treat leg ulcers is based on the properties associated with the risk factors present in patients with venous insufficiency. Most of the drugs used possess mechanisms of action which address one or more factors identified in the pathophysiology of venous ulceration. These have been successful using keratinocyte sheet cultures from the patient's own skin (autografts) for several years (18). Studies have used cultured autografts for chronic non-healing leg ulcers. The results of one study which applied cultured autografts to chronic non-healing leg ulcers showed healing of four of six chronic ulcers within 35 days of application, with closure for up to two years. Results of other studies are inconclusive (19, 20).

Allografts

Recently, grafts derived from an unrelated donor source have been used. Various studies by Phillips and colleagues have shown that allografts tend to provide a host stimulus to wound healing in difficult leg ulcers, and that more than two thirds of ulcers studied healed within eight weeks, with a mean healing time of 3.3 weeks (21, 22). It is believed that the allograft acts as a temporary wound covering and, with time, the grafted keratinocytes are replaced by the host keratinocytes (22).

The use of grafts may provide pain relief and appear to accelerate healing. Due to the complex nature of harvesting, the grafts should be reserved for wounds which have failed to heal by conservative treatment measures.

Growth factors

Over the past few years there has been a significant increase in research on the relationship of growth factors to wound healing. Many of these growth factors have been found to have effects on skin and potential effects on wound healing. In many animal studies, epidermal growth factors (EGF) and drugs have been introduced to improve haemodynamic parameters and reduce fibrin build-up.

Pentoxifylline (Trental) is thought to assist venous ulcer healing. The drug is used in the treatment of intermittent claudication through increasing erythrocyte flexibility (23). Other claimed actions include increased oxygen delivery, decreased cytotoxicity, decreased fibrinogen levels, enhanced fibrinolytic activity, and decreased platelet aggregation. This drug would be expected to facilitate healing and introduce a potential for ulcer recurrence. More evidence is needed to substantiate improvements in wound closure claimed for these treatments.

Anabolic steroids, such as stanozolol, are believed to stimulate fibrinolysis and encourage return of tissue to normal by decreasing fibrin barrier formation and reduce ulceration (24–26). Reduction of fibrin would be expected to improve oxygen and nutrient exchange between tissue and blood vessels.

Other drugs such as vasodilators including calcium-channel blockers, serotonin antagonists, and prostaglandins are still controversial in their actual effect on wound repair. The use of diuretics may have a place in the treatment of leg ulcers, but are only appropriate when given as a short course to patients with severe oedema.

Each of the above mentioned drugs have contraindications which must be weighed carefully against benefits prior to its use. The significance of systemic medications for treatment of venous insufficiency needs more extensive testing in order to clarify and support the use of systemic medications in venous ulcer treatment and prophylaxis.

Summary

Ulcers may occur due to venous insufficiency and lower extremity calf pump failure. The results may be ensuing oedema, trapping of white blood cells with release of damag-

ing free radicals, and pericapillary fibrin deposition. Acute smaller lesions are usually treated and resolve through adequate compression and occlusive dressings. Non-surgical treatment of larger and more chronic wounds mandate the use of some form of external compression. Appropriate occlusive dressings address the wound environment problem and are most effective when used simultaneously with compression therapy. Additional studies into the use of sequential compression devices and long term fibrinolysis are needed to determine their therapeutic and prophylactic value in venous ulcerations. The long term use of compression devices may be needed to prevent further ulcer recurrence. The wound manager must obtain a thorough review of the patient's overall medical status, drugs, and nutrition, and be familiar with the systemic factors affecting venous disease. A review of all available treatment modalities suggests that a combination offers the best means of attaining wound closure.

Non-venous leg ulceration

Epidemiology

It is estimated that approximately 1 per cent of the United Kingdom population suffer from chronic leg ulcers (27) with one quarter of these being open and requiring treatment. Population studies have defined the point prevalence at between 1.5 and 1.8 per 1000 (27, 28), though this rises to 3 per 1000 in the 61–70 age range, and up to 20 per 1000 in those over 80 years old (28). This amounts to some 400 000 sufferers, incurring a cost to the National Health Service of £150–£600 million per annum, similar to the cost of tobacco-related disease (29). Incidences in other parts of the world vary slightly. A well performed study in Freemantle, Western Australia produced a figure of 1.1 per 1000 (30). This was not easily explained by population demographics and may represent a genuine geographical variation. Higher incidences, however, have been reported in the USA and Sweden with rates of 2 and 3 per 1000 respectively (31, 32), though these differences were thought to be attributable to a more elderly and more compliant population (32).

All studies of leg ulcer incidence demonstrate an increased incidence in females, with male:female ratios ranging from 1:1.9 in Australia to 1:2.8 in Scotland. This difference is largely attributable to the fact that a far greater proportion of the elderly population is female, men having a shorter life expectancy. The incidence of leg ulceration in those under 40 years old is equal between the sexes (33). Little data are available on leg ulcer prevalence across ethnic groups, though a survey in Brazil of hospital attendees found that 3.6 per cent had had an ulcer at some time (34).

Aetiology

The causes of leg ulceration are many and varied. A full list is shown in Table 10.1. Clinical studies have consistently shown venous disease to be the most common cause with between 67 and 81 per cent of patients having some degree of venous insufficiency (28, 30, 35, 36). Venous insufficiency is thought to be the primary cause of ulceration in 52–58 per cent of leg ulcers (30, 36, 37). Arterial disease is present in 28–40 per cent of patients with 8.8–12 per cent of ulcers being of primarily ischaemic origin. Other causes of ulceration reported in population surveys include immobility (32 per cent), obesity (48 per cent), rheumatoid arthritis (9 per cent), diabetes (2.5 per cent), and vasculitis (2 per cent). Many patients presenting with an ulcerated leg have several factors, not least advanced age and concurrent systemic illness, contributing to the aetiology of their ulcer. Some authors have stated that most leg ulcers are indeed multifactorial (35).

The diversity of conditions which may present as leg ulcers and the fact that any individual patient may be endowed with more than one aetiological factor makes a structured and systematic approach to each patient and to each individual lesion essential. It is only when the correct diagnosis has been made that the correct treatment can be given.

Clinical assessment

History

It is essential in addressing the problem of a chronically ulcerated leg to take an adequate history, not only of the ulcer itself but from the patient as a whole. Illnesses and operations the patient has suffered in the past may give vital clues as to the underlying cause of the ulcer. If, for example, the patient had previously had a colectomy for ulcerative colitis, the prospect of a related cutaneous vasculitis should spring to mind. Patients may also be taking numerous prescribed drugs, some of which may have known dermatological side-effects and be causing the problem, or may potentially interact with treatments such as antibiotics.

The history of the ulcer itself should include its duration, whether it is a recurrence of a previous lesion, and its current progress. Venous ulcers are often of long duration and are recurrent in 66 per cent of cases (38). Ischaemic ulcers, however, are more likely to be of recent onset. Symptoms associated with the ulcer may also give a clue as to its aetiology. Pain is a characteristic feature of acute vasculitis, though any ulcer, if infected, may also be painful locally. This should not be confused with the pain of ischaemia, which though not related to the ulcer itself usually affects the whole of the foot and lower leg. Obvious causative events such as trauma or a burn should also be sought in the history.

Examination

Examination should start with the patient as a whole, looking for signs of systemic disease. Though not directly causative of leg ulceration there are many factors which may be contributing to poor wound healing which, if treated appropriately, would improve the chances of a successful outcome. These are listed in Table 10.3 and are discussed more fully in Chapter 6. Examination of the ulcer itself follows the basic principles of any other skin lesion. First, the site of the ulcer should be noted, not just for descriptive purposes but as it relates significantly to the underlying aetiology. Venous ulcers classically affect the gaiter area, typically just above the medial malleolus. Ulcers of the feet, however, are far less likely to be due to venous disease and are more likely to be due to diabetes, arterial disease, or both (30). Vasculitides typically affect

Table 10.3 Systemic disease leading to poor wound healing

Primary metabolic diseases	Diabetes
	Hypothyroidism
Liver disease	Jaundice
	Cirrhosis
	Malignant infiltration
	Hypoproteinaemia
Renal disease	Uraemia
	Nephrotic syndrome – hypoproteinaemia
Anaemia	Myelodysplasia
	Iron deficiency/blood loss
	Chronic disease

the front of the shin though lesions can occur anywhere on the body. Ulcer size should be documented so that the progress of treatment can be monitored. Though subjective, a lot can be gained from study of the ulcer shape and the characteristics of its edge. Vasculitic and hypertensive (Martorell's) ulcers tend to be circular and punched out with a clean border. Most venous ulcers have an irregular border and are often associated with the surrounding skin changes of lipodermatosclerois. An irregular, heaped up, or rolled border should always raise the suspicion of malignancy. The colour of an ulcer may give clues to a clinician of the progress towards healing and the presence of complications. The best way to judge wound colour is with experience, though photographic methods do exist which are able to quantify this (39). A healthy granulating wound bed should appear bright pink with little or no contact bleeding. The hyperaemia caused by bacterial infection, particularly by staphylococci, produces reddening and a tendency to bleed when touched. The ulcer bed may also be tender. Infection by *Pseudomonas* species produces a characteristic blue-green hue in the wound exudate and an odour which is readily recognized by an experienced health care worker. Slough is usually yellow and may build up in an ulcer bed leading to delayed wound healing and recurrent infection. Black colouration of an ulcer is indicative of necrosis, either of tissue or slough. This will impede ulcer healing and should be removed, either by sharp debridement or using a hydrocolloid dressing.

Investigation

The majority of leg ulcers can be diagnosed correctly by an experienced doctor or nurse without recourse to expensive and time-consuming investigations. Some baseline procedures are, however, mandatory for the efficacious and safe management of a patient with leg ulceration. Blood should be taken for haematological and biochemical assessment to exclude concurrent illness which may adversely affect healing. These assessments should include meaurement of serum urea and electrolytes, to look for renal and metabolic disease; glucose to eliminate diabetes; albumin, billirubin, and liver enzymes to exclude liver disease. A full blood count will pick up anaemia and may show evidence of infection with a raised white cell count and a neutrophilia. A swab of the wound should be taken for bacteriological culture. X-ray radiographs of the affected limb are not always indicated though they should always be performed, to exclude osteomyelitis in diabetics with foot problems, ulcers secondary to trauma (limb fracture), or where the ulcer is over a bony prominence. The final and perhaps most important routine investigation which should be performed on every presenting patient is the measurement of the ankle and brachial systolic blood pressure and the calculation of the ankle:brachial pressure index (ABPI). This investigation assesses the adequacy of the peripheral circulation. It is as important to know that arterial disease is absent as that it is present and may be causing the ulcer. This is because the mainstay of treatment of the most common type of ulcer, the primary venous ulcer, involves compression therapy of some kind, either using a bandage, elastic stocking, or mechanical device. Application of compression in the presence of significant arterial disease can tip the balance of the blood supply to the leg and lead to distal necrosis occasionally precipitating leg amputation (40).

The technique of ABPI measurement is uncomplicated and easily learned by both doctors (41) and nurses (42) after appropriate training. Using a hand-held Doppler (HHD) ultrasound device, a foot vessel, the dorsalis pedis, posterior tibial, or peroneal artery is located. A sphygmomanometer cuff around the calf is then inflated to abolish the Doppler signal. The same process is repeated with a brachial artery and the cuff around the upper arm. The leg pressure is then divided by the arm pressure to give the ankle:brachial pressure index (ABPI). In health, the leg pressure should be higher than that in the arm. Studies of healthy individuals produced a mean ABPI of 1.1 with a standard deviation of 0.08 (43). Thus an ABPI of greater than 0.9 is within two standard deviations of the normal population and has been used as the cut-off point for excluding significant arterial disease (40).

This regimen of systematic patient assessment will enable a doctor or nurse to diagnose and appropriately treat the majority of leg ulcers presenting to them. Specific investigations for venous disease are discussed earlier in this chapter. Some specific ulcer aetiologies require special tests to confirm the diagnosis.

Vascular disease

Disorders anywhere in the vascular tree from the aortic valve of the heart to the capillaries of the skin and the draining veins of a limb can cause ulceration. Venous disorders account for the greatest proportion of leg ulcers and are described earlier in this chapter.

Arterial disease

The correct diagnosis of peripheral vascular occlusive disease in a patient presenting with a leg ulcer may save the patients limb if not their life. Between 20 and 40 per cent of patients with leg ulcers will have some degree of arterial disease (28, 30, 35, 36), which is the primary cause of the ulcer in around 10 per cent (28, 30, 36, 37). A primary arterial ulcer is usually the result of severe vascular disease. The patient usually has a history of gradually worsening symptoms over many years. Intermittent claudication should be sought in the history. Classically, pain occurs in the calf after walking a specific distance. Symptoms occur earlier if the patient is walking uphill. To satisfy the criteria for claudication, however, the pain must resolve with rest and then recur with continued exercise. Worsening of the occlusive disease shortens the claudication distance to a degree that it begins to interfere with the patient's normal activities. Eventually the foot may be so ischaemic that pain may occur at rest. This rest pain is usually located in the foot, being the most distal and therefore most poorly perfused part of the limb. Rest pain is characteristically worse at night when the foot is elevated. Patients, if questioned, often admit to sleeping with the affected leg hanging out of the bed to help reduce their pain. They are, in effect, using gravity to increase the perfusion pressure of the leg and improve flow, thereby reducing their symptoms. Patients should be asked about family history of vascular disease, and whether they smoke, as treatment of familial hyperlipidaemia and cessation of smoking are important in arresting the progress of arterial disease.

Ulcers due to arterial disease are most likely be situated on the foot. Of ulcers below the ankle, 74 per cent are due to arterial disease (30). Often the tip of, or a whole toe, becomes ulcerated. Ulcers may also break out as a result of minor trauma to the leg or over bony prominences. The nature of an ischaemic ulcer means that it is poorly nourished with blood with resulting necrosis and slough formation. The bed of the ulcer rarely develops granulation tissue and tendon or even bone may be visible. The ischaemic leg is cooler than the other with a slow capillary return and dry, hairless skin. Peripheral pulses should be palpated from the groins down, and documented. They may, however, be impalpable due to oedema, and an experienced surgeon may feel a weak pulse even in the presence of severe disease (40).

Investigation should include blood tests to exclude anaemia and other systemic disease. Aetiological factors leading to the development of peripheral vascular disease should be screened for. Blood should be taken for erythrocyte sedimentation rate, autoantibodies, and cryoglobulins to exclude autoimmune vasculitis and hyperviscosity syndromes. Fasting blood should be analysed for glucose to exclude diabetes and serum lipids to diagnose hyperlipidaemia. The principal investigation which establishes the diagnosis is the ankle:brachial pressure index. For practical purposes, an ABPI of greater than 0.8 or 0.9 is used as the cutoff point to exclude arterial disease. With an ABPI of 0.7 one would expect a patient to have symptoms of intermittent claudication, although this level of ischaemia is rarely severe enough to cause ulceration alone. An ABPI of 0.4 to 0.5, however, denotes more severe disease. The patient may well complain of rest pain and is at risk of spontaneous ulceration. Below 0.4 the limb can be regarded as being critically ischaemic and may have altered sensation and skin necrosis and requires urgent consideration for revascularization (Chapter 9).

More patients have a degree of arterial disease than have primary arterial ulcers. Once the diagnosis of vascular insufficiency has been made, the further management of the patient will depend upon not only the severity of the arterial disease but the general condition of the patient and the suitability of therapeutic interventions to improve the circulation. In general, this decision is best made by the vascular surgeon who will have the full armamentarium of investigative tools available, such as colour Duplex ultrasound, digital subtraction, and magnetic resonance angiography and will be able to discuss the pros and cons of the various options with the patient.

The management of ischaemic ulcers is essentially to correct the underlying cause and reperfuse the foot. Trials of vasoactive drugs have been so far only marginally effective in improving symptoms (44–46) but not limb survival (47). The options available therefore remain largely surgical. Duplex ultrasound scanning or angiography may reveal a significant short stenosis amenable to percutaneous transluminal angioplasty. More commonly, the degree of vessel occlusion is more severe and requires bypass surgery to restore limb perfusion. If these interventions are deemed unfeasible, either for technical reasons or that the patient is too frail, symptomatic relief can be obtained by performing a chemical lumbar sympathectomy. This, in effect, destroys the sympathetic vasomotor tone to the affected limb and can lead to an improvement in blood flow.

Care of the ulcer itself requires the selection of an appropriate dressing to control exudate or hydrate slough as necessary. Signs of infection should always be looked out for as the combination of ischaemia and infection can lead to rapidly spreading cellulitis and limb loss within hours.

Acute ischaemia

This is rarely a problem for a wound manager, as the majority of acutely ischaemic limbs present to the casualty department or directly to a vascular surgeon. Acute ischaemia is characterized by a recent sudden onset of pain, accompanied by paraesthesiae (pins and needles) and occasionally anaesthesia. The skin may be mottled or have a fixed unblanching appearance which indicates established necrosis. The patient may also be unable to move the affected limb. The differential diagnosis is between an embolus or acute thrombosis. The difference is usually apparent from the history. A history of heart disease and atrial fibrillation would suggest an embolus, whereas previous claudication, a thrombosis. Arteriography is mandatory if there is pre-existing vascular disease as an emergency bypass may be necessary. Intra-arterial thrombolysis is the treatment of choice.

Martorell's ulcer

In 1945 Martorell described a series of four cases of leg ulceration associated with hypertension (48). Since then the description of these ulcers as a specific disease entity has been challenged (49), although the term is still in use. The ulcers are characteristically on the anterolateral aspect of the leg at the junction of the middle and distal thirds of the tibia. They may be bilateral and symmetrical. There is no evidence of peripheral arterial occlusive disease or any pathology other than persistently elevated diastolic blood pressure. The ulcers are thought to be caused by local ischaemia following microvascular obliteration by thickening of the walls of the cutaneous arterioles. Various treatments have been described from topical application of 'brilliant green' (50) to lumbar sympathectomy (51).

Vasculitis

The reported incidence of vasculitis as a cause of leg ulceration is poorly documented. Two studies have included it as a primary cause of leg ulceration which accounts for 2–4 per cent of ulcers (30, 37). The vasculitides are a heterogeneous group of disorders whose only common link is that they cause focal inflammation of the walls of blood vessels. They can affect any vessel in the body and produce varied symptoms dependent on the site and severity of inflammation. Groups of symptoms and signs commonly associated with each other have been collected together into an array of syndromes, usually named after the person who first described them. Despite this, much of the pathophysiology of vasculitis remains unclear making a structured approach to these diseases difficult. Classification according to underlying aetiology (Table 10.4) is the most widely used system, being based on clinical syndromes. Most vasculitic leg ulcers arise in association with connective tissue disease (rheumatoid arthritis) or as a result of a drug reaction or inflammatory bowel disease (pyoderma gangrenosum).

The diagnosis of vasculitis requires an index of suspicion. The ulcers are usually on the shin and often appear clean, shallow, and otherwise healthy, although slough and necrosis may be present in the acute phase. Many of the patients are frail and may be taking long-term steroids for a systemic connective tissue disease. The ulcer may be surprisingly painful despite the absence of infection. Blood tests may show an elevated ESR. Depending on the cause of the vasculitis serum autoantibodies may be elevated. The final diagnosis, however, is a histological one and the most important investigation is therefore an ulcer biopsy. Though invasive, biopsies are easily taken in the clinic. The ulcer edge should be infiltrated with lignocaine and a piece of tissue taken from the margin, incorporating skin and granulation tissue. A 6 mm biopsy punch is the most convenient instrument to use. The specimen is placed in formalin and sent to the pathology department for processing. The defect left by the biopsy closes quickly and does not adversely affect ulcer healing.

Table 10.4 Aetiological classification of vasculitis

Non-infective systemic vasculitis	Polyarteritis nodosa
	Giant cell arteritis
	Takayasau's disease
	Wegener's granulomatosis
	Buerger's disease
Infective systemic vasculitis	Rickettsial, fungal, and other causes
	Syphilis
Vasculitis in other diseases	Associated with connective tissue disease
	Henoch–Schönlein purpura
	Serum sickness vasculitis
	Miscellaneous (drugs, malignancy, cryoglobulinaemia)
	Churg–Strauss syndrome
	Kawasaki disease (mucocutaneous lymph node syndrome)

Table 10.5 Histological classification of vasculitis

Leucocytoclastic vasculitis	Fibrinoid necrosis of media, polymorph infiltrate Immune complex disease SLE, PAN, erythema multiforme, drug reactions, septicaemia
Mononuclear vasculitis	Rare, occasional medial necrosis, no polymorphs, endothelial swelling Drug reaction, chronic urticaria Pityriasis lichenoides, chilblain
Granulomatous vasculitis	Epithelioid granulomas, multinucleate giant cells Wegener's granulomatosis

SLE, systemic lupus erythematosus; PAN, Polyarteritisnodosa.

Histologically, vasculitis is classified into three groups according to the immunological processes at work (Table 10.5). This classification is probably the most useful as it tells us something of the mechanisms of tissue damage and may allow effective treatments to be developed.

Leucocytoclastic or immune complex vasculitis is characterized by fibrinoid necrosis of the tunica media of the blood vessels accompanied by a heavy infiltrate of neutrophil polymorphs. This is usually associated with immune complex disease. Circulating immune complexes cause endothelial damage and increased vascular permeability due to release of platelet-derived factors and IgE-mediated reactions. Immune complexes become trapped on the exposed basement membrane, activating the complement system. The resulting release of chemotacic factors C3a, C5a, and C567 complex causes accumulation of neutrophil polymorphs in the vessel wall which release lysosomal enzymes causing vessel wall necrosis and thrombosis.

Mononuclear or cell-mediated vasculitis is triggered by an antigen, often a drug or similar allergen encountering a sensitized lymphocyte. This results in the release of macrophage migratory inhibiting factors which recruit and activate macrophages to the affected area. These phagocytose the offending antigen, releasing lysosomal enzymes in the process. This causes some vessel wall damage though medial necrosis is rare. If the antigen persists the macrophage can undergo epithelioid transformation and form a chronic granuloma. Granulomatous vasculitis results from the persistence of the cell-mediated response outlined above. It is most often seen in Wegener's granulomatosis where granulomas containing multinucleate giant cells are a characteristic feature.

Management of vasculitic ulcers is often disappointing with a high proportion of lesions remaining open, despite prolonged treatment (52). The ulcer itself should be dressed according to the general principles of moist wound healing. Specific treatments for the vasculitis itself are currently far from satisfactory. Systemic steroids can be of benefit as can cytotoxic therapy (53). More recently, improved results have been obtained by giving 'pulsed' therapy involving short term, high dose drugs with or without a lower background dose (54–56).

Diabetes

Diabetes itself does not cause leg ulcers. The systemic effects of diabetes, however, can be devastating and often contribute to the aetiology of an ulcer or delay healing. The effects of diabetes in promoting leg ulceration are mediated through damage to the arterial nervous and immune systems as well as the wound environment itself. Between 2 and 5 per cent of leg ulcers are due to diabetes (30, 35, 37), with 2.2 per cent of diabetics having an ulcer at any one time (57). Most diabetic ulcers are confined to the foot (30).

Diabetes is an aetiological factor in the development of peripheral vascular disease and many diabetics present with primarily ischaemic ulcers as described above. The pattern of vascular disease in these patients is somewhat different, however. Over recent years, the concept of diabetics being plagued by unreconstructable microvascular disease has been challenged (58). Many diabetics display a particular pattern of arterial disease with sparing of more proximal vessels and occlusion in the calf with reconstitution at the foot. Good results have been reported of distal bypass surgery in this group of patients (59).

Perhaps the most devastating effect of diabetes is its associated peripheral neuropathy. This usually presents in a 'stocking' distribution and can lead to problems with ulceration in two ways. The first and most obvious is that the anaesthetic skin of the foot becomes prone to injury, usually as a result of ill-fitting shoes leading to a chronic pressure ulcer. Secondly, the lack of sensation leads to orthopaedic problems and joint deformities. These 'Charcot's' feet develop abnormally high pressures under the deformed weight-bearing areas, again leading to local pressure necrosis.

As well as producing local problems with the vascular and neural supply to the foot, the effect of diabetes on other organ systems also contributes to poor healing. Infection, though not directly the cause of ulceration, is particularly devastating. The high glucose and often low oxygen content of the tissues creates an ideal environment for bacterial proliferation. This can rapidly lead to abscesses, spreading cellulitis, and eventually limb loss. Susceptibility to infection is also compounded by the decreased chemotatic and inflammatory response displayed by the neutrophils of diabetic patients. Occasionally wound healing may be significantly impaired by uraemia or nephrotic syndrome secondary to diabetic kidney disease.

Management of diabetic ulcers or 'the diabetic foot' is becoming almost a speciality in itself (60). Evaluation is best performed in a multidisciplinary diabetic foot clinic with access to medical diabetologists and vascular surgeons as well as specialist nurses, podiatrists, and orthotists. Once significant vascular disease has been excluded or maximally treated, management should consist of aggressive debridement of the often hypertrophic keratinous edges of the ulcers, off-weighting of the ulcer using appropriate or custom-made footwear, and strict diabetic control.

Infection

Bacterial infection usually arises in a pre-existing ulcer from other causes. Infection in an ulcer is characterized by pain, an increase in the ulcer exudate, and usually an accompanying smell. Assessment of colour can also be used to diagnose infection, as mentioned previously. Most ulcers are colonized by skin commensals such as coagulase-negative staphylococci, non-haemolytic streptococci, and coryneforms. This does not usually affect ulcer healing and may even contribute to the normal inflammatory processes involved. Clinical infection with *Staphylococcus aureus* and particularly group A streptococci can rapidly increase the size of the ulcer and lead to spreading cellulitis and systemic upset. If suspected, swabs should be taken from the ulcer bed and the patient treated empirically with systemic antibiotics. Topical antibacterials have little role to play in the management of ulcer infection other than the use of silver sulphadiazine in the treatment of *Pseudomonas aeruginosa*.

Occasionally synergistic infections can arise spontaneously giving rise to rapidly spreading gangrene or even necrotizing fasciitis. This should be treated by rapid hospital admission, systemic antibiotics, and urgent and aggressive surgical debridement of the affected tissue. Fungal infections are rare, other than in immunocompromised patients, and should be treated by identification of the organism and appropriate antibiotics. Parasitic infestation is virtually unheard of in the western nations as a cause of leg ulceration, although they are more common in Africa where guinea worm is still endemic.

Neuropathy

There are many causes of lower limb neuropathy but the mechanism of ulceration is essentially the same. As in diabetics, anaesthesia leads to direct and sometimes chronic injury, eventually leading to skin breakdown and ulceration. Joint deformity leads to pressure over weight-bearing areas with a subsequent risk of necrosis. Particular causes of neuropathy also contribute additional problems. Diabetics, as described above, often have associated vascular disease making their skin more prone to breakdown. Paralysis, whether from birth in spina bifida, or acquired by spinal injury or disease such as multiple sclerosis, brings with it inherent leg immobility often leading to leg dependency and oedema. Problems may also be encountered particularly in younger patients with acquired disease who justifiably resent their disability and are occasionally difficult to motivate to the importance of caring for their damaged limb. Whatever the cause of the neuropathy, the management is the same. Off-weighting and protecting the ulcerated skin, ensuring an adequate blood supply, and education to prevent recurrence.

Oedema

Oedema from whatever cause can contribute to the pathogenesis of leg ulceration. Primary congenital lymphoedema (Milroy's syndrome) is uncommon, and though thought to be due to congenital abnormalities of lymph drainage, does not usually present until early adulthood. The main differential diagnosis is venous occlusion which should be excluded by duplex ultrasound or venography. Treatment is with a firm (class 3) compression stocking (Chapter 11). Acquired lymphoedema usually results from disruption of the lymphatic chain in the femoral triangle either through tumour invasion or secondary to treatment such as surgery or radiotherapy. Deep venous thrombosis or occlusion should be excluded and treatment geared to the underlying cause. If malignant infiltration is thought to be responsible then local or systemic chemo- or radiotherapy is often effective. Steroids may also be of benefit.

Much of the oedema seen in the legs of patients with ulceration is secondary to their underlying ulcer aetiology. Venous lipodermatosclerosis is classically associated with thickened oedematous skin, as is the dependant ulceration found in the very immobile patient without venous disease. Many of the patients presenting with ulcers also have cardiovascular disease with mild ankle oedema secondary to congestive cardiac failure. The temptation when presented with limb oedema possibly resulting in ulceration is to prescribe a diuretic to 'reduce the fluid'. Other than in congestive cardiac failure this rarely achieves more than inducing electrolyte imbalance and disturbing the patient's sleep. The correct treatment of limb oedema is its underlying cause. If this is not amenable to treatment then graded compression bandaging or class two compression stockings (if the ABPI is greater than 0.9) will effectively shift the fluid into the vascular compartment from where most patients will be able to excrete the excess without pharmacological help.

Malignancy

Most primary skin lesions are easily recognized and referred for appropriate surgical or dermatological treatment. Confusion can arise, however, where a patient, usually elderly, presents with an ulcerating lesion of long duration which may have been refractory to other treatments. Occasionally the classical rolled, pearly edge with surrounding telangiectasia may give away a basal cell carcinoma, though these are uncommon on the leg. More commonly, the lesion will be scaly and slowly enlarging, with an ulcerated sloughy centre characteristic of a squamous carcinoma. Both of these lesions are malignant although metastasis is uncommon. They should be excised with a minimum 0.5 cm margin, and the defect closed primarily or with a skin graft. More serious is the malignant melanoma which may present in many guises and should be excised with a minimum 1–2 cm margin, and carefully followed up for signs of recurrence. Occasionally, malignancy can occur in the base of a pre-existing (usually venous) ulcer. Called a Marjolin's ulcer, this is essentially a squamous cell carcinoma and should be treated as such by excision and grafting. The danger is that there are many 'non healing' venous ulcers which only occasionally will harbour a malignancy. Diagnosis will be assured by maintaining a high index of suspicion when dealing with long-standing ulcers and by performing an ulcer biopsy (61).

Trauma

Traumatic tissue loss resulting in a skin defect cannot be classed as a leg ulcer, as the situation has more in common with acute wounding than the development of a chronic leg ulcer. Usually the patient is healthy with no underlying disease and the defect heals in the normal way. The complications of trauma can, however, lead to longer term problems resulting in chronic ulceration.

The incidence of deep vein thrombosis following leg trauma or surgery approaches 30 per cent without heparin prophylaxis (62). Venous insufficiency may result and lead to lipodermatosclerosis and ulceration. Open fractures may become infected. The resultant osteomyelitis may be difficult to eradicate, particularly if associated with prosthetic plates and screws. These chronic infections are a source of misery to the patient, who typically suffers recurrent sinus formation over the fracture site. The only effective treatment is removal of all prosthetic material and bone sequestra, and long term antibiotics.

Occasionally an ulcer may develop due to chronic self-inflicted trauma. These 'factitious' ulcers are often difficult to diagnose as all organic pathology must be excluded first. Various strategies have been suggested for these difficult-to-treat patients, including confrontational approaches as well as psychotherapy.

Wound bacterial colonization and infection

All burn wounds and many other traumatically injured tissues are colonized with microorganisms at some time during the process of healing. The effect that these organisms have on the outcome of the wound depends not only upon the virulence and invasiveness of the organism, but also upon the immunological status of the host involved (see Chapter 7). These important relationships have been outlined elsewhere (63). This section addresses the historical aspects of wound monitoring for colonization and infection, the methods for quantifying organisms in the wound, some of the organisms involved, and how some techniques designed to be beneficial in wound healing may not have the desired effect.

The wound

It should be appreciated that acute traumatic wounds and the immediate inflammatory mediator release associated with them are different from chronic wounds or from chronic, infected wounds. The presence of bacteria in or on a wound should be weighed against clinical signs and symptoms which might interfere with wound healing. Wound healing and the wound response to microorganisms may be altered by other pathologic processes such as ageing, diabetes, ischaemia, and malnutrition (Chapter 6). These processes may occur alone or may occur in concert. Wound management must then become an organized series of protocols tailored for each individual type of wound and disease process encountered.

In this section some bias will be more towards the acute traumatic wound, but discussion of chronic wounds will be included.

Wound monitoring

Wound monitoring is performed for a variety of reasons which include the determination of wound organisms, the degree of wound colonization, and the proper therapy to avoid infection and achieve rapid wound healing. An accepted method of monitoring, to include all wound types and situations, continues to be a matter for debate. A recent survey of burn care facilities in the United States (64) revealed that wound monitoring was routinely practised in 90 per cent of those facilities (Table 10.6). This survey revealed that the swab culture was the most often employed method to monitor burn wounds. The swab culture, however, has been questioned as a valid technique by some, as it is qualitative rather than quantitative and addresses only colonization.

Elek in 1956 (65) established the concept that numbers of organisms in the wound might have importance. Elek showed that staphylococci in numbers greater than 10^6 would cause pustules in normal skin and that if an inflammatory response was introduced before colonization, this number was reduced to 10^3. A year earlier it had been shown that skin grafts in rabbits would be destroyed by the introduction of 10^5 or more staphylococci, streptococci, or pseudomonads into the wound (66). The term 'burn wound sepsis' was derived from the work of Teplitz and his colleagues (67, 68) who showed that there was a direct relationship between numbers of bacteria in the wound and systemic sepsis. Their work with rats showed that numbers of pseudomonas greater than 10^5/gram of tissue, and invasion into adjacent viable tissue, were directly related to systemic sepsis (67, 68). These historic experiments linking organism numbers to invasion and sepsis led some physicians to redefine the relationship between host, organism, and wound. An interesting fact is that these experiments established 10^5 as a 'magic number' which has since been universally applied to all organisms and to all wounds.

Following these classic experiments, the quantitative

Table 10.6 Usual methods for monitoring burn wounds for microbial flora

Method	Number ($n = 55$)	Percentage
Surface swab	20	36.4
Quantitative biopsy	16	29.1
Swab, quantitative biopsy, and histological biopsy	5	9.1
Swab or quantitative biopsy	5	9.1
Other	3	5.5
Swab or histological biopsy	1	1.8
Swab or bath water	1	1.8
Contact plates	1	1.8
Quantitative and histological biopsy	1	1.8

wound biopsy was adopted by many investigators as a useful tool in predicting wound therapy and outcome. Robson and colleagues showed that successful wound closure was inhibited in wounds populated with microorganisms exceeding 10^5/gram of tissue (69). Parks and his colleagues showed that surgical intervention in wounds shown by biopsy to be heavily colonized was not only safe, but also beneficial (70).

As the quantitative biopsy gained in popularity, other investigators explored ways to provide data showing tissue invasion in a faster, more economical fashion. These experiments led to the rapid slide (71), rapid paraffin slide (72), and frozen section techniques (73).

The biopsy, however, was considered by some clinicians as too invasive for all applications, and other less invasive, quantitative techniques have been explored. These techniques include the capillary gauze methods (74), the quantitative swab (75, 76), and the absorbent disc (77). The laboratory at the University of Michigan Medical Center has recently compared the quantitative swab with the quantitative biopsy for monitoring burn wounds and found a positive correlation between the two techniques (Table 10.7). Although these techniques are valuable in selected cases, they do not address the issue of sepsis by invasion of microorganisms into viable, healthy tissue.

The quantitative biopsy is still used in Michigan for monitoring full thickness wounds in burns, ulcerative wounds, and trauma, and the quantitative swab for monitoring superficial wounds. Other laboratories have a differing opinion. Holder (78), for example, states 'We have not used quantitative culturing for a decade and do not feel that its elimination has had negative impact on overall patient care or survival from infection'.

Regardless of methods employed, it remains a fact that some physicians want to know if microorganisms are in the wound, some want to know how many there are, and if they are in viable tissue, and most feel that wound monitoring in some form is important. But, is it important to monitor all wounds? Is the presence of bacteria in, or on any wound to be equated with sepsis or the failure of the wound to heal? There are investigators who have determined that some wounds harbour so few organisms, and have such a low risk for infection, that routine microbiology is not warranted (79). (Likewise, routine microbial monitoring of small superficial burn wounds, or limited skin graft donor sites, may be misuse of resources in these days of cost containment.

Protocols (80) which take into account the wound (deep or superficial, presence or absence of necrosis), the patient's immune status and medical history, the organisms involved, and the clinical signs and symptoms, may be more reliable in the prediction of sepsis than wound monitoring alone.

Wound organisms

The usual colonizers of burn and traumatic wounds are those organisms immediately available to the wound, such as skin staphylococci or streptococci, or the ubiquitous opportunists, such as *Pseudomonas*. Before the development of adequate resuscitation techniques, the seriously injured did not survive to become colonized with other Gram-negative organisms or fungi. Advances in care, accompanied by prolonged hospitalization, have exposed the debilitated patient to environmental microorganisms not usually encountered. The clinical course of ensuing infections depends not only on the factors outlined above, such as environment and immune status, but also on the disruption of natural protective flora by treatment regimens designed to be therapeutic.

The group A, beta-haemolytic *Streptococcus* was the major threat to burn patients prior to World War II (81). This organism was also responsible for as much as 50 per cent of postpartum mortality (82). Although carried by approximately 5 per cent of the population as respiratory flora, this organism has been well controlled by penicillin and is easily treated when recognized. It should be cautioned that group A, beta-haemolytic *Streptococcus* continues to cause wound cellulitis and in some areas of the world is responsible for fulminant and fatal sepsis in the newborn (83).

Streptococcus faecalis (enterococcus) is becoming more important as a wound pathogen. Stone and others (84) have shown this organism to be the predominant cause of wound infection in 44 per cent of clean and 43.5 per cent of contaminated wounds. In a review of intra-abdominal infections, Shires and Dineen (85) showed enterococci to be the second most often isolated organisms (21 per cent) after *Escherichia coli* (31 per cent). A more recent study has associated this organism in wound and respiratory infection with the use of cephalosporin antibiotics (86). In the University of Michigan Medical Center, this organism has increased from 5 per cent in 1984 to 19 per cent in 1987 as a significant wound organism (Fig. 10.2).

Coagulase-positive *Staphylococcus* continues to be a significant wound organism in the burn patient population and accounts for approximately 30 per cent of the significant wound cultures. Half of those organisms are methicillin resistant (MRSA). Reports of problems associated with MRSA infections were frequent between 1977 and 1988 (87–90), and although the organism continues to be present, successful management protocols have been developed.

Changing patterns of antimicrobial susceptibility have been common for the Gram-negative bacteria as well. *Pseudomonas* has become increasingly resistant to antimicrobials. *Pseudomonas* and staphylococci have alternated as predominant wound flora in some burn units (81, 91)

Table 10.7 Correlation between swab and biopsy for the quantification of burn wound microflora

Swab	Biopsy (Organisms per g of tissue)						
	NG	10^2	10^3	10^4	10^5	10^6	10^7
NG	39	7	1	0	0	0	0
1+	7	1	1	0	0	0	0
2+	8	7	6	2	0	0	0
3+	1	0	3	8	1	0	0
4+	0	1	2	4	8	3	17

NG = no growth; 1+ = 1–4 organisms; 2+ = 5–10 organisms; 3+ = 11–29 organisms; 4+ = >30 organisms.

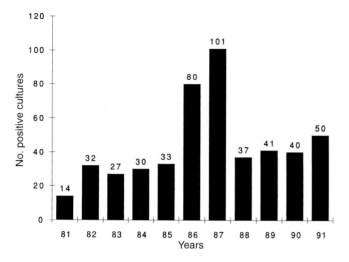

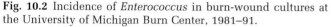

Fig. 10.2 Incidence of *Enterococcus* in burn-wound cultures at the University of Michigan Burn Center, 1981–91.

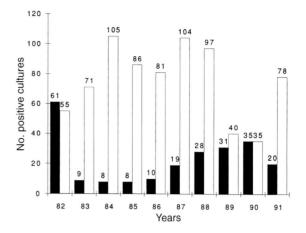

Fig. 10.3 Incidence of *Enterobacter cloacae* (filled bars) and *Pseudomonas aeruginosa* (open bars) in burn wounds at the University of Michigan Burn Center.

and have had varying susceptibility patterns. From 1987 to 1990 in the University of Michigan Medical Center, wound cultures with *Pseudomonas aeruginosa* decreased. This decrease in *Pseudomonas* infection was also noted by McManus (92) who attributed this decline at his institution to improved patient isolation. However, following a gradual decline in Michigan, *Pseudomonas* is again on the increase (Fig. 10.3).

Other Gram-negative organisms have made their appearance with a certain degree of impact. In Michigan, *Proteus*, *Klebsiella* and *Serratia* are currently on the decline in acute wounds (Fig. 10.4), while wound colonization by *Enterobacter* is on the increase (Fig. 10.3). The appearance of these Gram-negative organisms has been regional or cyclic. Their increasing resistance patterns to antimicrobials has led to two more recently observed organisms with inordinately resistant susceptibility patterns. *Acinetobacter calcoaceticus antitratus* may assume broad antibicrobial resistance through transduction and has caused great concern in some health care facilities (93, 94). *Xanthomonas maltophilia* is another highly resistant Gram-negative organism to emerge. Originally classified as a pseudomonad, this organism is adept at enzymatic degradation of antimicrobials and, although not as yet causing any mortality in the patient population in Michigan, has been cause for concern.

Reasons for this ecological progression of acute wound flora is based on a number of factors which include type and duration of topical and systemic antimicrobials used as well as the type of surgical approach to the wound. It has been shown that choices of wound treatment may favour one organism type over another. Some examples include the growth of fungi subsequent to the use of mafenide acetate (85), the overgrowth of *Staphylococcus* with povidone–iodine use (95), and the overgrowth of *Pseudomonas* associated with enzymatic debridement (96).

A review of the past six months' data from chronic wounds monitored in the University of Michigan Medical Center laboratory showed that 70 per cent (23/33) grew organisms in significant numbers. The predominant organisms recovered

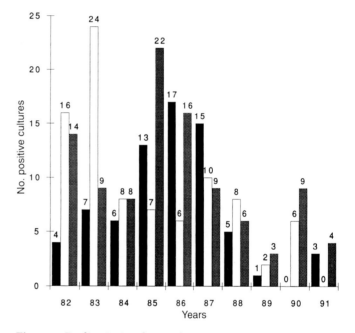

Fig. 10.4 Decline in incidence of *Serratia* (filled bars), *Klebsiella* (open bars), and *Proteus* (shaded bars) in burn wounds at the University of Michigan Burn Center.

were staphylococci and enterococci (Table 10.8). Twelve of the 23 wounds (52 per cent) grew mixed flora.

Where Gram-negative and Gram-positive wound flora have been controlled, opportunistic yeast and fungi may become wound colonizers. The most common of these has been *Candida* (97, 98) followed by *Rhyzopus*, *Mucor*, and *Aspergillus*. Again, the use of broad spectrum antimicrobials may lead to such superinfections. The role of translocation in *Candida* pathogenicity for traumatized patients remains controversial and unclear. From 1986 through to 1987, there was an outbreak of *Candida* in acute wounds at the University of Michigan Medical Center which was associated with the

Table 10.8 Organisms recovered from 23/33 chronic wounds

Organism	Number of wounds positive
Staphylococcus	15
Enterococcus	9
Enteric Gram-negative	5
Pseudomonas	5
Bacillus	2
Diphtheroids	2
Peptococcus	1
Candida	1

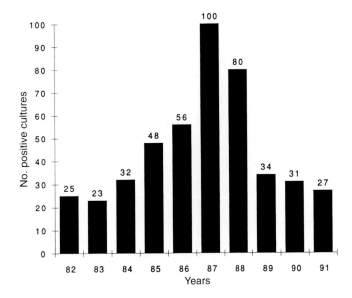

Fig. 10.5 Incidence of *Candida* in burn wounds at the University of Michigan Burn Center.

dic surgical wounds has been reported and has had an associated mortality of 10 per cent (102).

A review of the literature by Murray and Finegold (103) revealed several case reports of anaerobic burn wound infection as well as synergism between anaerobic and aerobic organisms in burn wound sepsis. This incidence of mixed anaerobic/aerobic organisms has been shown to be as high as 80 per cent in abdominal abscess with the predominant aerobes being *Escherichia coli* and streptococci (101). Mixed infections have also been associated with necrotizing fasciitis. A study of 16 patients revealed that 81 per cent of wounds grew mixed flora containing 29 species (104).

Wound dressings

The question of which wound dressing to use is directly related to numbers of bacteria in the wound, as well as the type of wound. Wounds which harbour large numbers of microorganisms and necrotic tissue have led to abscess formation when occluded by dressing (105). Therefore, it would seem unwise to occlude a wound that has no epidermal component, contains dead, necrotic tissue, and is heavily colonized. This fear of closed abscess formation led to the use of the exposure method for wounds, but total exposure resulted in desiccation and infection which delayed wound healing. The use of semiocclusive gauze dressings was thought to have the greatest chance of avoiding infection by wicking away purulence and bacteria (106).

Since 1962, there has been a growing body of evidence that superficial wounds may re-epithelialize faster under moist conditions (107). Further, recent evidence suggests that large populations of bacteria which colonize, but do not invade the wound may not have a negative influence on wound healing when under occlusive dressings (108–111). At least two burn surgeons have concluded that the presence of bacteria under occlusive dressings on acute wounds should not be correlated with infection (112). Likewise, Witkowski and Parish (113) have expressed a similar view for chronic wounds. A review of the literature (111) has shown an overall infection rate of 2.05 per cent for occluded wounds compared to 5.36 per cent for non-occluded wounds. It appears that occlusion leads to more rapid wound healing and less infection. Reasons for this may be numerous and could include an environment which selects for epithelial growth over bacterial growth (113–115), fewer dressing changes with associated mechanical disruption of epithelial growth (116), or absence of antimicrobial preparations which may retard epithelial cell division (117). Regardless, it seems that moist wounds heal faster than dry wounds and bacterial numbers do not always equate with infection.

occupation of the new facility. This outbreak appeared to be environmental and has since declined (Figure 10.5). A recent review of fungal infection from the Army Institute for Surgical Research showed a marked decline in bacterial wound infection, but not in fungal wound infection (99). In that survey, *Aspergillus* caused 71 per cent of infections, *Candida* 19 per cent, and *Mucor*, *Rhyzopus*, and *Fusarium* combined caused 10 per cent.

Surgical infections caused by the anaerobic bacteria clostridia and *Bacteroides* are well documented. Shires and Dineen (85) reviewed burn, trauma, and intra-abdominal wound infections and showed in a series of intra-abdominal infections that *Bacteroides* accounted for 48 per cent and clostridia for 17 per cent of anaerobic isolates. A review of biliary surgery in 1892 patients from the Mayo Clinic showed an overall incidence of anaerobic infection of 5 per cent (100). In that study, *Bacteroides* was more often associated with serious pathology than the clostridia. A more recent study of anaerobic, intra-abdominal, post-surgical, wound infection showed anaerobes alone in 13 per cent of all specimens and in 16 per cent of abscesses; the predominant organism recovered was *Bacteroides* (101). Anaerobic septic arthritis in orthopae-

Summary

It appears that wound infection continues to be a major concern in the traumatized patient. Likewise, healing of chronic wounds may be impaired if necrosis persists and if organism numbers and species are not in control. Causative organisms in wounds seem to change from time to time and from institution to institution, and some are becoming more serious because of their limited susceptibility patterns and related mortality. The proper technique for microbial wound monitoring is a matter of choice, and most clinicians find it worthwhile. The argument continues concerning colonization versus invasion based solely on numbers of organisms. It may be more practical to predict infection based on several clinical signs and symptoms, using microbiology as a part of the equation leading to optimal decision making. The implication is that control of wound infection is multifactorial and should include improved antimicrobials, improved early surgical intervention, improved temporary or permanent wound closure, immune modulation, and improved nutrition.

References

1. Fronek, A. (1989). *Non-invasive diagnostics in vascular disease.* McGraw-Hill, New York.
2. Coleridge-Smith, P. (1990). Non-invasive venous investigations. *Vas. Med. Rev.*, **1**, 139–66.
3. Warwick, R. and Williams, P. L. (eds) (1975). *Gray's anatomy*, (35th edn), pp. 704–6. W. B. Saunders, Philadelphia.
4. Draver, D. J. (1986). *Anatomy of the lower extremity*, pp. 206–10. Williams and Wilkins, Baltimore.
5. Thomas, P. R. S., Nash, G. B., and Dormandy, S. A. (1988). White cell accumulation in the dependent legs of patients with venous hypertension: a possible mechanism for trophic changes in the skin. *Br. Med. J.*, **295**, 296–9.
6. Scurr, J. H. and Coleridge-Smith, P. D. (1997). Venous disease; a role for the microcirculation. *Wounds.* (In Press.)
7. Hendericks, W. H. and Swallow, R. T. (1988). Management of stasis leg ulcers with Unna's boots versus elastic support stockings. *J. Am. Acad. Derma.*, **12**, 90–98.
8. Lewis, C. E. J., Antoine, J., Mueller, C., Talbot, W. A., Swaroop, R., and Edwards, W. S. (1976). Elastic compression in the prevention of venous stasis. *Am. J. Surg.*, **132**, 739–43.
9. Caprini, J. A., Chucker, J. L., Zuckerman, L., Wagner, J. P., Franck, C. A., and Culten, S. E. (1983). Thrombosis prophylaxis using external compression. *Surg. Gyna. Obstet.*, **116**, 599–609.
10. Harman, T. J., Pugh, J. L., Smith, R. D., Robertson, W. W., Yost, R. P., and Janssen, H. F. (1982). Cyclic sequential compression of the lower limb in prevention of deep venous thrombosis. *J. Bone Joint Surg.*, **64**, 7, 1059–62.
11. Buckley, A., Davidson, J. M., and Damareth, C. D. (1987). Epidermal growth factors increase granulation tissue formation dose dependency. *J. Surg. Res.*, **45**, 322–8.
12. Laato, N., Niinkiski, J., and Gerbin, B. (1986). Stimulation of wound healing by epidermal growth factor. *Ann. Surg.*, **203**, 279–81.
13. Brown, G. L., Nanney, L. B., and Griffen, J. (1989). Enhancement of healing by topical treatment with epidermal growth factor. *New Engl. J. Med.*, **321**, 76–9.
14. Brown, G. L., Curtsinger, L. J., and White. M. (1988). Acceleration of tensile strengths of incisions treated with EGF and TGF-beta. *Ann. Surg.*, **208**, 788–94.
15. Falanger, V., Eaglestein, W., Bucali, B., Kutz, M., Harris, B., and Carson, P. (1992). Topical use of human recombinant epidermal growth factor (h-EGF) in venous ulcers. *J. Derm. Surg. Onc.*, **18**, 604–6.
16. Brown, G. L., Nanney, L. B., and Griffen, J. (1989). Enhancement of healing by topical treatment with epidermal growth factor. *New Engl. J. Med.*, **321**, 76–9.
17. Phillips, T. J. and Dovcer, J. S. (1991). Leg ulcers. *Journal of the Am. Acad. Derm.*, **25**, 968–87.
18. Phillips, T. (1988). Cultured skin grafts: past, present, future. *Arch. Derm.*, **124**, 1035–8.
19. Heffon, S. A., Castwell, D., and Biozes, D. G. (1986). Grafting of skin ulcers with cultured autologous epidermal cells. *J. Am. Acad. Derm.*, **14**, 399–405.
20. Leight, I. M. and Purkis, P. E. (1986). Cultured grafted leg ulcers. *Clinics in Experimental Dermatology*, **11**, 650–3.
21. Phillips, T. and Gilchrist, B. A. (1990). Cultured epidermal grafts in the treatment of leg ulcers. *Adv. Derm.*, **5**, 33–50.
22. Phillips, T., Kehinde, O., and Green H. (1989). Treatment of skin ulcers with cultured epidermal allografts. *J. Am. Acad. Derm.*, **21**, 191–9.
23. Browse, N. L., Jarrett, P. E. M., Morland, M., and Burnand, K. G. (1977). Treatment of lipodermatosclerosis of the leg by fibrinolytic enhancement, a preliminary report. *Br. Med. J.*, **ii**, 434.
24. Davidson, J. F., Lockhuw, M., McDonald, G. A., and McNicol, G. P. (1972). Fibrinolytic enhancement by stanozolol: a double blind trial. *Br. J. Haem.*, **22**, 543–59.
25. Burnand, K. G., Clemenson, G., Morland, M., Jarret, P. E. M., and Browse, N. L. (1980). Venous lipodermatosclerosis treatment enhancement and elastic compression. *Br. Med. J.*, 280–7.
26. Browse, N. L. (1986). Aetiology of venous ulceration. *J. Surg.*, **10**, 938–43.
27. Callam, M. J., Ruckley, C. V., Harper, D. R., *et al.* (1985). Chronic ulceration of the leg: extent of the problem and provision of care. *Br. Med. J.*, **290**, 1855–6.
28. Cornwall, J. V., Dore, C. J., and Lewis, J. D. (1986). Leg ulcers: epidemiology and aetiology. *Br. J. Surg.*, **73**, 693–6.
29. Wilson, E. (1989). Prevention and treatment of venous leg ulcers. *Health Trends*, **21**, 97.
30. Baker, S. R., Stacey, M. C., Sing G., *et al.* (1992). Aetiology of chronic leg ulcers. *Eur. J. Vasc. Surg.*, **6**, 245–51.
31. Coon, W. W., Willis III, P. W., and Keller, J. B. (1973). Venous thromboembolism and other venous disease in the Tecumesh community health study. *Circulation*, **48**, 839–46.
32. Nelzen, O., Bergqvist, D., Lindhagen, A., *et al.* (1991). Chronic leg ulcers: an underestimated problem in primary health care among elderly patients. *J. Epid. Comm. Health.*, **45**, 184–7.
33. The Alexander House Group (1992). Consensus paper on venous leg ulcers. *Phlebology*, **7**, 48–58.
34. Maffei, F. H. A., Magaldi, C., Pinho, S. Z., *et al.* (1986). Varicose veins and chronic venous insufficiency in Brazil: prevalence among 1755 inhabitants of a country town. *Int. J. Epid.*, **15**, 210–17.
35. Ruckley, C. V., Dale, J. J., Callam, M. J., *et al.* (1982). Causes of chronic leg ulcer. *Lancet*, **ii**, 615–16.
36. Nelzen, O., Bergqvist, D., and Lindhagen, A. (1991). Leg ulcer aetiology – a cross sectional population study. *J. Vasc. Surg.*, **14**, 557–64.
37. Salaman, R. A. and Harding, K. G. (1994). Aetiology and prognosis of chronic leg ulcers. Proceedings of fourth conference on advances in wound management, Copenhagen, 1994. Macmillan, London.
38. Callam, M. J., Harper, D. R., Dale, J. J., *et al.* (1987). Chronic ulcer of the leg: clinical history. *Br. Med. J.*, **294**, 1389–91.
39. Boardman, M., Melhuish, J., Palmer K., *et al.* (1993). Hue, saturation and intensity in the healing wound image. Proceeding of the Third European Conference on Advances in Wound Healing, Harrogate, 1993, pp. 45–8. Macmillan Magazines, London.
40. Callam, M. J., Harper, D. R., Dale J. J., *et al.* (1987). Arterial disease in chronic leg ulceration: an underestimated hazard? Lothian and Forth Valley leg ulcer study. *Br. Med. J.*, **294**, 929–31.

41. Ray, S. A., Srodon, P. D., Taylor R. S., *et al.* (1994). Reliability of ankle:brachial pressure index measurement by junior doctors. *Br. J. Surg.*, **81**, 188–90.

42. Cameron, J. (1991). Using Doppler to diagnose leg ulcers. *Nursing Standard*, **5**, 25–7.

43. Bernstein, E. F. and Fronek, A. (1982). Current status of non invasive tests in the diagnosis of peripheral arterial disease. *Surg. Clin. North Am.*, **3**, 473–88.

44. Trubestein, G., Bohme, H., and Heidrich, H. (1984). Naftidrofuril in chronic arterial disease. Results of a controlled multicenter study. *Angiology*, **35**, 701–8.

45. Porter, J. and Cutler, B. S. (1982). Pentoxifylline efficacy in the treatment of intermittent claudication: Multicenter controlled double blind trial with objective assessment of chronic arterial disease patients. *Am. Heart. J.*, **104**, 66.

46. Antiplatelet trialists collaboration. I: Prevention of death, myocardial infarction and stroke by prolonged antiplatelet therapy in various categories of patients. *B. Med. J.*, **308**, 81–106.

47. Strandness, E. D. (1987). Vascular diseases of the extremities. In *Principles of internal medicine*, (ed. E. Braunwald and K. J. Isselbacher), pp. 1040–6. McGraw-Hill, New York.

48. Martorell, F. (1945). Las ulceras supramaleolares por arteriolitis de las grandes hipertensas. *Actas del I Policlinico*, December.

49. Leu, H. J. (1992). Hypertensive ischaemic leg ulcer (Martorell's ulcer): a specific disease entity? *Int. Ang.*, **11**, 132–6.

50. Alonso, T. (1954). Diastolic arterial hypertension and ulcer of the leg. Martorell's syndrome. *Lancet*, **i**, 1059.

51. Monserrat, J. (1958). Diastolic arterial hypertension and ulcer of the leg – Martorell's syndrome. *Lancet*, 226–7.

52. Salaman, R. A. (1994). What is vasculitis? Proceedings of 4th European Conference on Advances in Wound Management, 1994. Macmillan Magazines, London.

53. Fauci, A. S., Katz, P., Haynes B. F., *et al.* (1979). Cyclophosphamide therapy of severe systemic necrosing vasculitis. *N. Engl. J. Med.*, **301**, 235–8.

54. Pandya, A. G. and Sontheimer, R. D. (1992). Treatment of pemphigus vulgaris with pulse intravenous cyclophosphamide. *Arch. Dermatol.*, **128**, 1626–30.

55. Roach, B. A. and Hutchinson G. J. (1993). Treatment of refractory systemic lupus erythematosus-associated thrombocytopenia with intermittent low-dose intravenous cyclophosphamide. *Arth. Rheum.*, **36**, 682–4.

56. Mevorach, D., Leibowitz, G., Brezis M., *et al.* (1992). Induction of remission in a patient with Takayasau's arteritis by low dose pulses of methotrexate. *Ann. Rheum. Dis.*, **51**, 904–5.

57. Boulton, A. J. M. (1993). The diabetic foot. *Med. Int.*, 271–4.

58. Stephenson, B. M., Salaman, R. A., Shute, K., *et al.* (1994). Infrainguinal revascularisation in the diabetic patient. *Br. J. Surg.*, **81**, 150.

59. Isaksson, L. and Lundgren, F. (1994). Vein bypass surgery to the foot in patients with diabetes and critical ischaemia. *Br. J. Surg.*, **81**, 517–20.

60. Edmonds, M. E., Blundell, N. P., and Morris, H. E. (1986). Improved survival of the diabetic foot: the role of a special foot clinic. *Q. J. Med.*, **232**, 763–71.

61. Ackroyd, J. S. and Young, A. E. (1983). Leg ulcers that do not heal. *Br. Med. J.*, **286**, 207–8.

62. Berqvist, D. (1983). *Postoperative thromboembolism.* Springer, Berlin.

63. Thomson, P. D. (1984). Host defenses: basic physiology and management. In *Life support systems in intensive care*, (ed. R. H. Bartlett, W. M. Whitehouse, and J. G. Turcotte), pp. 169–86. Yearbook Medical, Chicago.

64. Taddonio, T. E., Thomson, P. D., Smith, D. J., and Prasad, J. K. (1990). A survey of wound monitoring and topical antimicrobial therapy. *J. Burn Care Rehabil.*, **11**, 423–7.

65. Elek, S. D. (1956). Experimental staphylococcal infections in the skin of man. *Ann. NY Acad. Sci.*, 65–85.

66. Liedberg, N. C. F., Reiss, E., and Artz, C. P. (1955). Effects of bacteria on take of split thickness skin grafts in rabbits. *Annals Surg.*, 142–92.

67. Teplitz, C., Davis, D., Mason, A. D., and Moncrief, J. A. (1964). Pseudomonas burn wound sepsis I. Pathogenesis of experimental burn wound sepsis. *J. Surg. Res.*, **4**, 200–16.

68. Teplitz, C., Davis, D., Walker, H. L., *et al.* (1964). Pseudomonas burn wound sepsis II. Haematogenous infection at the junction of the burn wound and the unburned hypodermis. *J. Surg. Res.*, **4**, 217–22.

69. Robson, M. C., Lea, C. E., Dalton, J. B., and Heggers, J. P. (1968). Quantitative bacteriology and delayed wound closure. *Surg. Forum*, **XIX**, 501–2.

70. Parks, D. H., Linares, H. A., and Thomson, P. D. (1981). The surgical management of burn wound sepsis. *Surg. Gynaecol. Obstet.*, **153**, 374–6.

71. Robson, M. C., Duke, W. F., and Krizek, T. J. (1973). Rapid bacterial screening in the treatment of civilian wounds. *J. Surg. Res.*, **14**, 426–30.

72. Magee, C., Haury, B., Rodeheaver, G., Fox, J., Edgerton, M. T., and Edlich, R. F. (1977). A rapid technique for quantitating wound bacterial count. *Am. J. Surg.*, **133**, 760–2.

73. Kim, S. H., Hubbard, G. B., McManus, W. F., Mason, A. D., and Pruitt, B. A. (1985). Frozen section technique to evaluate early burn wound biopsy. A comparison with the rapid section technique. *J. Trauma*, **25**, 1134–7.

74. Brentano, L. and Gravens, D. L. (1967). A method for the quantitation of bacteria in burn wounds. *Appl. Microbiol.*, **15**, 670.

75. Georgiade, N. G., Lucas, M. C., and Osterhout, S. (1969). A comparison of methods for quantitation of bacteria in burn wounds. II Clinical evaluation. *Am. J. Clin. Pathol.*, 3–40.

76. Levine, N. S., Lindberg, R. B., Mason, A. D., and Pruitt, B. A. (1976). The quantitative swab culture and smear: a quick, simple method for determining the number of viable aerobic bacteria on open wounds. *J. Trauma*, **16**, 89–94.

77. Williams, H. B., Breidenbach, W. C., Callaghan, W. B., Richards, G. K., and Prentis, J. J. (1984). Are burn wound biopsies obsolete? A comparative study of bacterial quantitation in burn patients using the absorbent disc and biopsy technique. *Annals Plast. Surg.*, **13**, 388–95.

78. Holder, I. A. (1988). The burn wound: microbiological aspects. In *Burns in children*, (ed. H. F. Carvajal and D. H. Parks), pp. 213–22. Yearbook Medical, Chicago.

79. Marshall, K. A., Edgerton, M. T., Rodeheaver, G. T., Magee, C. M., and Edlich, R. F. (1976). Quantitative microbiology: its application to hand injuries. *Am. J. Surg.*, **131**, 730–3.

80. Carvajal, H. F., Feinstein, R., Traber, D. L., Parks, D. H., Kiker, R., Larson, D. L., and Whorton, E. B. (1981). An objective method for early diagnosis of gram negative septicaemia in burned children. *J. Trauma*, **21**, 221–7.

81. Alexander, J. W. (1979). The body's response to infection. In *Burns – a team approach*, (ed. C. P. Artz, J. A. Moncrief, and B. A. Pruitt), pp. 107–19. W B Saunders, Philadelphia.

82. Frobisher, M., Sommermeyer, L., and Blaustein, E. H. (eds). (1964). Staphylococcal and streptococcal infections. In *Microbiology for nurses*, pp. 267–85. W B Saunders, Philadelphia.

83. Wannamaker, L. W. and Ferrieri, P. (1975). Streptococcal infections – updated. *Disease Monthly*, Oct., 1–40.

84. Stone, A. M., Tucci, V. J., Isenberg, H. D., and Wise, L. (1976).

Wound infection: a prospective study of 7519 operations. *Am. Surg.*, **42**, 849–52.

85. Shires, G. T. and Dineen, P. (1982). Sepsis following burns, trauma and intra-abdominal infections. *Arch. Int. Med.*, **142**, 2012–22.

86. Leoung, G. S., Chaisson, R. E., and Mills, J. (1987). Comparison of nosocomial infections due to *Staphylococcus aureus* and enterococci in a general hospital. *Surg. Gynecol. Obstet.*, **165**, 339–42.

87. Crossley, K., Landesman, B., and Zaske, D. (1979). An outbreak of infections caused by strains of *Staphylococcus arueus* resistant to methicillin and aminoglycosides II. Epidemiologic studies. *J. Infect. Dis.*, **139**, 280–7.

88. Locksley, R. M., Cohen, M. L., Quinn, T. C., Tomkins, L. S., Coyle, M. B., Kirihara, J. M., and Counts, G. W. (1982). Multiply antibiotic resistant *Staphylococcus aureus*: introduction, transmission and evolution of nosocomial infection. *Ann. Int. Med.*, **97**, 317–24.

89. Thompson, R. L., Cabezude, I., and Wenzel, R. P. (1982). Epidemiology of nosocomial infections caused by methicillin-resistant *Staphylococcus aureus*. *Ann. Int. Med.*, **97**, 309–17.

90. Hunt, J. L., Purdue, G. F., and Tuggle, D. W. (1988). Morbidity and mortality of an epidemic pathogen: methicillin resistant *Staphylococcus aureus*. *Am. J. Surg.*, **156**, 524–8.

91. Thomson, P. D., Berlin, W. M., and Reinarz, J. A. (1977). Incidence of *Pseudomonas aeruginosa* infections from an open burn ward. (Abstract.) *Proc. Am. Soc. Microbiol.*, **56**, 124.

92. McManus, A. T. (1989). *Peudomonas aeruginosa*: a controlled burn pathogen? *Antibiot. Chemother.*, **42**, 103–8.

93. Sjerertz, R. K. and Sullivan M. L. (1985). An outbreak of infection with *Acinetobacter calcoaceticus* in burn patients: contamination of patient's mattress. *J. Infect. Dis.*, **151**, 252–8.

94. Zaer, F. and Deodhar, L. (1989). Nosocomial infections due to *Acinetobacter calcoaceticus*. *J. Postgrad. Med.*, **35**, 14–16.

95. Moncrief, J. A. (1979). Topical antibacterial treatment of the burn wound. In *Burns – a team approach*, (ed. C. P. Artz, J. A. Moncrief, and B. A. Pruitt), p. 250. W B Saunders, Philadelphia.

96. Krizek, T. J., Robson, M. C., and Grobkin, M. G. (1974). Experimental burn wound sepsis, evaluation of enzymatic debridement. *J. Surg. Res.*, **17**, 219.

97. Spebar, M. J. and Pruitt, B. A. (1981). Candidiasis in the burn patient. *J. Trauma*, **21**, 237–9.

98. Prasad, J. K., Feller, I., and Thomson, P. D. (1987). A ten year review of *Candida* sepsis and mortality in burn patients. *Surg*, **101**, 213–16.

99. Becker, W. K., Cioffi, W. G., McManus, A. T., Kim, S. H., McManus, W. F., Mason, A. D., and Pruitt, B. A. (1991). Fungal burn wound infection. A ten year experience. *Arch. Surg.*, **126**, 44–8.

100. Bourgault, A. M., England, D. M., Rosenblatt, J. E., Forgacs, P., and Bieger, R. C. (1979). Clinical characteristics of anaerobic bacticilia. *Arch. Int. Med.*, **139**, 1346–9.

101. Brook, I. (1989). A twelve year study of aerobic and anaerobic bacteria in intra-abdominal and post-surgical abdominal wound infections. *Surg. Gynecol. Obstet.*, **169**, 387–92.

102. Fitzgerald, R. H., Rosenblatt, J. E., Teeney, J. H., and Bourgault, A. M. (1982). Anaerobic septic arthritis. *Clin. Orthop.*, **164**, 141–8.

103. Murray, P. M. and Finegold, S. M. (1984). Anaerobes in burn-wound infections. *Rev. Infect. Dis.*, **1S**, 184–6.

104. Giuliano, A., Lewis, F., Hadley, K., and Blaisdell, F. W. (1977). Bacteriology of necrotizing fasciitis. *Am. J. Surg.*, **134**, 52–7.

105. Bennett, R. G. (1982). The debatable benefit of occlusive dressings for wounds. *J. Derm. Surg. Oncol.*, **8**, 166–7.

106. Syme, J. (1837). *The principles of surgery*, (2nd edn). John Stark, Edinburgh.

107. Winter, G. D. (1962). Formation of the scab and rate of epithelialisation of superficial wounds in the skin of the young domestic pig. *Nature*, **193**, 293–4.

108. Mertz, P. M. and Eaglstein, W. M. (1984). The effect of a semiocclusive dressing on the microbial population in superficial wounds. *Arch. Surg.*, **119**, 287–98.

109. Mulder, G. D., Kissil, M. T., and Mahr, J. J. (1989). Bacterial growth under occlusive and non-occlusive wound dressings. *Wounds*, **1**, 63–9.

110. Gilchrist, B. and Reed, C. (1989). The bacteriology of chronic venous ulcers treated with occlusive hydrocolloid dressings. *Br. J. Dermatol.*, **121**, 337–44.

111. Hutchinson, J. J. (1990). The rate of clinical infection in occluded wounds. In *International forum on wound microbiology*, (ed. J. W. Alexander, P. D. Thomson, and J. J. Hutchinson, pp. 27–34. Excerpta Medica, Princeton.

112. Madden, M. R., Nolan, E., Finkelstein, J. L., Yurt, R. W., Smeland, J., Goodwin, C. W., *et al.* (1989). Comparison of an occlusive and semi-occlusive dressing and the effect of the wound exudate upon keratinocyte proliferation. *J. Trauma*, **29**, 924–30.

113. Witkowski, J. A. and Parish, L. C. (1992). Rational approach to wound care. *Int. J. Derm.*, **31**, 27–8.

114. Lilly, H. A. (1990). *Pseudomonas aeruginosa* under occlusive dressings. In *International forum on wound microbiology*, (ed. J. W. Alexander, P. D. Thomson, and J. J. Hutchinson), pp. 12–17. Excerpta Medica, Princeton.

115. Hermans, M. H. (1990). The incidence of infections under dressings: a prospective comparative trail of a hydrocolloid dressing DuoDERM CGF versus conventional dressings in the treatment of leg ulcers, burns and donor sites: an interim report. In *International forum on wound microbiology*, (ed. J. W. Alexander, P. D. Thomson, and J. J. Hutchinson), pp. 35–41. Excerpta Medica, Princeton.

116. Madden, M. R., Finkelstein, J. L., Smeland, J., Pesce, L., Goodwin, C. W., Staiano-Coico L., and Shires, G. T. (1990). The fate of cultured epidermal allografts on burn wounds. (Abstract.) *Proc. Am. Burn. Assoc.*, **22**, 72.

117. Lineaweaver, W., Howard, R., Souey, D., McMorris, S., Freeman, J., Crain, C., *et al.* (1985). Topical antimicrobial toxicity. *Arch. Surg.*, **120**, 267–70.

Further reading: bacterial colonization and infection

Waldstrom, T., Eliasson, I., Holder, I., and Ljungh, A. (ed.) (1990). *Pathogenesis of wound and biomaterial-associated infections.* Springer, London.

Alexander, J. W., Thomson, P. D., and Hutchinson, J. J. (ed.) (1990). *International forum on wound microbiology.* Excerpta Medica, Princeton.

11

Wound dressings

S. THOMAS and I. M. LEIGH

The ideal dressing should provide an environment at the surface of the wound in which healing may take place at the maximum rate consistent with the production of a healing wound with an acceptable cosmetic appearance (1).

Introduction

For centuries, man has applied a variety of substances to his wounds to stem bleeding, ease pain, or provide protection for newly formed tissue. Many of these agents were simple absorbents that were used to remove exudate and produce a dry wound, an essential prerequisite for rapid and uneventful healing – or so it was believed. It was not until the work of George Winter, in the early 1960s, that this view was challenged and the advantages of moist wound healing finally became recognized. Winter identified 19 characteristics he believed that a surgical dressing should exhibit (2). His recommendations stimulated a great deal of research from which many sophisticated new dressings have evolved that are variously designed to absorb exudate, combat odour, prevent infection, or produce and maintain an environment at the wound surface which facilitates debridement, granulation, or epithelialization.

Major changes take place within a healing wound, and these can have an important influence on dressing selection. During the early stages of treatment of a pressure sore, for example, a product that facilitates debridement may be required. If the cleansed wound then produces large volumes of exudate, a dressing with significant fluid handling capacity may be necessary; but as exudate production diminishes, a product that retains moisture at the wound surface may be required to facilitate epithelialization. Therefore, the aim of the practitioner should be to select – from the range of dressings available – the product that is most appropriate (ideal) for the treatment of a particular wound at *a specific stage in the healing process.*

It is currently believed that in order for healing to proceed at the optimum rate, a wound should be:

- moist with exudate but not macerated;
- free of clinical infection and excessive slough;
- free of toxic chemicals, particles, or fibres released by the dressing;
- at the optimum temperature;
- undisturbed by frequent or unnecessary dressing changes;
- at the correct pH.

The aim of this chapter is to identify the major properties and performance characteristics of the dressings in common use and indicate how these contribute to the clinical use of the products concerned by providing the optimal healing environment as defined above.

Surgical absorbents

Probably the earliest material to be manufactured specifically for use as a wound dressing was lint. First used in about the

14th century, it was produced by scraping the surface of old rags with sharp blades to produce a mass of soft fibres similar in appearance to modern cotton wool. This fibrous material was used for about 400 years to pack wounds and cavities, and as such was a mainstay of surgical practice. In the beginning of the 19th century, however, sheet lint was developed, although this was still produced by hand until the invention of the power-driven linting machine in 1856. Lint was originally produced from linen cloth, but in the early 1900s, linen fabric was gradually replaced by cotton which, after linting, was sometimes medicated with agents such as boric acid, iodoform, or cyanide of zinc and mercury. Although lint is still used in significant quantities for domestic first-aid purposes, it is now rarely used as a surgical absorbent in the hospital environment. For these applications, an alternative fabric, absorbent cotton gauze, is more commonly used.

The origins of the surgical use of 'gauze' are obscure, but it is known that Lister used absorbent pads made from a muslin cloth of open texture which were often washed and reused many times. Gauze, like lint, was sometimes impregnated with antiseptics such as carbolic acid or iodoform, but in the last decade of the 19th century, pressurized steam began to be used for the sterilization of surgical absorbents, and as a result the popularity of the medicated gauzes gradually declined.

Surgical swabs are prepared from rolls of absorbent cotton gauze that are slit to width, cut, and folded to the required size. The cutting and slitting process results in cut edges that are a potential source of particles and loose fibres. The loss of debris can be minimized by careful folding to ensure that no cut edges are exposed, but this does not provide a complete solution to the problem as individual fibres can still become detached form the threads or yarns from which the gauze is constructed.

The clinical significance of the loss of fibrous material from gauze is not always fully appreciated. Fibres from a dressing may predispose a wound to infection (3), or become embedded in the granulation tissue where they may disrupt the normal healing pattern and adversely affect the quality of the healed wound (4). Cellulose residues, in common with other particulate and fibrous materials, can also lead to the formation of granulomas and the development of fibrous intra-abdominal adhesions (5–8), which in turn can produce intestinal obstruction (9). In one study (10), it was reported that foreign body reactions were detected in biopsies of adhesions from 61 per cent of 309 patients who had undergone repeated surgical procedures. Of these, adhesions in 26 per cent of patients were shown to result from gauze lint. The remainder were due to talc, which was used as a dusting powder for surgical gloves in the 1940s and 1950s. More serious reactions to cellulose fragments used to reinforce aneurysms have also been described (11).

Alternatives to cotton gauze swabs, manufactured from non-woven fabrics, are now available for both topical and surgical use. These have less propensity to shed particles and fibres and may eventually replace woven cotton gauze for most applications (12, 13).

Cotton gauze was one of the components of the first commercial dressing pads described by Gamgee (14) in 1880. They were made from a mass of bleached cotton fibres covered with a fine gauze fabric developed from that used by nurserymen to stretch under the roofs of conservatories. Although still used as a secondary dressing or as a padding for orthopaedic purposes, Gamgee tissue has been largely replaced by other more sophisticated pads with non-woven coverstocks.

Because simple gauze or non-woven pads have a tendency to adhere to the wound surface, dressings with low-adherent wound contact layers have been developed. These include perforated plastic films (e.g. Melolin™, Telfa™, and Release™), heat-calendered non-woven fabrics made from hydrophobic fibres, and dressings coated with metallic aluminium.

Primary wound contact materials

Absorbent dressing pads without a low-adherent face should be used in conjunction with an appropriate primary wound contact layer. This must be sufficiently porous to allow the free passage of fluid from the surface of the wound into the secondary dressing in order to prevent maceration of the underlying tissue.

The dressing most commonly used for this purpose is 'tulle gras,' developed by Lumière during World War I. The original formulation contained Balsam of Peru but this was found to induce skin reactions in some patients (15) and was subsequently omitted. Tulle dressings containing a variety of other medicaments such as local anaesthetic agents, sulphonamides, antibiotics (including penicillin), vitamins, and honey were also produced, but the use of these declined when it was recognized that the topical application of antibiotics could cause sensitivity reactions in some patients or lead to the emergence of resistant strains of microorganisms. It was therefore recommended that only antibiotics such as framycetin (which are too toxic or otherwise unsuitable for systemic administration) should be applied to the skin (16). Framycetin is a broad-spectrum antibiotic which is active against both Gram-positive and Gram-negative bacteria, including common skin pathogens such as *Staphylococcus aureus*, *Escherichia coli*, and *Pseudomonas aeruginosa*. It is the active ingredient in Sofra-Tulle™ which was first used in the 1960s (17–19), when it was claimed to reduce the risk of sepsis and promote healing (20–22). Although it was initially claimed that framycetin did not cause hypersensitivity reaction, 70 cases of contact dermatitis due to neomycin or framycetin were recorded over a two year period by Kirton and Munro-Ashman (23) who argued that these materials should be used with considerable restraint.

Fucidin-Intertulle™ which contains 2 per cent sodium fusidate, is highly active against *S. aureus*, including strains which are resistant to other antibiotics. Fucidin is used in the systemic treatment of serious infections, and concerns have been expressed about its use as a topical preparation (24). Fucidin-Intertulle, unlike Sofra-Tulle, does not appear to cause skin sensitization (25, 26).

To avoid the problems of skin sensitivity and bacterial resistance, some manufacturers have produced dressings containing antimicrobial agents such as chlorhexidine acetate, e.g. Bactigras™. Chlorhexidine is a potent antiseptic agent with a broad spectrum of activity (27) which does not appear to induce bacterial resistance in normal use (28). It has a low incidence of skin sensitization (29), but one instance of anaphylaxis has been reported following the application of a dressing containing chlorhexidine. The patient, who had suffered from asthma as a child, had previously been exposed to chlorhexidine for treatment of a burn (30).

Doubts have been expressed concerning the bioavailability of chlorhexidine from hydrophobic ointment base following a series of *in vitro* tests, which suggested that the dispersed powder cannot readily be extracted from the dressing by serum or wound exudate. It was therefore concluded that the dressing was unlikely to exert any significant antimicrobial effect *in vivo* (31, 32), although this has been the subject of some debate (33–36).

Bioavailability problems do not occur with an alternative preparation Inadine™, which consists of a knitted viscose fabric impregnated with water-soluble polyethylene glycol (PEG) containing 10 per cent povidone–iodine, equivalent to 1 per cent available iodine. Unlike chlorhexidine acetate, the povidone–iodine is easily extracted from the hydrophilic base by serum or exudate and this imparts pronounced (though short-term) antibacterial activity to the dressing (32), which has been claimed to have some practical advantages over chlorhexidine tulle in the treatment of burns (37).

The semiocclusive nature of paraffin gauze dressings can cause maceration of the skin surrounding a heavily exuding wound but on drier wounds it is by no means uncommon to find that the dressing becomes firmly attached to the surface, or is incorporated into the granulation tissue. If this occurs, removal can cause trauma and result in pain that may be severe enough to require the use of opiate analgesia (38).

More modern alternatives to the paraffin gauze dressings include the simple knitted viscose fabric products, the non-adherent NA™ dressing, and Tricotex™. A recent development of these, silicone NA™ has, as the name suggests, a layer of silicone polymerized on to the fabric to further reduce the possibility of adherence.

Tegapore™ presents a new approach to the development of a non-adherent wound contact layer. It consists of a fine polyamide net, the surface of which has been heat treated to render it totally smooth. The pores in the net, although large enough to allow the passage of exudate, are too small to prevent the ingress of granulation tissue.

As a result the dressing can be left in place for extended periods. The use of this material means that simple absorbent pads can be used as secondary dressings and these can be changed as frequently as required with no danger of adherence or the possibility that cellulose fibres or particles may find their way into the wound.

Foam dressings

Not all absorbent dressings are cellulose in origin. In recent years a number of foam products have been introduced which have many desirable properties. Specifically, they provide thermal insulation, do not shed fibres or particles, are easily cut or shaped, and help to maintain a moist environment at the surface of the wound. They are also gas permeable, relatively non-adherent, light, and comfortable to wear and in some cases they are able to cope with significant volumes of exudate.

Silastic foam is a room-temperature vulcanizing, silicone foam dressing that is produced *in situ* from two components which are mixed together and poured into the wound. Once set, the dressing (or stent) can be left in position in a deep wound without the need for bandages or secondary dressings. One stent may be used for a week, or even longer, provided a simple routine of wound toilet is adopted, and it has been found that many patients are able to manage their own wounds using this material.

Silastic foam was first used as a dressing for the treatment of 40 pilonidal sinus excision cavities in 1972–73 (39). Since then it has been used in the management of various types of granulating wounds (40–42), particularly donor sites (43), pressure sores (44), amputation stump wounds (45), enterocutaneous (46) and oro-cutaneous fistulae (47), hidradentitis suppurative (48–50), scar control (51), pinnaplasty (52, 53), epidermoid cancer of the cheek (54), penile dressings (55, 56), fungating breast wounds (57), and skin graft fixation (58).

Lyofoam consists of a soft, hydrophobic, open-cell polyurethane foam sheet, one surface of which has been heat-treated to collapse the cells of the foam, allowing them to take up liquid by capillary action. The dressing is permeable to gases and water vapour but resists the penetration of liquids owing to the hydrophobic nature of the unmodified foam. When brought into contact with blood or exudate, fluid is drawn up into the wound contact surface by capillary action and transferred, by this means, laterally across the face of the dressing. The aqueous component of the absorbed fluid is lost as water vapour through the back of the dressing.

An early account of the use of Lyofoam was published in 1977 (59), and it has been used for the treatment of leg ulcers (60). More detailed use of Lyofoam for leg ulcers was reported by Mayerhausen and Kreis (61). Hughes and colleagues (62) described a community study, involving 200 patients with superficial injuries, in which Lyofoam compared favourably with a perforated plastic film dressing.

Allevyn consists of a hydrophilic polyurethane foam sheet, backed with a moisture vapour-permeable polyurethane membrane, and faced with an apertured polyurethane net. The dressing is indicated for the treatment of leg ulcers and other exuding lesions. The foam is capable of absorbing and retaining large volumes of fluid even under pressure, but on a drier wound, the polyurethane backing layer reduces moisture vapour loss and thus helps to prevent dehydration of the wound surface.

The absorbent properties of Allevyn foam have been utilized in the formation of Allevyn 'cavity wound dressing' which consists of chips of foam encapsulated within a thin layer of a conformable, perforated polymeric film. The dressing, which is available in a range of shapes and sizes, has been developed as an alternative to Silastic foam for the management of cavity wounds.

Spyrosorb and Spyroflex are thin sheets of self-adhesive

foam which have limited absorbency, but are very permeable to moisture vapour. They are intermediate, in performance terms, between the products described above and the semipermeable polyurethane films.

Semipermeable film dressings

In contrast to the dressings described previously, the principal function of which is to absorb or otherwise facilitate the removal of exudate, semipermeable film dressings prevent the loss of wound fluid which is therefore retained at the surface of the wound.

Although films made from isinglass and collodion were applied to wounds during the last quarter of the 19th century, the first use of a film made from 'modern' polymer was reported in 1945 by Bloom (63) who described the application of 'Cellophane' to 55 patients with burns, following his experiences with the material in an Italian prison camp during World War II. Soon after, in 1948, Bull and colleagues (64) described a dressing which had a semipermeable Nylon window supported in an adhesive polyvinyl frame; the clinical applications of this dressing were reported some two years later by Schilling and colleagues (65).

Winter (66) and Hinman and colleagues (67), in a classic series of experiments carried out in the early 1960s, demonstrated that compared with dry dressings, the application of a film appeared to promote rapid wound healing. Unfortunately, it was also found that the impermeable nature of some of the products they used caused skin maceration and bacterial proliferation. This problem was overcome in 1971 by the introduction of Opsite™, an adhesive film made from polyurethane which was permeable to water vapour. Other products soon followed including Bioclusive™ and Tegaderm™. These differ from Opsite, and each other, principally in their method of application, but there are other differences in their physical properties which may have implications for their clinical performance.

In a comparative laboratory-based comparison of the properties of six film dressings (68), their moisture vapour permeability was found to range from 436 to 862 g/m²/24 h. However, as the water vapour loss from uncovered wounds has been reported to vary from 3400 to 5200 g/m²/24 h (69), such relatively small variations are unlikely to be significant in this context, for even with the most permeable of the products, large volumes of exudate often accumulate beneath the dressing.

In contrast, intact skin transpires water vapour at a rate which varies between 10 and 80 g/m²/h. At the lower end of this range, the more permeable dressings may be able to cope with the moisture produced, but with a less permeable product, or a higher transpiration rate, some liquid will become trapped beneath the film (70). An accumulation of sweat and skin secretions may lead to failure of the adhesive bond or the formation of wrinkles, through which bacteria may reach the dressing, may cause irritant dermatitis (71), or tissue maceration associated with an increase in the bioburden of the skin, thereby increasing the possibility of wound infection. It is in this context that the differences in the moisture vapour permeability of the various adhesive films may become important.

More recently, developments in plastics technology have resulted in the production of new types of polyurethane films that have greatly enhanced moisture vapour permeability. One such is Opsite™ IV 3000, which is manufactured from a hydrophilic polyurethane with a permeability of 3000 g/m²/24 h and developed for use as an IV cannula dressing. Preliminary studies suggest that this new material appears to be superior to standard adhesive films in preventing accumulation of moisture on the skin surfce and the build-up of microflora (72).

Other developments in this area include Omiderm™, a thin non-adhesive hydrophilic polyurethane membrane on to which has been grafted acrylamide and hydroxyethylmethacrylate side chains. Although the film is relatively inelastic when dry, it rapidly absorbs water or exudate and becomes very elastic and comfortable when wet. It is very permeable to moisture vapour (in the order of 5000 g/m²/24 h), and also permits the passage of water-soluble antimicrobial agents (73). The use of Omiderm has been described in the treatment of donor sites, chronic wounds, ulcers, and burns (74, 75).

In addition to moisture vapour permeability, other factors which may influence the clinical performance of film dressings include their permeability to oxygen and carbon dioxide and their ability to provide an effective barrier to bacteria. In his early work, Winter (76) compared the rate of epidermal wound healing in wounds dressed with films of varying oxygen permeability, and concluded that, for rapid epithelialization, a dressing with high oxygen permeability is required.

Apparently conflicting results were reported by Sirvio and Grussing (77) who found that shallow wounds on domestic pigs dressed with a highly permeable silicone film healed more slowly than comparable wounds dressed with a less permeable polyurethane film. They proposed that healing was inhibited by an increase in wound pH caused by the loss of carbon dioxide through the silicone. No differences in healing rate were detected between wounds dressed with the polyurethane and Saran, a film that is virtually impermeable to oxygen. The authors concluded, however, that their results do not preclude the possibility that topical oxygen could enhance epithelialization in less well perfused wounds in which oxygen tension may fall below the value required for normal epidermal cell function.

The ability of different dressings, including a semipermeable film, to form an effective bacterial barrier *in vivo* was investigated in an animal study in which Opsite™, Vigilon™, and Granuflex™, applied to standard wounds on a pig, were repeatedly challenged with suspensions of *S. aureus* and *P. aeruginosa* (71). The inefficacy of the dressings was considered to be due to bacteria gaining access from the edge of the dressing (through wrinkles or channels formed beneath the film), rather than by direct penetration through the film itself.

Film dressings have been used in the treatment of burns and donor sites (78–83), decubitus ulcers (84), and postoperative wounds (85, 86), and for the management of arterial and venous catheter sites (87–89).

In recent years, the development of additional new types of dressings has led to the decline or more selective use of film dressings. Many, particularly the more permeable products, are used to dress catheter sites; others are used prophylactically to prevent damage to fragile skin of bedridden patients. They are now rarely used for the management of exuding or chronic wounds. For these applications, the hydrocolloids or alginates are generally preferred.

Alginate dressings

Alginic acid and its salts are obtained in commercial quantities from certain species of brown seaweeds (Phaeophyceae) which are found in coastal waters in many areas of the world. Alginates have a complex structure, consisting of mannuronic acid and guluronic acid residues which form an essentially linear polysaccharide polymer. They absorb exudate or serous fluid and react chemically with it to form a hydrophilic gel, the rheological and ion exchange properties of which depend upon a number of factors. These include the relative proportions of mannuronic and guluronic acid residues and the method of sterilization of the final dressing. Those made from fibres rich in mannuronic acid form soft amorphous gels that partially dissolve or disperse in solutions containing sodium ions but dressings rich in guluronic residues tend to swell in the presence of sodium ions whist retaining their basic structure (90). The gelled dressing provides a moist covering to the surface of the wound which is generally believed to facilitate normal healing. It has been suggested that calcium alginate may actually stimulate or accelerate the wound healing process as the material has been shown to promote the growth of mouse fibroblasts in culture (91), but this effect has yet to be demonstrated *in vivo*. The fate of alginate fibres or residues remaining in the wound after removal of the dressing is uncertain, for although it is generally assumed that they are enzymatically degraded to monosaccharides and eliminated, this has not bee confirmed experimentally (92, 93).

Calcium alginate was first used clinically in the 1940s following preliminary investigations carried out by Blaine (94). The haemostatic properties were utilized during dental, aural, and neurosurgical procedures, and compared with those of other haemostatic agents in a further study reported by Blaine in 1951 (95).

For a number of reasons, alginate dressings failed to become commercially successful until the mid 1980s when two new dressings were introduced. Sorbsan™ is manufactured from fibres of calcium alginate rich in mannuronic acid whilst Kaltostat™ is manufactured from the mixed sodium/ calcium salts of alginic acid rich in guluronic acid. A third dressing, Tegasorb™, is made from the same alginate as Sorbsan but with a structure resembling that of a non-woven swab.

Different forms of alginate dressings are available: sheets for application to superficial or surface wounds and rope or ribbon for packing cavities and sinuses. Composite dressings have also been developed. Sorbsan Plus™, which is used for the management of heavily exuding wounds, consists of an absorbent viscose pad faced with a layer of alginate fibre. Sorbsan SA consists of a piece of alginate fleece applied to a thin sheet of self-adhesive foam forming an island dressing for use in lightly exuding wounds. In a further development, Kaltocarb™, alginate has been combined with activated charcoal cloth to form a dressing for the treatment of malodorous wounds. The differences in the chemical composition and structure of the two principal alginate dressings have important implications for their performance and method of use which have been discussed in detail previously (96).

In the mid 1980s a number of papers were published which described the use of Sorbsan and Kaltostat in the treatment of donor sites (97, 98), diabetic ulcers, and other problem wounds (99–102). The financial implications of the use of alginate dressings were discussed following a community study involving 64 patients in which the healing rates of leg ulcers dressed with Sorbsan were compared with those dressed with paraffin gauze (103).

Fanucci and Seese (104) also described the use of calcium alginate in the management of traumatic, chronic, and surgical wounds and concluded that the material consistently produced dramatic and cost-effective wound healing. The haemostatic properties of the new alginate dressings have been considered again (105, 106).

The presence of pathogenic organisms in a wound does not necessarily preclude the use of an alginate dressing, but in such situations, daily changes should be considered. The use of alginates may help to prevent or overcome wound infection (107); cavity wounds dressed with alginate in this study were less painful, contained fewer organisms, and healed faster than those dressed with gauze and proflavine. Further anecdotal evidence has come from a national survey of medical and nursing staff involved in the management of patients with fungating wounds. The results of this survey revealed that Sorbsan is considered to be the dressing of choice when such wounds become infected (108). For this application it is preferred even to medicated products such a tulles or dressings containing povidone–iodine. A possible explanation for the reported benefit that resulted from the use of Sorbsan in infected wounds may be found in the work of Barnett and Varley (109), who showed that wounds dressed with Sorbsan contained elevated numbers of polymorphs which contribute to wound cleansing and the removal of bacteria.

Alginate dressings may also exert a mechanical cleansing action by taking up and entrapping bacteria within the gel which are removed when the dressing is changed. Topical antibiotics or antimicrobial agents should not be used with alginate dressings for some of the excipients used in their formulation may inhibit the gelling process.

One of the principal advantages of alginate dressings is that they have a high degree of patient acceptability, for they can usually be removed without causing pain or trauma to new tissue (38). However, alginates may induce a transient burning sensation due to partial dehydration of the wound bed by the hydrophilic alginate fibre, when applied to a relatively dry wound.

No sensitivity reactions to alginate dressings have been reported and the dressings may generally be used successfully on some patients who have reacted badly to other products (101).

Hydrogel dressings

A hydrogel is formed when insoluble polymers with hydrophilic sites bind or react chemically together to form pores that absorb or otherwise take up significant volumes of water. The polymers themselves may be prepared from synthetic or semisynthetic materials or a combination of the two and the properties of the resultant gel may be varied by changing the degree of cross-linking of the structure. In the dry state these polymeric species are sometimes described as xerogels.

The potential value of hydrogels in medicine was first recognized by Wichterle and Lim (110), who described a family of products based upon glycol methacrylates. Two basic types of gel dressing are currently used in wound management. The first group of products has a fixed three-dimensional macrostructure and is usually presented in the form of beads such as Debrisan™, Intrasite™, and Iodosorb™; or thin flexible sheets such as Geliperm™ and Vigilon™. Dressings of this type do not change their physical form as they absorb fluid, although they may swell and increase in volume. The swelling process will continue until the gel becomes fully saturated or until equilibrium is reached.

Hydrogel bead dressings

Debrisan is made from an insoluble material with a cross-linked structure prepared from dextran, a linear polymer of glucose. The dressing is presented in the form of hydrophilic spherical beads, 0.1–0.3 mm in diameter, that can absorb about four times their own weight of liquid. When placed upon a wound the beads initially take up exudate by capillary action. Water and low molecular weight material is then absorbed into their internal structure, causing them to swell, although a significant proportion of the asborbed liquid-containing material with a molecular weight greater than about 5000 Da is held in the spaces between. As the beads in contact with the wound become saturated, excess exudate together with bacteria and cellular debris is drawn progressively away from the surface of the wound into the drier layers behind (111). This process continues until all the beads become saturated, at which point the movement of exudate will cease and bacteria, which have been transported to the outer layer of the dressing, may start to spread back downwards again.

Because of practical problems associated with the use of the dressing, an alternative presentation, Debrisan paste, was devised in which the beads are mixed with polyethylene glycol 600 and water. In a further development, this paste was enclosed in a non-woven textile bag to facilitate its removal from the surface of the wound.

All three formulations are used primarily for the treatment of wounds containing pus, debris, and soft yellow necrotic tissue, although one study has suggested that the use of the beads may also have a positive effect upon the formation of granulation tissue (112).

Debrisan does not appear to cause allergic reactions, even in patients who are sensitive to one or more components of commonly used topical preparations (113). Implantation studies with Debrisan, involving rabbits and guinea pigs (114), revealed that unchanged beads were present up to three years after implantation, loosely encapsulated by connective tissue; but no granuloma formation was detected.

Debrisan has been used in the treatment of burns (115), particularly those of the hand (116, 117); leg ulcers (118, 119); pressure areas (120, 121); infected wounds (122); and other miscellaneous wound types. In comparative studies, the beads were found to be superior to Eusol and paraffin in the treatment of infected surgical wounds (123), and more effective than streptokinase–streptodornase (Varidase™) (124) and saline soaks (125). When compared with Silastic foam in the treatment of 50 open surgical wounds, it was reported that the cost of Debrisan was considerably higher than that of the silicone foam.

Iodosorb, which is similar in appearance and mode of action to Debrisan, contains 0.9 per cent w/w of iodine in beads formed from a hydrophilic three-dimensional network of cadexomer-cross-linked starch chains. In the presence of water or aqueous solutions, the beads swell and the iodine is slowly liberated. When applied to an exuding wound, any liberated iodine is carried away from the damaged tissue, forming a concentration gradient with the lowest levels at the surface of the wound.

Two new presentations of Iodosorb have recently been developed, Iodosorb Ointment™, an inert ointment base containing 0.9 per cent w/w iodine, and Iodoflex™, which consists of a layer of the ointment sandwiched between two layers of fabric. Both preparations are intended for the treatment of chronic leg ulcers.

Unlike Debrisan, Iodosorb is biodegradable and is hydrolysed by an α-amylase to low molecular weight fractions which consist mainly of maltose and glucose. Iodosorb is promoted for the management of sloughy and infected wounds such as pressure sores (126), and leg ulcers (127–130).

Hydrogel sheet dressings

Geliperm™ is most commonly used in the form of a flexible transparent hydrated sheet, which contains 96 per cent water, 1 per cent agar, and 3 per cent polyacrylamide. It is also available in a dry sheet form that must be hydrated prior to application. The gel is impermeable to bacteria (131), but permeable to water vapour and gases, and will allow the passage of solutes with a molecular weight of up to about 1×10^3 kDa. For this reason, Geliperm, particularly the dry sheet form, in common with some other hydrogels, can be used as delivery system for topical antiseptic agents and growth factors (132–134). Geliperm has also been used as a coupling agent for ultrasound in the treatment of fractures (135) and soft tissue injuries (136).

Vigilon, also known as Spenco™, consists of a radiation cross-linked, high molecular weight polyethylene oxide copolymer containing 96 per cent water supported on a net of low density polyethylene. The dressing is supplied with both surfaces covered with a perforated sheet of polyethylene film. One piece of film must be removed prior to application of the dressing, but depending upon the amount of exudate present, the second sheet may be left in place or removed as required. Like Geliperm, the gel (with both plastic layers removed) is permeable to water vapour and gases, but impermeable to bacteria.

Because they have a limited absorbent capacity, hydrogel sheets should be reserved for the treatment of lightly exuding wounds – such as dermabrasions (137) and minor burns. They also have a useful role in the management of skin that has been damaged by radiotherapy, as in the management of breast cancer (108). Gel dressings are cool and soothing and have a high degree of patient acceptability. For minor burns, they may be refrigerated before use. Provided that they are not allowed to dry out, hydrogel sheets can be applied and removed without causing secondary trauma or pain.

Hydrogel sheets can be difficult to retain and they have a tendency to dry out on lightly exuding wounds; applied to heavily exuding wounds they can cause maceration. Experimental wounds infected with *Pseudomonas* spp. can deteriorate very rapidly when treated with sheet hydrogels such as Geliperm and Vigilon (138, 139).

Amorphous hydrogels

Because of their poor fluid handling characteristics and relatively high cost, the use of hydrogel sheets is limited. This is in marked contrast to the amorphous hydrogel Intrasite™. Unlike the sheet presentations, Intrasite does not have a fixed three-dimensional macrostructure. As the dressing absorbs fluid, it progressively decreases in viscosity until, ultimately, it becomes a dispersion of polymer in water. Intrasite is a colourless, transparent, aqueous gel, containing 2 per cent polymer, 78 per cent water, and 20 per cent propylene glycol (as a preservative and humectant). Intrasite is widely used for the treatment of many types of wound, particularly those covered with slough or necrotic tissue. It is believed that the gel facilitates autolytic debridement of rehydrating dead tissue and promotes phagocytic and enzymatic activity.

The wound cleansing properties of Intrasite were compared with those of Debrisan paste in a controlled trial involving 29 patients with grade 3 or 4 pressure sores. The gel was found to clean wounds faster and more cost-effectively than the Debrisan paste, which is licensed for this indication (140).

Intrasite can also be used as a carrier for topical medicaments, particularly metronidazole which is incorporated into the gel at a concentration of 0.8 per cent w/w. Topical metronidazole is an extremely effective adjunct to systemic treatment for wounds infected with sensitive microorganisms and is particularly effective in reducing the odour associated with extensive or infected pressure areas (141) and fungating carcinomas (108). Laboratory studies suggest that at 0.8 per cent metronidazole is active against a range of microorganisms, not just the anaerobic species with which it is most generally associated (142).

The use of Intrasite gel was compared with Iodosorb in the treatment of leg ulcers in a comparative trial involving 98 patients (143). Although no significant differences were detected between the two therapies in terms of healing rate, odour formation, or granulation tissue, the authors concluded that, although an acceptable healing rate was achieved with both materials, Iodosorb was significantly more expensive in use.

Intrasite has also been used with advantage in the management of extravasation injuries in neonates (144). For this application the gel is applied liberally to the affected area and enclosed in a sterile plastic bag, specially shaped to form a boot or glove. The treatment offers a number of significant advantages over more traditional techniques, resulting in a healed wound with a highly acceptable cosmetic appearance.

Hydrocolloid dressings

In scientific terms, a 'colloid' is produced when very small, submicroscopic particles of one material are dispersed uniformly in another. If solid particles are dispersed in a liquid phase a 'sol' or hydrophilic colloid (hydrocolloid) is produced. In recent years this description has been applied to a family of dressings, but it is doubtful if these products comply strictly with this definition as most form hydrogels rather than hydrocolloids when hydrated.

Hydrocolloid dressings take up wound fluid to form a moist gel on the wound surface which facilitates healing but does not cause maceration of the surrounding skin. Depending upon the product concerned, this gelling process may occur very rapidly (within hours) or take several days to complete. The resultant gel may be a viscous mobile fluid or it may be contained within the structure of the dressing itself, resulting in a thicker more cohesive mass that maintains its integrity as it swells. The semi-liquid gel produced by some of the dressings has a very unpleasant odour and bears a superficial resemblance to pus. Although the dressings currently available differ in composition and construction, most consist of a carrier, typically a thin sheet of foam or a semipermeable film, coated with an absorbent mass containing sodium carboxymethylcellulose (NaCMC) together with other gel-forming agents, elastomers, and adhesives.

Granuflex™ (Duoderm™) is composed of gelatin, pectin, and sodium carboxymethylcellulose (NaCMC), dispersed in an adhesive mass of polyisobutylene. This is applied to a thin layer of a semi-open-cell polyurethane foam bonded on to a polyurethane film to act as a carrier.

A second generation product, Granuflex E, also contains gelatin, pectin, and NaCMC, but here the absorbents and gel-forming agents are contained in a cross-linked matrix. As a result, the gel that is formed as the dressing absorbs liquid is not free running, but remains confined within the structure of the dressing. When first produced, Granuflex E was claimed to be more absorbent than the original formulation and thus more suitable for the management of heavily exuding wounds. Results of laboratory tests, however, do not appear to support this claim, an observation that has formed the subject of some debate (145, 146). Granuflex E is also available in a bordered form, in which the edges of the carrier project past the margin of the adhesive mass. This gives the dressing a profiled edge and reduces the possibility of it becoming displaced in use.

A further development of Granuflex E is Granuflex E Extra Thin™, which consists of a thin coating of the same adhesive used on Granuflex E, applied directly to a piece of polyurethane film. This dressing, which is marketed as an alternative to the semipermeable film dressings of the British Pharmacopoeia, can be used in the treatment of minor wounds, superficial pressure sores, and post-surgical wounds.

Biofilm™, although similar to Granuflex in terms of the chemical composition of the adhesive base, is backed with a non-woven polyester fabric sheet. Like the other hydrocolloids, in the dry state, Biofilm dressing is virtually impermeable to water vapour, but as it takes up fluid and forms a gel, the dressing becomes highly permeable.

Comfeel Ulcer Dressing™ consists of a semipermeable polyurethane film bearing a cross-linked flexible elastic mass made from a styrene–isoprene block copolymer together with polycyclopentadine dioctyladipate which contains 42 per cent NaCMC as the principal gel-forming agent. Like Granuflex E, the dressing forms a firm cohesive mass that retains its integrity as it absorbs exudate and swells.

Tegasorb™ consists of an oval shaped piece of polyurethane film, coated with a layer of an acrylic adhesive. The film extends past the border of a hydrocolloid mass composed of polyisobutylene, in which are dispersed hydrophilic gelable polysaccharide particles, the identity of which has not been disclosed. All the dressings are self-adhesive and available in a range of sizes to suit different types of wounds. Some manufacturers also produce the absorbent component of the dressing in the form of granules or pastes for the treatment of small cavities.

Young and colleagues, in a controversial publication, reported that in pig studies, gel residues from hydrocolloid dressings appeared to cause a prolonged inflammatory reaction, and that particulate material (which had become incorporated into the wound bed and hypodermis) was still apparent beneath the surface of the healed wound six months after injury (147). The clinical relevance of these findings in human wounds has yet to be determined.

The volume of exudate that can be handled by a hydrocolloid dressing depends upon the composition of the adhesive mass and the moisture vapour permeability of the backing layer. In their intact state, all the hydrocolloid dressings are impermeable to moisture vapour but when fully hydrated, as a result of the absorption of wound exudate, the permeability increases so that a proportion of the aqueous component of exudate that collects under the dressing may pass out through the back in the form of moisture vapour. The results of a detailed investigation of the gel-forming properties and fluid-handling characteristics of six hydrocolloid dressings have been published (148).

The majority of hydrocolloid dressings, but not all, are backed with a continuous plastic film which renders them impervious to liquids and bacteria. The impermeable nature of this film has been confirmed *in vivo* by challenge tests which have shown that the dressings can prevent organisms from the external environment reaching the surface of the wound (149). The resulting barrier properties of the dressings have been used in the past to prevent the spread of epidemic methicillin resistant *Staphylococcus aureus* (EMRSA) from infected wounds (150).

One product, Biofilm, has a backing layer made of a non-woven fabric. This is permeable to moisture vapour, but is also hydrophobic and thus resists the penetration of aqueous solutions or wound exudate under normal conditions of use. If, however, the fully hydrated dressing is occluded or subjected to significant pressure, it is possible that strike-through may occur, allowing bacteria to pass through the backing. This possibility was investigated by Lawrence and Lilly (151), who described a laboratory test which showed that bacteria were able to pass through the dressing in 24 h. Their work stimulated a considerable amount of interest and subsequent correspondence, regarding both the suitability of the test method and the relevance of their results to the clinical situation (152–159).

Hydrocolloids are relatively easy to use, require infrequent changing, and do not cause trauma upon removal. They also appear to promote the growth of granulation tissue, possibly by producing a hypoxic environment within the wound (160). Because of the relatively impermeable nature of the intact hydrocolloid sheets, they facilitate rehydration of the skin surrounding the wound and thus bring about a marked improvement in its appearance and texture. It has also been shown *in vitro* that extracts of some hydrocolloid dressings possess fibrinolytic activity (161). It has been postulated that this effect may have some clinical benefits, aiding the removal of the extravascular pericapillary fibrin cuffs which are often associated with venous ulceration. These are believed to prevent diffusion of oxygen from the affected vessels, causing local tissue necrosis and death. The clinical relevance of these findings has been questioned by Samuelson and Nielsen (162), who showed, using standard chromogenic assay techniques, that the activation of tissue-plasminogen activator (t-PA) by extracts of hydrocolloids is very weak compared with that produced by fibrin, a natural constituent of the tissue repair process.

Hydrocolloid dressings have been used successfully in the management of burns (163) and donor sites (164), but they are mainly used for the treatment of chronic wounds such as leg ulcers (165, 166, 167) and pressure sores (168, 169). Their use has also been reported in the management of epidermolysis bullosa (170) and following surgery for excision of perianal hidradenitis suppurativa (171). If applied to small necrotic wounds, such as black heels, the relatively impermeable nature of the intact dressing prevents the loss of moisture vapour from the dead tissue causing it to become rehydrated and thus more easily removed by autolysis.

It has been noted that wounds dressed with hydrocolloids sometimes overgranulate (172), although no causal relationship has been demonstrated. If this occurs, a change to a more permeable dressing may allow the problem to resolve. If not, the short-term daily application of a cream containing a low potency corticosteroid will usually cause the excess granulation tissue to subside but this should only be used under medical supervision.

Most hydrocolloids can be cut or shaped to fit areas that are difficult to dress, and they also provide a protective function, preventing contamination of the wound from external sources. Because hydrocolloid dressings are relatively thin, they can be applied beneath compression hosiery and normal clothing and their impermeable nature means that patients can bathe or shower with the dressings in position.

Hydrocolloid sheet dressings are generally reserved for the

treatment of superficial or relatively flat wounds; they should not be used to cover empty cavities as this may lead to the accumulation of exudate or necrotic material. Small cavities may be dressed with hydrocolloid pastes held in place with a hydrocolloid sheet.

The apparently occlusive nature of the hydrocolloid dressings sometimes gives rise to concern that their use may predispose a wound to infection. However, a detailed review of nearly 70 published studies relating to the use of occlusive dressings (173) indicates that the prevalence of infections in wounds dressed with these materials is less than half that of wounds dressed with conventional products. It has been suggested that this is due, at least in part, to the efficient action of host defence mechanisms in the moist environment produced beneath the dressing (174). It has also been demonstrated that some hydrocolloids produce an acidic environment at the wound surface, causing the pH to fall to a minimum of 5.6 after 24 h (175), and such conditions are known to inhibit the growth of some bacteria *in vitro*. Although no evidence has been published to suggest that the use of hydrocolloid dressings is likely to contribute to the formation of anaerobic wound infections, in one leg ulcer study (176) it was shown that their use led to an increase in the total number of wounds which contained facultative anaerobes. These did not impair healing and there was no statistical difference between the healing rates of ulcers which contained anaerobes and those which did not. In the same study it was shown that although there was generally little change in the bacterial flora of the wound, in every case where *Pseudomonas* spp. were present initially, these declined in numbers under the hydrocolloid dressing and in all cases were eventually eliminated altogether. It has also been demonstrated that unlike truly occlusive products such as impermeable tapes, the use of hydrocolloids (and semipermeable films) does not lead to an increase in bacterial numbers on normal skin (177). All the available evidence therefore suggests that hydrocolloids are unlikely to cause or promote wound infection.

Hydrocolloid sheets are easy to use. A dressing should be selected which is large enough to cover the wound completely and overlap on to the surrounding skin by about 2 cm. The backing layer is removed and the dressing pressed firmly into position. Once in place it may sometimes be left undisturbed for up to a week, but more frequent changes will be required if the wound is exuding heavily.

Although there are no absolute contraindications to the use of hydrocolloid sheets, other than proven sensitivity to one of the ingredients, it is generally currently recommended that they should be used with caution in the treatment of clinically infected wounds. In these situations systemic antibiotic cover should be considered and the condition of the wound monitored on a regular and frequent basis. The literature produced by each manufacturer should be consulted for more detailed advice in this area.

The role of bandages in wound management

Bandages have a history stretching back thousands of years to the time of the ancient Egyptians who used simple woven fabrics coated with adhesives, resins, and other medicaments to aid wound healing. Simple non-extensible bandages continued to be widely used well into the first half of the 20th century and many nursing texts published around this time contain detailed and complex diagrams illustrating the application of flannel, Domette, or white open wove bandages. Considerable skill was required on the part of the user to ensure that these bandages were applied correctly because of their inextensible nature and poor conformability but as newer, extensible and more conformable products were introduced, application technique became less critical and the art of bandaging no longer formed a major part of a nurse's education. Finally, with the development of tubular bandages which require virtually no expertise on the part of the user, training in bandaging virtually ceased altogether.

Recently, however, interest in both the science and art of bandaging has been reawakened, particularly in relation to the importance of compression in the treatment and prevention of venous leg ulcers, for it is generally agreed that conservative treatment of this condition should be directed at increasing the transfer of tissue fluid from the interstitial spaces back into the vascular and lymphatic compartments, and achieving a maximal increase in deep venous velocity in order to reduce pooling of blood in the calf veins. Both of these aims may be met by the application of external compression. The degree of pressure required depends upon the condition to be treated, and remains a matter of some debate, although it is accepted that a pressure gradient should be produced along the leg, with the highest pressure being exerted at the ankle.

Traditional cotton bandages are unable to sustain elevated levels of graduated compression (178–180), but a technique involving the application of four different bandages that has been claimed to produce and maintain clinically effective levels of graduated compression has been described by Backhouse and colleagues (181). Known as the 'four-layer' system, it consists of a layer of orthopaedic wadding, followed by a standard crêpe, a lightweight elastomeric bandage, Elset™, held in place with a layer of cohesive bandage (Coban™). Using this system the authors achieved average pressures of 42 mmHg (5.6 kPa) at the ankle, reducing to 17 mmHg (2.3 kPa) just below the knee.

Although none of the bandages used by Backhouse and colleagues is individually able to produce high levels of pressure, when applied in combination they are able to achieve the desired results. However, a similar effect can also be achieved at lower cost by the use of a single competent compression bandage.

The consequences of the inappropriate or excessive application of pressure have been described by Callam and colleagues (182), who recorded that the injudicious use of compression – by the use of bandages, compression hosiery, or anti-embolism stockings – in limbs with occult arterial disease had apparently led to severe skin necrosis and, in a few instances, amputation. As a result, they recommended that, unless distal pulses of good volume could be detected, Doppler pressures should be measured in the ankle before treatment with compression.

A multidisciplinary working party has recently classified

extensible bandages into groups according to their performance when tested by a new laboratory method that has since become the subject of a draft British Standard. This classification recognizes three basic types of bandages as described below.

Type 1: Lightweight conforming stretch bandages

These are products that have a simple dressing retention function. They usually incorporate lightweight elastomeric threads, which impart a high degree of elasticity, but little power, to the bandage.

Type 2: Light support bandages

These bandages, which include the familiar crêpe-type products of the British Pharmacopoeia, may be used to prevent the formation of oedema, and give support in the management of mild sprains and strains. They have limited extensibility and elasticity, and tend to 'lock out' at relatively low levels of extension. It is this feature that enables the bandages to be applied firmly over a joint to give support without generating significant levels of pressure.

When applied firmly over the calf region, they will also provide a relatively rigid covering that tends to resist the changes that occur in the geometry of the calf during walking. This in turn generates intermittent increases in sub-bandage pressure which may help to reinforce the action of the calf muscle pump. Because the pressure generated beneath these bandages is produced at least in part by the action of walking, it follows that they are not suitable for applying sustained compression in immobile patients or for reducing existing oedema, although they may be suitable for application to patients who have venous disorders associated with some degree of arterial insufficiency where the use of powerful compression bandages would be contraindicated.

Type 3: Compression bandages

The true compression bandages are further divided into four sub-groups according to the levels of pressure that they are able to maintain.

1. Type 3a bandages, wich are broadly equivalent in performance terms to class 1 compression hosiery of the Drug Tariff, are able to provide and maintain low levels of pressures, up to 17 mmHg (2.3 kPa) on an ankle of average dimensions.

2. Type 3b, which are broadly equivalent to class 2 compression hosiery of the Drug Tariff, may be used to apply moderate to high levels of compression (up to about 24 mmHg or 3.2 kPa on an ankle of average dimensions).

3. Type 3c, similar to class 3 compression hosiery of the Drug Tariff, can apply and maintain of the order of 35 mmHg (4.7 kPa) on an ankle of average dimensions. It is products in this group, such as Tensopress™ and Setopress™, that are generally used for the treatment of venous ulcers.

4. Type 3d bandages are capable of applying pressures up to 50 mmHg (6.7 kPa) or even higher, and their power is such that they can be expected to apply and sustain these pressures on even the largest and most oedematous limbs for extended periods.

All the pressures referred to above are based on the assumption that the bandage has been applied in the form of a spiral with a 50 per cent overlap between turns, effectively producing a double layer of bandage at any point on the limb. The use of an alternative technique may produce pressures that are significantly higher than those quoted. The pressure profiles produced by different types of bandaging regimen were compared in a later paper by Callam and colleagues (183) who concluded that elastic compression bandages are more effective than minimal stretch systems for producing sustained compression.

The ability of a bandage to perform in the required fashion is largely determined by its elastic properties, although the thickness, weight, and conformability of the fabric are also important.

Sub-bandage pressure, which is a function of the tension induced in the fabric during application and the radius of curvature of the limb, can be calculated from Laplace's law as follows:

$$p = \frac{t}{rw}$$

where p = pressure (in Pa); t = bandage tension (in N); r = radius of curvature of the limb (in m); and w = bandage width (in m). In more practical units, this equation may be rewritten as

$$p = \frac{t \times 4630}{cw}$$

where p = pressure (in mmHg); t = bandage tension (in kgf); c = circumference of the limb (in cm); w = bandage width (in cm). As the effects of additional layers of bandage are additive, two turns applied with constant tension will give virtually twice the pressure of a single turn.

The relationship between tension and extension can be measured in the laboratory and expressed as load–extension curves, the shape and slope of which can be used to provide much useful information on the anticipated performance of the products concerned.

Dressing retention bandages should have long, shallow extensibility curves, which allow them to stretch and conform, without restricting movement; but bandages that are required to apply significant levels of pressure should have good regain characteristics, and a load–extension curve that rises smoothly but not too rapidly over the working range.

Bandages whose primary function is one of support should have a degree of extensibility, to facilitate application, but should resist excessive extension when subjected to further tension.

Because sub-bandage pressure is inversely proportional to the radius of curvature of the limb, it follows that bandage applied with constant tension to a normal leg will tend to exert higher pressures at the ankle than at the calf thus producing a pressure gradient. It should be recognized, however, that differences exist in the radius of curvature at various points around the circumference. Over the tibia, for example, where the radius of curvature is relatively small, very high pressures may be generated.

The technique of the operator is also very important, as sub-bandage pressure is controlled by both the tension produced in the banage during application, and the number of turns applied. Most medical and nursing staff apply a compression bandage at the tension that they consider to be appropriate to the size and condition of the limb. However, this target value varies from one person to another and, as a result, the levels of pressure applied by different individuals can be very different. A number of attempts have been made to overcome this problem by manufacturers, who have printed geometrical designs upon their bandages which change shape when a predetermined level of tension is achieved. In this way it is possible to exert some control over the application tension and thus the sub-bandage pressure that is produced.

The use of cultured keratinocytes for skin grafting

The epidermis is a self-renewing tissue, with a progenitor population deriving from the basal cell layer of keratinocytes in interfollicular skin (184). In a steady state, the self-renewal balances corneocyte shedding at the epidermal surface, but there is a huge capacity for proliferation on demand and this produces an altered state of differentiation (185). When the epidermis is wounded, keratinocytes at the wound edge are activated to migrate across the wound surface and to divide rapidly to provide an expanded population (186–188). When epidermal keratinocytes are isolated from each other, by enzymic digestion of the skin, the expansion potential of the keratinocytes can be harnessed to provide rapidly expanding colonies on a tissue culture dish, by providing the correct growth support medium and a suitable substrate to support their attachment and growth. The keratinocytes divide frequently and migrate rapidly until the colonies meet to cover the dish then stratification produces a multilayered epidermis (189). Understanding of the growth of keratinocytes was limited until 1975, when Rheinwald and Green (190) described the use of 3T3 feeder cells and mitogens to encourage keratinocyte growth. Cyclic AMP elevating agents (including cholera toxin, ref. 191) and epidermal growth factor (EGF, refs 192, 193) were found to stimulate growth and lateral migration of colonies, and the importance of calcium in obtaining stratified rather than monolayer cultures of keratinocytes was noted (194, 195). Thus it became possible to use defined media to determine the growth of large numbers of keratinocytes *in vitro* (196).

Once optimal growth conditions were established, the clinical use of cultured sheets to provide skin grafts in patients needing skin expansion techniques to cover major burns or developmental naevi, was explored (197, 198). Although it was clear from early studies that keratinocyte grafts could be used to replace skin permanently in badly burned patients (199–202), later wider use produced mixed clinical results,

with reports of graft take varying from 0 to 100 per cent but being generally lower than with conventional skin grafts (203). The range of conditions treated increased, with congenital naevi, leg ulcers, tattoos, and other surgical wounds receiving grafts (204, 205). Keratinocytes were also used to treat chronic secretory otitis with mastoid cavities that required relining with epithelium (206). Oral keratinocytes are readily cultured under conditions identical to those for epidermal keratinocytes and have been used to treat cleft palate wounds, cancer defects, and submucosal fibrosis (207, 208). Cultured urothelial cells can also be used to treat hypospadias (209). The clinical results of keratinocyte autografting are difficult to analyse systematically, largely being anecdotal, and there are many factors which could influence graft outcome: stage of keratinocyte culture, infection, use of antiseptics (210), dressing technique, type of backing dressing, depth and type of wound, and state of the wound bed. There is a consensus, however, that wounds remain fragile for some months following keratinocyte autografting, due to the slow maturation of the basement membrane zone (211) and limited regeneration of a neodermis (212, 213).

The role of keratinocytes as active members of the skin's immune system has only recently been recognized (214). In addition to the production of immunological cytokines (215), keratinocytes can express adhesion molecules and HLA class II molecules following activation by skin disease or wounding *in vivo*, probably mediated by TNF and gamma interferon (214, 216). *In vitro*, gamma interferon induces class II and ICAM-1 expression. Skin allograft rejection has been thought to be mediated by the passenger leucocytes, particularly the antigen presenting cells of the skin, the dendritic Langerhans cells (217). As cultures of keratinocytes lose Langerhans cell markers and the ability to elicit a mixed epidermal cell lymphocyte response (218, 219), it was proposed that keratinocyte allografts would survive transplantation. Early clinical reports of keratinocyte allografts in burns suggested this to be the case (220), and further support came from work in donor sites (221, 222). However, other studies showed keratinocyte allograft rejection (223), albeit after prolonged survival, and more recent DNA-based techniques have shown evidence of non-survival of keratinocyte allografts early (1 week) after treatment of burns (224), tattoos (225), donor sites (226), and leg ulcers (227). It may be that imperceptible replacement of keratinocyte allografts with autologous cells occurs, without a frank rejection response (228, 229). Animal models have been used to analyse the fate of keratinocyte allografts and most studies in mouse, rat, and pig have shown rejection, whic is delayed compared to grafting with intact skin (230). However, conflicting data were reported for keratinocyte allografts in mouse, with no rejection at 70 days (231). There remains a logistic problem in biopsying human wounds very early after grafting as dressing changes are very likely to damage the graft, which is very susceptible to shearing forces, making the fate of keratinocytes early after grafting difficult to determine. The use of keratinocyte allografts in chronic wounds, particularly leg ulcers, has highlighted the effects of keratinocyte grafting without graft take. Many groups have noted the effect of keratinocyte allografts (and presumably autografts) in promoting wound healing from the ulcer edge, or from islands of epithelium within the ulcer (232–234).

The production by keratinocytes of many growth factors (235, 236), basement membrane (237), and extracellular matrix proteins (211) can obviously play a role in stimulating keratinocyte migration and mitosis. These factors, which can be purified or produced by recombinant DNA technology, clearly have a potential as wound treatments (238–240). However, further studies of the roles of growth factors in normal wound healing are required. For example, in view of the role of transforming growth factor beta (TGFβ) in promoting scarring (240) and the reduction in adult scarring obtained by using antibody to TGFβ (241), it may be more appropriate to block some growth factors than enhance them.

Keratinocytes exhibit poor stratification and differentiation when under optimal growth stimulating conditions, as differentiation is sacrificed to achieve high growth rates (189, 242). Normal skin has a complex dermis which appears to play an important directive or permissive role in epidermal differentiation, both in development and in adult life (243). Therefore attempts have been made to enhance keratinocyte differentiation. The use of collagen-coated dishes (244) to promote differentiation developed into using isolated collagenous matrices; the 'living skin equivalent' (245) involved contracting a collagen gel by the incorporation of dermal fibroblasts, then seeding keratinocytes on to the surface, or incorporating small fragments of skin. In this 'living skin equivalent,' optimal cornification was obtained by raising the culture to an air–liquid interface. These collagen gels are susceptible to proteolysis and therefore work is continuing to produce stable dermis equivalents either by incorporating extra ingredients into the gel, such as chondroitin sulphate (246, 247), or by cross-linking, as in chitosan cross-linked human collagens (248).

Cadaver skin has been widely used as a burn dressing and can be treated with the enzyme dispase to remove the epidermis. This de-epidermalized dermis can be used as a substrate for the culture of keratinocytes (249), and promotes differentiation with cornitication obtained by raising to an air–liquid interface. Skin equivalents of all sorts require previous culture of the cellular components: keratinocytes and fibroblasts, once established, cannot be easily passaged in culture, therefore have a more limited expansion potential than keratinocyte grafts alone. Clinical experience with skin equivalents is currently largely anecdotal but seems to suggest that graft maturation may occur more readily than with intact skin and has been successfully reported in treatment of junctional epidermolysis bullosa (250), leg ulcers (251), tattoos (252), and burns (253). However, the presence of proteolytic enzymes in the wound bed causes problems with the stability of the dermal graft.

An appreciation of the role of dermis in keratinocyte differentiation has led to a re-examination of the role of the dermis in keratinocyte autograft take. Although few comparative studies have been made, it is clear that the use of cadaver skin as a wound dressing, whilst waiting for a keratinocyte graft to take, may have an important effect. In the mid 1980s, Cuono and others showed that two-stage grafting, first with cadaver dermis followed by abrasion of the epidermis and application of cultured keratinocytes, gave a good clinical and morphological result (254–256). This is now being widely and formally tested. Animal studies (pig) have shown that there is still considerable dermal degeneration in two-stage grafting with autologous dermis and autologous keratinocytes, but normal collagen bundles reform rapidly and the basement membrane structure is good (257). In addition, nerve regeneration occurs underneath the keratinocytes but not under denuded areas (257). There is no biological evidence that allogenic keratinocytes and fibroblasts within skin equivalents will survive transplantation.

There is thus a compelling need to continue to improve the clinical results from both keratinocyte autografts and autologous skin equivalents for those life-threatening situations where there is extensive skin loss. This improvement can probably be made by attention to and rigorous evaluation of all the factors influencing graft take, including dermal equivalent production, perhaps with added pleomorphic cell populations containing heterogeneous fibroblasts and endothelial cells. Once the results equate to the performance of intact skin grafts, then the clinical applications can be widened. The wound healing effect of keratinocyte grafts as dressings may be replaced by the use of purified growth factors and matrix proteins, but as yet the full complement of keratinocyte-derived growth factors has not been identified, nor have their complex interactions. An exciting start has been made, to be followed by the long and less sensational path to clinical validation.

References

1. Thomas, S. (1990). *Wound management and dressings*. Pharmaceutical Press, London.
2. Winter, G. D. (1975). Epidermal wound healing. In *Surgical dressings in the hospital environment*, (ed. T. D. Turner and K. R. Brain), Conference Proceedings, Cardiff, March 1975, pp. 47–81. Surgical Dressings Research Unit, Welsh School of Pharmacy, Cardiff.
3. Elek, S. D. (1976). Experimental staphylococcal infections in the skin of man. *Ann. N. Y. Acad. Sci.*, **65**, 85–90.
4. Wood, R. A. B. (1976). Disintegration of cellulose dressings in open granulating wounds. *Br. Med. J.*, **i**, 1444–5.
5. Saxen, L. and Myllarniemi, H. (1968). Foreign material and post-operative adhesions. *New Engl. J. Med.*, **279**, 200–2
6. Weibel, M. A. and Majno, G. (1973). Peritoneal adhesions and their relation to abdominal surgery. *Am. J. Surg.*, **126**, 345–53.
7. Tinker, M. A., Burdman, D., Deysine, M., Teicher, I., Platt, N., and Aufses, A. H. (1974). Granulomatous peritonitis due to cellulose fibres from disposable surgical fabrics: laboratory investigation and clinical implications. *Ann. Surg.*, **180**, 831–5.
8. Tinker, M. A., Teicher, I., and Burdman, D. (1977). Cellulose granulomas and their relationship to intestinal obstruction. *Am. J. Surg.*, **133**, 134–9.
9. Ellis, H. (1983). Introduction. In *Adhesions the problems*, (ed. H. Ellis and M. Lennox), Conference Proceedings, pp. 1–5. Westminster Hospital Medical School, London.
10. Myllarniemi, H. (1983). Adhesion formation due to foreign material. In *Adhesions: the Problems*, (ed. H. Ellis and M. Lennox), Conference Proceedings, pp. 22–6. Westminster Hospital Medical School, London.

11. Chambi, I., Tasker, R. R., Gentill, F., Lougheed, W. M., Smyth, H. S., *et al.* (1990). Gauze induced granuloma (gauzoma): an uncommon complication of gauze reinforcement of berry aneurysms. *J. Neurosurg.*, **72**, 163–70.

12. Thomas, S., Loveless, P., Hay, N. P., and Toyick, N. (1993). Comparing non-woven, filmated and woven gauze swabs. *J. Wound Care*, **2**, 35–41.

13. Burgess, N. A., Moore, H. E., Thomas, S., Shukla, H., and Lewis, M. H. (1992). Evaluation of a new non-woven theatre swab. *J. Roy. Coll. Surg. Edin.*, **37**, 191–3.

14. Gamgee, S. (1880). Absorbent and medicated surgical dressings. *Lancet*, **i**, 127–38.

15. Trevethick, R. A. (1957). Sensitization to tulle gras dressings. (Letter.) *Br. Med. J.*, **2**, 883–4.

16. D'Arcy, P. F. (1972). Drugs on the skin: a clinical and pharmaceutical problem. *Pharm. J.*, **209**, 491–2.

17. Lunn, J. A. (1962). Controlled trial of a wound dressing: Sofra-Tulle. *Practitioner*, **188**, 527–8.

18. Jackson, P. W. (1962). Sofra-Tulle in the treatment of minor wounds. *Practitioner*, **189**, 675–8.

19. Currie, J. P. and Sinclair, D. M. (1963). Framycetin in the treatment of cutaneous injuries. *Practitioner*, **190**, 112–3.

20. Ramirez, A. T., Lansigan, N., and Posuncuy, C. J. N. (1969). Topical framycetin in the treatment of burns. *Philippine J. Surg. Special.*, **24**, 1–14.

21. Smith, R. A. (1972). The treatment of burns: a clinical evaluation of Sofra-Tulle. *Clin. Trials J.*, **9**, 37–40.

22. Wicks, C. J. and Peterson, H. I. (1972). Medicated wound dressings – a historical review. *Opusc. Med.*, **17**, 90–5.

23. Kirton, V. and Munro-Ashman, D. (1965). Contact dermatitis from neomycin and framycetin. *Lancet*, **ii**, 138–9.

24. Martindale (1989). *The extra pharmacopoeia*, (29th edn), (ed. J. E. F. Reynolds), p. 235. Pharmaceutical Press, London.

25. Ritchie, I. C. (1968). Clinical and bacteriological studies of a new antibiotic tulle. *Br. J. Clin. Pract.*, **22**, 15–16.

26. McCormack, B. L., Nathan, M. S., and Fernandez, A. (1968). Practical evaluation of a new sodium fusidate (Fucidin) wound dressing. *J. Ir. Med. Ass.*, **61**, 137–41.

27. Davies, G. E., Francis, J., Martin, A. R., Rose, F. L., and Swain, G. (1954). 1,6-Dichlorophenyldiguanidohexane ('Hibitane'): laboratory investigation of a new antibacterial agent of high potency. *Br. J. Pharmac. Chemother.*, **9**, 192–6.

28. Longworth, A. R. (1971). Chlorhexidine. In *Inhibition and destruction of the microbial cell*, (ed. W. B. Hugo), pp. 95–106. Academic Press, London.

29. Senior, N. (1972). Some observations on the formulation and properties of chlorhexidine. *J. Soc. Cosmet. Chem.*, **11**, 1–19.

30. Evans, R. J. (1992). Letter. *Br. Med. J.*, **304**, 686.

31. Thomas, S. and Russell, A. D. (1976). An *in vitro* evaluation of Bactigras, a tulle dressing containing chlorhexidine. *Microbios. Lett.* **2**, 169–77.

32. Thomas, S., Dawes, C. E., and Hay, N. P. (1983). Improvements in medicated tulle dressings. *J. Hosp. Infect.*, **4**, 391–8.

33. Andrews, J. K., Buchan, I. A., and Horlington, M. (1982). An experimental evaluation of a chlorhexidine medicated tulle gras dressing. *J. Hosp. Infect.*, **2**, 149–57.

34. Thomas, S. (1982). An experimental evaluation of a chlorhexidine medicated tulle gras dressing. (Letter.) *J. Hosp. Infect.*, **2**, 399–400.

35. Andrews, J. K., Buchan, I. A., and Horlington, M. (1982). Letter. *J. Hosp. Infect.*, **2**, 401.

36. Lawrence, J. C. (1977). Minor burns. *Nurs. Mirror*, **144**, 58–60.

37. Han, K. H. and Maitra, A. K. (1989). Management of partial skin thickness burn wounds with Inadine dressings. *Burns*, **15**, 399–402.

38. Thomas, S. (1989). Pain and wound management. *Nurs. Times* (*Community Outlook Suppl.*), **85**, 11–15.

39. Wood, R. A. B. and Hughes, L. E. (1975). Silicone foam sponge for pilonidal sinus: a new technique for dressing open granulating wounds. *Br. Med. J.*, **3**, 131–3.

40. Wood, R. A. B., Williams, R. H. P., and Hughes, L. E. (1977). Foam elastomer dressing in the management of open granulating wounds: experience with 250 patients. *Br. J. Surg.*, **64**, 554–7.

41. Smith, R. C., Flynn, P. N., Gillett, D. J., Guiness, M. D., and Levey, J. M. (1981). Treatment of granulating wounds with Silastic foam dressings. *Australia N Z J. Surg.*, **51**, 35–57.

42. Macfie, J. and McMahon, M. J. (1980). The management of the open perineal wound using a foam elastomer: a prospective clinical trial. *Br. J. Surg.*, **67**, 85–9.

43. Harding, K. G., Richardson, G., and Hughes, L. E. (1980). Silastic foam dressings for skin graft donor sites: a preliminary report. *Br. J. Plast. Surg.*, **33**, 418–21.

44. Macfie, J. (1979). A liquid alternative to gauze. *Nurs. Mirror*, **149**, 30–2.

45. Stewart, C. P. U. (1985). Foam elastomer dressing in the management of a below-knee amputation stump with delayed healing. *Prosthet. Orthot. Int.*, **9**, 157–9.

46. Streza, G. A., Laing, B. J., and Gilsdorf, R. B. (1977). Management of enterocutaneous fistulas and problem stomas with silicone casting of the abdominal wall defect. *Am. J. Surg.*, **134**, 772–6.

47. Regnard, C. F. B. and Meehan, S. E. (1982). The use of a Silicone foam dressing in the management of malignant oral-cutaneous fistula. *Br. J. Clin. Pract.*, **36**, 6–8.

48. Morgan, W. P., Harding, K. G., Richardson, G., and Hughes, L. E. (1980). The use of Silastic foam dressing in the treatment of advanced hidradenitis suppurativa. *Br. J. Surg.*, **67**, 277–80.

49. Cook, P. J. and Devlin, H. B. (1985). Boils, carbuncles and hidradenitis suppurativa. *Surgery*, **19**, 440–2.

50. Miller, L. A. (1982). Hidradenitis suppurativa. *Nurs. Times*, **78**, 524–5.

51. Malick, M. H. and Carr, J. A. (1980). Flexible elastomer molds in burn scar control. *Am. J. Occup. Ther.*, **34**, 603–8.

52. Bandey, S. A., Atkins, J., and Neil, W. F. (1986). Silastic foam dressing in pinnaplasty. *J. Laryng. Otol.*, **100**, 201–2.

53. Ross, J. K., Matti, B., and Davies, D. M. (1987). A Silastic foam dressing for the protection of the post-operative ear. *Br. J. Plast. Surg.*, **40**, 213–14.

54. Shukla, H. S. (1982). Cosmetic and functional advantages of foam elastomer dressing in the management of epidermoid cancer of the cheek. *Br. J. Surg.*, **69**, 435–6.

55. DeSy, W. A. and Oosterlinck, W. (1982). Silicone foam elastomer: a significant improvement in post-operative penile dressing. *J. Urol.*, **128**, 39–40.

56. Whitaker, R. H. and Dennis, M. J. S. (1987). Silastic foam dressing in hypospadias surgery. *Ann. R. Coll. Surg.*, **69**, 59–60.

57. Bale, S. and Harding, K. G. (1987). Fungating breast wounds. *J. Distr. Nurs.*, **5**, 4–5.

58. Groves, A. R. and Lawrence, J. C. (1985). Silastic foam dressing: an appraisal. *Ann. R. Coll. Surg.*, **67**, 116–18.

59. Baccari, G. and Boschetti, E. (1977). Ferite, ustioni e piaghe medicate con spugnoa di poliuretano. Communication to the Sixth National Congress of the Società Italiana di Chirurgia d'Urgenze e Pronto Soccorso, Padua, 9–11 June 1977.

60. Creevy, J. (1985). Lyofoam – use in the treatment of leg ulcers. In *Advances in wound management*, (ed. T. D., Turner, R. J., Schmidt, and K. G. Harding), pp. 39–40. John Wiley, London.

61. Mayerhausen, W. and Kreis, M. (1987). Ulcus cruris. *Arzt. Prax.*, **5**, 2033–5.

62. Hughes, L. E., Harding, K. G., Bale, S., and McPake, B. (1989). Wound management in the community – comparison of Lyofoam and Melolin. *Care Science and Practice*, **7**, 64–7.

63. Bloom, H. (1948). Cellophane dressing for second degree burns. *Lancet*, **ii**, 559.

64. Bull, J. P., Squire, J. R., and Topley, E. (1948). Experiments with occlusive dressings of a new plastic. *Lancet*, **ii**, 213–15.

65. Schilling, R. S. F., Roberts, M., and Goodman, N. (1950). Clinical trial of occlusive plastic dressings. *Lancet*, **i**, 293–6.

66. Winter, G. D. (1962). Formation of the scab and the rate of epithelization of superficial wounds in the skin of the young domestic pig. *Nature*, **193**, 293–4.

67. Hinman, C. D. and Maibach, H. (1963). Effect of air exposure and occlusion on experimental human skin wounds. *Nature*, **200**, 377–9.

68. Thomas, S., Loveless, P., and Hay, N. P. (1988). Comparative review of the properties of 6 semipermeable film dressings. *Pharm. J.*, **240**, 785–9.

69. Lamke, L. O., Nilsson, G. E., and Reithner, H. L. (1977). The evaporative water loss from burns and water vapour permeability of grafts and artificial membranes used in the treatment of burns. *Burns*, **3**, 159–65.

70. May, R. S. (1983). Physiological activity from an occlusive wound dressing. In *Wound healing symposium*, (ed. J. C. Lawrence), pp. 35–49. Proceedings of a Symposium, Birmingham, 1982. Oxford Medicine Publishing Foundation.

71. Mertz, P. M., Marshall, D. A., and Eaglstein, W. H. (1885). Occlusive wound dressings to prevent bacterial invasion and wound infection. *J. Am. Acad. Derm.*, **12**, 662–8.

72. Maki, D. G., Wheeler, S., and Stolz, S. M. (1990). Study of a novel highly-permeable polyurethane dressing for IV catheters. Poster presented at the Hospital Infection Society International Meeting, London, 2–6 Sept. 1990.

73. Behar, D., Juszynski, M., Ben-Hur, N., Golan, J., Eldad, A., Tuchman, Y., *et al.* (1986). Omiderm, a new synthetic wound covering: physical properties and drug permeability studies. *J. Biomed. Mat. Res.*, **20**, 731–8.

74. Golan, J., Eldad, A., Rudensky, B., Tuchman, Y., Sterenberg, N., Ben-Hur, N., *et al.* (1985). A new temporary synthetic skin substitute. *Burns*, **11**, 274–80.

75. Cristofoli, C., Lorenzini, M., and Furlan, S. (1986). The use of Omiderm, a new skin substitute, in a burn unit. *Burns*, **12**, 587–91.

76. Winter, G. D. (1974). Epidermal regeneration studied in the domestic pig. In *Epidermal wound healing*, (ed. H. I. Maibach and D. T. Rovee), pp. 71–112. Year Book Medical, Chicago.

77. Sirvio, L. M. and Grussing, D. M. (1989). The effect of gas permeability of film dressings on wound environment and healing. *J. Invest. Dermatol.*, **93**, 528–31.

78. James, J. H. and Watson, A. C. H. (1975). The use of Opsite, a vapour permeable dressing, on skin graft donor sites. *Br. J. Plast. Surg.*, **28**, 107–10.

79. Bergman, R. B. (1977). A new treatment of split-skin graft donor sites. *Arch. Chir. Neerl.*, **29**, 69–72.

80. Dinner, M. I., Peters, C. R., and Sherer, J. (1979). Use of semipermeable polyurethane membrane as a dressing for split-skin donor sites. *Plast. Reconstr. Surg.*, **64**, 112–14.

81. Barnett, A., Berkowitz, R. L., Standord, R. M., and Vistnes, L. M. (1983). Comparison of synthetic adhesive moisture vapour permeable and fine mesh gauze dressings for split thickness skin donor graft sites. *Am. J. Surg.*, **145**, 379–81.

82. Conkle, W. (1981). Opsite dressing: new approach to burn care. *J. Emerg. Nurs.*, **7**, 148–52.

83. Neal, D. E., Whalley, P. C., Flowers, M. W., and Wilson, D. H. (1981). The effects of an adherent polyurethane film and conventional absorbent dressing in patients with small partial thickness burns. *Br. J. Clin. Pract.*, **35**, 254–7.

84. Braverman, A. M. and Nasar, M. A. (1981). The treatment of superficial decubitus ulcers. *Practitioner*, **225**, 1842–3.

85. Drake, D. (1984). Surgical wound management with adhesive polyurethane membrane. *Ann. Roy. Coll. Surg.*, **66**, 74–5.

86. Tinckler, L. (1983). Surgical wound management with adhesive polyurethane membrane: a preferred method for routine usage. *Ann. Roy. Coll. Surg.*, **65**, 257–9.

87. Bragg, V. and Martin, C. (1983). Polyurethane film dressing. *J. Enterostom. Ther.*, **10**, 185–6.

88. Peterson, P. J. and Freeman, P. T. (1982). Use of a transparent polyurethane dressing for peripheral intravenous catheter care. *National Intraven. Ther. Ass.*, **5**, 387–90.

89. Palidar, P. J., Simonowitz, D. A., Oreskovich, M. R., Dellinger, E. P., Edwards, W. A., Adams, S., and Karkeck, J. (1982). Use of Opsite as an occlusive dressing for total parenteral nutrition catheters. *J. Parent. Ent. Nutr.*, **6**, 150–1.

90. Thomas, S. P. J. and Loveless, P. J. (1992). Observations on the fluid handling properties of alginate dressings. *Pharm. J.*, **248**, 850–1.

91. Schmidt, R. J. and Turner, T. D. (1986). Alginate dressings. (Letter.) *Pharm. J.*, **236**, 36–7.

92. Schmidt, R. J. and Turner, T. D. (1986). Calcium alginate dressings. (Letter.) *Pharm. J.*, **236**, 578.

93. Cair Ltd (1986). Calcium alginate dressings. (Letter.) *Pharm. J.*, **236**, 578.

94. Blaine, G. (1947). Experimental observations on absorbable alginate products in surgery. *Ann. Surg.*, **125**, 102–14.

95. Blaine, G. (1951). A comparative evaluation of absorbable haemostatics. *Postgrad. Med. J.*, **27**, 613–20.

96. Thomas, S. P. J. and Loveless, P. J. (1992). Observations on the fluid handling properties of alginate dressings. *Pharm. J.*, **248**, 50–85.

97. Groves, A. R. and Lawrence, J. C. (1986). Alginate dressing as a donor site haemostat. *Ann. Roy. Coll. Surg.*, **68**, 27–8.

98. Attwood, A. I. (1989). Calcium alginate dressing accelerates graft donor site healing. *Br. J. Plast. Surg.*, **43**, 373–9.

99. Frase, R. and Gilchrist, T. (1983). Sorbsan calcium alginate fibre dressings in footcare. *Biomaterials*, **4**, 222–4.

100. Gilchrist, T. and Martin, A. M. (1983). Wound treatment with Sorbsan – an alginate fibre dressing. *Biomaterials*, **4**, 317–20.

101. Thomas, S. (1985). Use of calcium alginate dressing. *Pharm. J.*, **235**, 188–90.

102. Odugbesan, O. and Barnett, A. H. (1987). Use of a seaweed-based dressing in management of leg ulcers in diabetics: a case report. *Pract. Diabet.*, **4**, 46–7.

103. Thomas, S. and Tucker, C. A. (1989). Sorbsan in the management of leg ulcers. *Pharm. J.*, **243**, 706–9.

104. Fanucci, D. and Seese, J. (1991). Multi-faceted use of calcium alginates. *Ostomy/Wound Management*, **37**, 16–22.

105. Groves, A. R. and Lawrence, J. A. (1986). Alginate dressings as a donor site haemostat. *Ann. Roy. Coll. Surg.*, **68**, 27–8.

106. Blair, S. D., Backhouse, C. M., Mathews, J. L., and McCollum, C. N. (1988). Comparison of absorbable materials for surgical haemostasis. *Br. J. Surg.*, **75**, 969–71.

107. Gupta, R., Foster, M. E., and Miller, E. (1991). Calcium alginate in the management of acute surgical wounds and abscesses. *J. Tissue Viability*, **1**, 115–16.

108. Thomas, S. (1992). Current practices in the management of fungating wounds. *Surgical Materials Testing Laboratory*, Bridgend, Wales.

109. Barnett, S. E. and Varley, S. J. (1987). The effects of calcium alginate on wound healing. *Ann. Roy. Coll. Surg.*, **69**, 153–5.

110. Wichterle, O. and Lim, D. (1960). Hydrophilil gels for biological use. *Nature*, **185**, 117–18.

111. Jacobsson, S., Rothman, U., Arturson, G., Ganrot, K., Haeger, K., and Juhlin, I. (1976). A new principle for the cleansing of infected wounds. *Scand. J. Plast. Reconstr. Surg.*, **10**, 65–72.

112. Niinikoski, J. and Renvall, S. (1980). Effect of dextranomer on developing granulation tissue in standard skin defects in rats. *Clin. Ther.*, **3**, 273–9.

113. Fraki, J. E., Peltonen, L., and Hopsu-Havu, V. K. (1979). Allergy to various components of topical preparations in stasis dermatitis and leg ulcer. *Contact Dermatitis*, **5**, 97–100.

114. Falk, J. and Tollerz, G. (1977). Chronic tissue response to implantation of Debrisan: an experimental study. *Clin. Ther.*, **1**, 185–91.

115. Gang, R. K. (1981). Debrisan and saline dressing. *Chir. Plast.*, **6**, 65–8.

116. Paavolainen, P. and Sundell, B. (1976). The effect of dextranomer (Debrisan) on hand burns. *Ann. Chir. Gynaec.*, **65**, 313–7.

117. Arturson, G., Hakelius, L., Jacobsson, S., and Rothman, U. (1978). A new topical agent (Debrisan) for the early treatment of the burned hand. *Burns*, **4**, 225–32.

118. Floden, C. H. and Wilkstrom, K. (1978). Controlled clinical trial with dextranomer (Debrisan) on venous leg ulcers. *Curr. Ther. Res.*, **24**, 753–60.

119. Groenwald, J. H. (1980). An evaluation of dextranomer as a cleansing agent in the treatment of the post-phlebitic statis ulcer. *South African Med. J.*, **57**, 809–15.

120. McClemont, E. J. W., Shand, I. G., and Ramsay, B. (1979). Pressure sores: a new method of treatment. *Br. J. Clin. Pract.*, **33**, 21–5.

121. Nasar, M. A. and Morley, R. (1982). Cost effectiveness in treating deep pressure sores and ulcers. *Practitioner*, **226**, 307–10.

122. Soul, J. (1978). A trial of Debrisan in the cleansing of infected surgical wounds. *Br. J. Clin. Pract.*, **32**, 172–3.

123. Goode, A. W., Glazer, G., and Ellis, B. W. (1979). The cost effectiveness of dextranomer and eusol in the treatment of infected surgical wounds. *Br. J. Clin. Pract.*, **33**, 325 and 328.

124. Hulkko, A., Holopainen, Y. V. O., Orava, S., Kangas, J., Kuusisto, P., Hyvarinen, E., *et al.* (1981). Comparison of dextranomer and streptokinase–streptodornase in the treatment of venous leg ulcers and other infected wounds. *Ann. Chir. Gynaec.*, **70**, 65–70.

125. Goode, A. W., Welch, N. T., and Boland, G. (1985). A study of dextranomer absorbent pads in the management of infected wounds. *Clin. Trials. J.*, **22**, 431–4.

126. Moberg, S., Hoffman, L., Grennert, M. L., and Holst, A. (1983). A randomised trial of cadexomer iodine in decubitus ulcers. *J. Am. Geriat. Soc.*, **109**, 77–83.

127. Skog, E., Arnesjo, B., Troeng, T., Gjores, J. E., Bergljung, L., Gundersen, J., *et al.* (1983). A randomised trial comparing cadexomer iodine and standard treatment in the out-patient management of chronic venous ulcers. *Br. J. Derm.*, **109**, 77–83.

128. Ormiston, M. C., Seymour, M. T. J., Venn, G. E., Cohen, R. I., and Fox, J. A. (1985). Controlled trial of Iodosorb in chronic venous ulcers. *Br. Med. J.*, **291**, 303–10.

129. Harcup, J. W. and Saul, P. A. (1986). A study of the effect of cadexomer iodine in the treatment of venous leg ulcers. *Br. J. Clin. Pract.*, **40**, 360–4.

130. Lindsay, G., Latta, D., Lyons, K. G. B., Livingstone, E. D., and Thomson, W. (1986). A study in general practice of the efficacy of cadexomer iodine in venous leg ulcers treated on alternate days. *Acta Ther.*, **12**, 141–8.

131. Barzokas, C. A., Corkhill, J. E., and Makin, T. (1983). Microbiological studies on Geliperm. In *Geliperm: a clear advance in wound healing*, (ed. H. F. Woods and D. Cottier), pp. 39–47. Proceedings of Oxford Conference, 1983.

132. Butcher, G. and Woods, H. F. (1983). Geliperm as a molecular carrier. In *Geliperm: a clear advance in wound healing*, (ed. H. F. Woods and D. Cottier), pp. 77–87. Proceedings of Oxford Conference, 1983.

133. Burgos, H. (1987). Incorporation and release of placental growth factors in synthetic medical dressings. *Clin. Mat.*, 133–9.

134. Wokalek, H., Ruh, H., Vaubel, E., Schopf, E., and Kickhofen, B. (1983). Theoretical aspects and clinical experience on a new hydrogel wound dressing material. In *Geliperm: a clear advance in wound healing*, (ed. H. F. Woods and D. Cottier), pp. 3–33. Proceedings of Oxford Conference, 1983.

135. Breuton, R. N., Brookes, H., and Heatley, F. W. (1987). The effect of ultrasound on the repair of a rabbit's tibial osteotomy held in rigid external fixation. *Bone Joint Surg.*, **69**, 494.

136. Breuton, R. N. and Campbell, B. (1987). The use of Geliperm as a sterile coupling agent for therapeutic ultrasound. *Physiotherapy*, **73**, 653–4.

137. Mandy, S. H. (1983). A new primary wound dressing made of polyethylene oxide gel. *J. Derm. Surg. Oncol.*, **9**, 153–5.

138. Brennan, S. S., Foster, M. E., Simpson, R. A., and Leaper, D. J. (1983). Infection and healing under hydrogel occlusive dressing. In *Geliperm: a clear advance in wound healing*, (ed. H. F. Woods and D. Cottier), pp. 49–62. Proceedings of Oxford Conference, 1983.

139. Leaper, D. J., Brennan, S. S., Simpson, R. A., and Foster, M. E. (1984). Experimental infection and hydrogel dressings. *J. Hosp. Infec.*, **5** (Suppl. A), 69–73.

140. Fear, M. and Thomas, S. (1991). Wound cleansing properties of Debrisan and Scherisorb gel: interim results of a clinical trial. *Proceedings of 1st European Conference on advances in wound management, 1991*, pp. 162–4. Macmillan Magazines, London.

141. Gomolin, I. H. and Brandt, J. L. (1984). Topical metronidazole therapy for pressure sores of geriatric patients. *J. Am. Geriat. Soc.*, **31**, 710–12.

142. Thomas, S. and Hay, N. P. (1991). The antimicrobial properties of two metronidazole medicated dressings used to treat malodorous wounds. *Pharm. J.*, **246**, 264–6.

143. Stewart, A. J. and Leaper, D. J. (1987). Treatment of chronic leg ulcers in the community: a comparative trial of Scherisorb and Iodosorb. *Phlebology*, **2**, 115–21.

144. Thomas, S., Rowe, H. N., Keats, J., Morgan, R. J. H., *et al.* (1987). A new approach to the management of extravasation injury in neonates. *Pharm. J.*, **239**, 584–5.

145. Lee, M. G., Haines-Nutt, F., and Thomas, S. (1991). Granuflex E. (Letter.) *Pharm. J.*, **246**, 350.

146. Lydon, M. (1991). Granuflex, E. (Letter.) *Pharm. J.*, **246**, 350.

147. Young, S. R., Dyson, M., Hickman, R., Lang, S., and Osborn, C. (1991). Comparison of the effects of semi-occlusive polyurethane dressings and hydrocolloid dressings on dermal repair: 1 cellular changes. *J. Invest. Dermatol.*, **97**, 586–92.

148. Thomas, S. and Loveless, P. (1991). A comparative study of the properties of six hydrocolloid dressings. *Pharm. J.*, **247**, 672–5.

149. Mertz, P. M. (1985). Occlusive wound dressings to prevent bacterial invasion and wound infection. *J. Am. Acad. Derm.*, **12**, 662–8.

150. Wilson, P., Burrough, S. D., and Dunn, L. J. (1988). Methicillin-resistant *Staphylococcus aureus* and hydrocolloid dressings. *Pharm. J.*, **241**, 787–8.

151. Lawrence, J. C. and Lilly, H. A. (1987). Are hydrocolloid dressings bacteria proof? *Pharm. J.*, **239**, 184.

152. Piercey, D. A. (1987). Are hydrocolloid dressings bacteria proof? (Letter.) *Pharm. J.*, **239**, 223.

153. Cherry, G. W. (1987). Are hydrocolloid dressings bacteria proof? (Letter.) *Pharm. J.*, **239**, 281.

154. Lawrence, J. C. (1987). Are hydrocolloid dressings bacteria proof? (Letter.) *Pharm. J.*, **239**, 310.

155. Thomas, S. and Hay, N. P. (1987). Are hydrocolloid dressings bacteria proof? (Letter.) *Pharm. J.*, **239**, 388–9.

156. Cherry, G. W. (1987). Are hydrocolloid dressings bacteria proof? (Letter.) *Pharm. J.*, **239**, 456.

157. Moores, J. (1987). Are hydrocolloid dressings bacteria proof? (Letter.) *Pharm. J.*, **239**, 486.

158. Lawrence, J. C. amd Lilly, H. A. (1987). Are hydrocolloid dressings bacteria proof? (Letter.) *Pharm. J.*, **239**, 486.

159. Johnson, A. (1987). Are hydrocolloid dressings bacteria proof? (Letter.) *Pharm. J.*, **239**, 486.

160. Cherry, G. W. and Ryan, T. J. (1985). Enhanced wound angiogenesis with a new hydrocolloid dressing. In *An environment for healing: the role of occlusion*, (ed. T. J. Ryan), pp. 61–8, International Congress and Symposium Series, No 88. Royal Society of Medicine, London.

161. Lydon, M. J., Hutchinson, J. J., Rippon, M., Johnson, E., Desousa, N., Scudder, C., *et al.* (1989). Dissolution of wound coagulum and promotion of granulation tissue under Duoderm. *Wounds*, **1**, 95–106.

162. Samuelsen, P. and Nielsen, D. E. (1990). Fibrinolysis and hydrocolloid dressings. Poster presentation, Clinical Dermatology in the year 2000, 22–25 May 1990, London.

163. Hermans, M. H. E. and Hermans, R. P. (1984). Preliminary report on the use of a new hydrocolloid dressing in the treatment of burns. *Burns*, **11**, 125–9.

164. Doherty, C., Lynch, G., and Noble, S. (1986). Granuflex hydrocolloid as a donor site dressing. *Care Crit. Ill.*, **2**, 193–4.

165. Cherry, G. W., Ryan, T. J., and McGibbon, D. (1984). Trial of a new dressing in venous leg ulcers. *Practitioner*, **288**, 1175–8.

166. Van Rijswijk, L., Brown, D., Freidman, S., *et al.* (1985). Multicentre clinical evaluation of a hydrocolloid dressing for leg ulcers. *Cutis*, **35**, 173–6.

167. Patrizi, P., Silvagni, M., Fiori, S. D., and Morgant, I. (1984). The treatment of superficial trophic ulcerations with Comfeel Ulcus. *Clin. Eur.*, **23**, 19–26.

168. Yarkony, G. M., Kramer, E., King, R., Lukane, C., and Carle, T. V. (1984). Pressure sore management: efficacy of a moisture reactive occlusive dressings. *Arch. Phys. Med. Rehab.*, **65**, 597–600.

169. Neill, K. M., Conforti, C., Kedas, A., and Burris, J. F. (1989). Pressure sore response to a new hydrocolloid dressing. *Wounds*, **1**, 173–85.

170. Eisenberg, M. (1986). The effect of occlusive dressings on re-epithelialisations of wounds in children with epidermolysis bullosa. *J. Pediat. Surg.*, **21**, 892–4.

171. Michel, L. (1985). Use of hydrocolloid dressing following wide excision of perianal hidradentitis suppurativa. In *An environment for healing: the role of occlusion*, (ed. T. J. Ryan), pp. 143–8, International Congress and Symposium Series, No 88. Royal Society of Medicine, London.

172. Ryan, T. J., Given, H. F., Murphy, J. J., *et al.* (1985). The use of a new occlusive dressing in the management of venous stasis ulceration. In *An environment for healing: the role of occlusion*, (ed. T. J. Ryan), pp. 99–103, International Congress and Symposium Series, No 88. Royal Society of Medicine, London.

173. Hutchinson, J. J. (1989). Prevalence of wound infection under occlusive dressings: a collective survey of reported research. *Wounds*, **1**, 123–33.

174. Varghese, M. E., Balin, A. K., Carter, M., and Caldwell, D. (1986). Local environment of chronic wounds under synthetic dressings. *Arch. Derm.*, **122**, 52–7.

175. Henry, M., Byrne, P. J., and Dinn, E. (1988). Pilot study to investigate the pH of exudate on varicose ulcers under Duoderm. In *Beyond occlusion: wound care*, (ed. T. J. Ryan), pp. 67–70. Proceedings. Royal Society of Medicine, London.

176. Gilchrist, B. and Reed, C. (1989). The bacteriology of chronic venous ulcers treated with occlusive hydrocolloid dressings. *Br. J. Derm.*, **121**, 337–44.

177. Lawrence, J. C. and Lilly, H. A. (1985). Bacteriological properties of a new hydrocolloid dressing on intact skin of normal volunteers. In *An environment for healing: the role of occlusion*, (ed. T. J. Ryan), pp. 51–7, International Congress and Symposium Series, No 88. Royal Society of Medicine, London.

178. Thomas, S., Wilde, L. G., and Loveless, P. (1986). Performance profiles of extensible bandages. In *Phlebology 85*, (ed. D. Negus and G. Jantet), pp. 667–70, Proceedings of a symposium, Union Internationale de Phlebologie, London, 16–20 September 1985. John Libbey, London.

179. Raj, T. B., Goddard, M., and Makin, G. S. (1980). How long do compression bandages maintain their pressure during ambulatory treatment of varicose veins? *Br. J. Surg.*, **67**, 122–4.

180. Tennant, W. G., Park, K. G. M., and Ruckley, C. V. (1988). Testing compression bandages. *Phlebology*, **3**, 55–61.

181. Backhouse, C. M., Blair, S. D., Savage, A. P., Walton, J., and McCollum, C. N. (1987). Controlled trial of occlusive dressings in healing chronic venous ulcers. *Br. J. Surg.*, **74**, 626–7.

182. Callam, M. J., Ruckley, C. V., Dale, J. J., and Harper, D. R. (1987). Hazards of compression treatment of the leg: an estimate from Scottish surgeons. *Br. J. Surg.*, **295**, 1382.

183. Callam, M. J., Haiart, D., Farouk, M., Brown, D., Prescott, R. J., and Ruckley, C. V. (1991). Effect of time and posture on pressure profiles obtained by different types of compression. *Phlebology*, **6**, 79–84.

184. Potten, C. S. and Morris, R. J. (1988). Epithelial stem cells *in vivo*. *J. Cell. Sci.*, **10**, 45–62.

185. Fuchs, E. (1990). Epidermal differentiation. *Curr. Opin. Cell Biol.*, **2**, 1028–35.

186. Odland, G. and Ross, R. (1968). Human wound repair I: epidermal regeneration. *J. Cell. Biol.*, **39**, 135–51.

187. Krawczyck, W. S. (1971). A pattern of epidermal cell migration during wounds healing. *J. Cell. Biol.*, **49**, 247–63.

188. Clark, R. A. F. (1985). Cutaneous tissue repair: basic biologic considerations. *J. Am. Acad. Derm.*, **13**, 701–25.

189. Holbrook, K. A. and Hennings, H. (1983). Phenotypic expression of epidermal cells *in vitro*: a review. *J. Invest. Dermatol.*, **81**, s 11–24.

190. Rheinwald, J. G. and Green, H. (1975). Serial cultivation of strains of human epidermal keratinocytes: the formation of keratinizing colonies from single cells. *Cell*, **6**, 331–44.

191. Green, H. (1978). Cyclic AMP in relation to proliferation of the epidermal cell – a new view. *Cell*, **15**, 801–15.

192. Rheinwald, J. G. and Green, H. (1977). Epidermal growth factors and multiplication of cultured human epidermal keratinocytes. *Nature*, **265**, 421–4.

193. Barrandon, Y. and Green, H. (1987). Cell migration is essential for sustained growth of keratinocyte colonies: the roles of transforming factor-α and epidermal growth factor. *Cell*, **50**, 1131–37.

194. Boyce, S. T. and Ham, R. G. (1983). Calcium regulated differentiation of normal epidermal keratinocytes in chemically defined clonal culture and serum-free serial culture. *J. Invest. Dermatol.*, **81**, 33S–40S.

195. Morris, R. J., Tacker, K. C., Baldwin, J. K., Fischer, S. M., and Slaga, T. J. A. (1987). A new medium for primary cultures of adult murine epidermal cells: application to experimental carcinogenesis. *Cancer Letters*, **34**, 297–304.

196. Pittelkow, M. R. (1989). Cultured epidermal cells for skin replacement. *Perspectives of Plastic Surgery*, **3**, 101–7.

197. Phillips, T. (1988). Cultured skin grafts: past, present, future. *Arch. Dermatol.*, **124**, 1035–8.

198. Leigh, I. M., McKay, I., Carver, N., Navsaria, H., and Green, C. (1991). Skin equivalents and cultured skin: from the Petri dish to the patient. *Wounds*, **3**, 141–8.

199. O'Connor, N. E., Mulliken, J. B., Banks-Schlegel, S., Kehinde, O., and Green, H. (1981). Grafting of burns with cultured epithelium prepared from autologous epidermal cells. *Lancet*, **i**, 75–8.

200. Gallico, G. G., O'Connor, N. E., and Compton, C. C. (1984). Permanent coverage of large burn wounds with autologous cultured human epithelium. *New Eng. J. Med.*, **331**, 448–51.

201. Teepe, R. G. C., Ponec, M., Kreis, R. W., and Hermans, R. (1986). Improved grafting method for the treatment of burns with autologous cultured human epithelium. *Lancet*, **i**, 385.

202. Kumagai, N., Nishima, H., Tanabe, H., Hosaka, T., Ishida, H., and Ogina, Y. (1988). Clinical applications of autologous cultured epithelia for the treatment of burn wounds and burn scars. *Plast. Reconstr. Surg.*, **82**, 99–108.

203. de Luca, M., Albanese, E., Bondanza, S., Megna, M., Ugozzoli, L., Molina, F., et al. (1989). Multicentre experience in the treatment of burns with autologous and allogenic cultured epithelium, fresh or preserved in a frozen state. *Burns*, **15**, 303–9.

204. Gallico, G. G., O'Connor, N. E., Compton, C. C., Remensnyder, J. P., Kehinde, O., and Green, H. (1989). Cultured epithelial autografts for giant congenital naevi. *Plast. Reconstr. Surg.*, **84**, 1–9.

205. Hefton, J. M., Caldwell, D., Biozes, D. G., et al. (1986). Grafting of skin ulcers with cultured autologous epidermal cells. *J. Am. Acad. Derm.*, **14**, 399–405.

206. Premachandra, D. J., Woodward, B. M., Milton, C. M., Sergeant, R. J., and Fabre, F. W. (1990). Treatment of postoperative otorrhoea by grafting of mastoid cavities with cultured autologous epidermal cells. *Lancet*, **335**, 365–7.

207. Langdon, J. D., Williams, D., Navsaria, H., and Leigh, I. M. (1991). Autologous keratinocyte grafting: a new technique for intra oral reconstruction. *Brit. Dent. J.*, **171**, 87–90.

208. de Luca, M., Albanese, E., Megna, M., et al. (1990). Evidence that human oral epithelium reconstituted *in vitro* and transplanted onto patients with defects in the oral mucosa retains properties of the original donor site. *Transplantation*, **50**, 454–9.

209. Romagnoli, G., de Luca, M., Faranda, F., Bandelloni, R., Tito-Franzi, A., Cataliotti, F., and Cancedda, R. (1990). Treatment of posterior hypospadias by the autologous graft of cultured urethral epithelium. *New Eng. J. Med.*, **323**, 527–31.

210. Tatnall, F. M., Leigh, I. M., and Gibson, J. R. (1987). Comparative toxicity of antimicrobial agents on transformed human keratinocytes. *J. Invest. Dermatol.*, **89**, 316–8.

211. Woodley, D. T., Peterson, H. D., Herzog, S. R., Stricklin, G. P., Burgeson, R. E., Briggaman, R. A., et al. (1988). Burn wounds resurfaced by cultured epidermal autografts show abnormal reconstitution of anchoring fibrils. *JAMA*, **259**, 2566–71.

212. Compton, C. C., Gill, J. M., Bradford, D. A., Regauer, S., Gallico, G., and O'Connor, N. E. (1989). Skin regenerated from cultured epithelial autografts on full thickness burn wounds from 6 days to 5 years after grafting. *Lab. Invest.*, **60**, 600–12.

213. Woodley, D. T., Briggaman, R. A., Herzog, S. R., Meyers, A. A., Peterson, H. D., and O'Keefe, E. J. (1990). Characterisation of neo-dermis formation beneath cultured human epidermal autografts transplanted on muscle fascia. *J. Invest. Dermatol.*, **95**, 20–6.

214. Nickoloff, B. J., Vrani, J., and Mitra, R. S. J. (1991). Modulation of keratinocyte biology by gamma interferon: relevance to cutaneous wound healing. In *Clinical and experimental approaches to dermal and epidermal repair: normal and chronic wounds*, pp. 141–54.

215. Kupper, T. S., Horowitz, M., Birchall, N., Mizutani, H., Coleman, D., McGuire, J., et al. (1988). Haemopoietic, lymphopoietic and proinflammatory cytokines produced by human and murine keratinocytes. *Ann. NY Acad. Sci.*, **548**, 262–70.

216. Barker, J. N. W. N., Sarma, V., Mitra, R. S., Dixit, V., and Nickoloff, B. J. (1990). Marked synergism between tumour necrosis factor and interferon gamma in the regulation of keratinocyte derived adhesion molecules and chemotactic factors. *J. Clin. Invest.*, **85**, 605–8.

217. Stingl, G., Katz, S. I., Clement, L., Green, I., and Shevack, E. M. (1978). Immunological function of 1a-bearing epidermal Langerhans cells. *J. Immunol.*, **121**, 2005–10.

218. Morhenn, V. B., Benike, C. J., Cox, A. J., et al. (1982). Cultured human epidermal cells do not synthesize HLA-DR. *J. Invest. Dermatol.*, **78**, 32–7.

219. Hefton, J. M., Amberson, J. B., Biozes, D. G., and Weksler, M. E. (1984). Loss of HLA-DR expression by human epidermal cells after growth in culture. *J. Invest. Dermatol.*, **83**, 48–50.

220. Hefton, J. M., Madden, M. R., Finkelstein, J. L., and Shires, G. T. (1983). Grafting of burn patients with allografts of cultured epidermal cells. *Lancet*, **ii**, 428–30.

221. Thiovolet, J., Faure, M., Demidem, A., et al. (1986). Long term survival and immunological tolerance of human epidermal allografts produced in culture. *Transplantation*, **42**, 274–80.

222. Thiovolet, J., Faure, M., and Demidem, A. (1986). Cultured human epidermal allografts are not rejected for a long period. *Arch. Derm. Res.*, **278**, 252–4.

223. Aubock, J., Irschik, E., Romani, N., et al. (1988). Rejection after slightly prolonged survival time of Langerhans cell-free allogeneic cultured epidermis used for wound coverage in humans. *Transplantation*, **45**, 730–7.

224. Burt, A. M., Pallet, C. D., Sloane, J. P., O'Hare, M. J., Schafler, K. F., Yardeni, P., et al. (1989). Survival of cultured allografts in patients with burns assessed with probe specific for Y-chromosome. *Br. Med. J.*, **298**, 915–17.

225. Brain, A., Purkis, P., Coates, P., Hackett, M., Navsaria, H., and Leigh, I. M. (1989). Survival of cultured allogeneic keratinocytes transplanted to deep dermal bed assessed with probe specific for Y chromosome. *Br. Med. J.*, **298**, 917–19.

226. Karawach, W. F., Oliver, A. M., Weiler, Miltoft, E., Abromovich, D. R., and Rayner, C. R. (1991). Survival assessment of cultured epidermal allografts applied over partial thickness burn wounds. *Br. J. Plast. Surg.*, **44**, 321–4.

227. Roseeuw, D., De Coninck, A., Lissens, W., et al. (1990). Allogeneic cultured epidermal grafts heal chronic ulcers although the do not remain as proved by DNA analysis. *J. Derm. Sci.*, **1**, 245–52.

228. Gielen, V., van, Faure, M., Mauduit, G., and Thivolet, R. (1987). Progressive replacement of human cultured epithelial allografts by recipient cells as evidenced by HLA Class 1 antigen expression. *Dermatologica*, **175**, 166–70.

229. van der Merwe, A. E., Mattheyse, F. J., Bedford, M., et al. (1990). Allografted keratinocytes used to accelerate the treatment of burn wounds are replaced by recipient cells. *Burns*, **16**, 193–7.

230. Fabre, J. W. and Cullen, P. R. (1989). Rejection of cultured keratinocyte allografts in the rat. *Transplantation*, **48**, 306–15.

231. Hammond, E. J., Ng, R. L. H., Stanley, J. R. et al. (1987). Prolonged survival of cultured epidermal allografts in the nonimmunosuppressed mouse. *Transplantation*, **44**, 106–12.

232. Leigh, I. M., Purkis, P. E., and Navsaria, H. A. (1987). Treatment of chronic venous ulcers with sheets of cultured allogenic keratinocytes. *Brit. J. Dermatol.*, **117**, 591–7.

233. Phillips, T. J., Kehinde, O., Green, H., and Gilchrist, B. A. (1989). Treatment of skin ulcers with epidermal allografts. *J. Am. Acad. Derm.*, **21**, 191–9.

234. Teepe, R. G. C., Koebrugge, E. J., Ponec, M., and Vermeer, B. J. (1990). Fresh versus cryopreserved cultured allografts for the treatment of chronic skin ulcers. *Brit. J. Dermatol.*, **122**, 81–9.

235. McKay, I. A. and Leigh, I. M. (1991). Epidermal cytokines and their roles in cutaneous wound healing. *Br. J. Dermatol.*, **124**, 513–18.

236. Mackenzie, R. C. and Sauder, D. N. (1990). Keratinocyte cytokines and growth factors. *Dermatologic Clinics*, **8**, 649–61.

237. Stanley, J. R., Hawley-Nelson, P., Yaar, M., et al. (1982). Laminin and bullous pemphigoid antigen are distinct basement membrane proteins synthesized by epidermal cells. *J. Invest. Dermatol.*, **78**, 456–9.

238. Lynch, S. E., Colvin, R. B., and Antionades, H. N. (1989). Growth factors in wound healing. *J. Clin. Invest.*, **84**, 640–6.

239. van Brunt, J. and Klausner, A. (1988). Growth factors speed wound healing. *Bio/Technology*, **6**, 25–30.

240. Sporn, M. B., Roberts, A. B., Shull, J. M., Smith, J. M., Ward, J. M., and Sodek, I. (1983). Polypeptide transforming growth factors isolated from bovine sources and used for wound healing *in vivo*. *Science*, **219**, 1329–31.

241. Shah, M., Foreman, D. M., and Ferguson, M. W. F. (1992). Control of scarring in adult wounds by neutralising antibody to transforming growth factors isolated from bovine sources and used for wound healing *in vivo*. *Science*, **219**, 1329–31.

242. Holbrook, K. A. (1989). Biological structure and function: perspectives on morphological approaches to the study of the granular layer keratinocyte. *J. Invest. Dermatol.*, **92**, 84–104.

243. Mackenzie, I. C. and Hill, M. W. (1984). Connective tissue influences on patterns of epithelial architecture on keratinisation in skin and oral mucosa of the adult mouse. *Cell Tissue Res.*, **235**, 551–9.

244. Karasek, M. A. and Charlton, M. E. (1971). Growth of postembryonic skin epithelial cells on collagen gels. *J. Invest. Dermatol.*, **56**, 205–10.

245. Bell, E., Sher, S., Hull, B., Merrill, C., Rosen, S., Chamson, A., et al. (1983). The reconstruction of living skin. *J. Invest. Dermatol.*, **81**, 2S–10S.

246. Burke, J., Yannas, I., Quinby, W., Bondoc, C., and Jung, W. (1981). Successful use of a physiologically acceptable artificial skin in the treatment of extensive burn injury. *Ann. Surg.*, **194**, 413–28.

247. Boyce, S. T. and Hansborough, J. F. (1988). Biologic attachment, growth, and differentiation of cultured human epidermal keratinocytes on a graftable collagen and chondroitin-6-sulphate substrate. *Surgery*, **103**, 421–31.

248. Vascovali, C., Damour, D., Shababedin, L., et al. (1989). Epidermalisation of an artificial dermis made of collagen. *Ann. Mediterranean Buns. Club.* **2**, 137–9.

249. Pruneiras, M., Regnier, M., and Woodley, D. (1983). Methods of cultivation of keratinocytes at an air liquid interface. *J. Invest. Dermatol.*, **81**, 28–33.

250. Carter, N., Green, C. J., Navsaria, H. A., and Leigh, I. M. (1991). Treatment of junctional epidermolysis bullosa with epidermal autografts. *J. Am. Acad. Derm.*, **172**, 256–50.

251. Moll, M. A. E., Nanning, P. B., Van Eendenburg, J-P., et al. (1991). Grafting of venous ulcers; an intraindividual comparison between cultured skin quivalents and full thickness skin punch grafts. *J. Am. Acad. Derm.*, **2**, 77–82.

252. Nanchalal, J., Otto, W. R, Dover, R., and Dhital, S. K. (1989). Cultured composite skin grafts: biological skin equivalents permitting massive expansion. *Lancet*, **ii**, 191–3.

253. Hansborough, J. F., Boyce, S. T., Cooper, M. L., and Foreman, T. J. (1989). Burn wound closure with cultured autologous keratinocytes and fibroblasts attached to a collagen–glycosaminoglycan substrate. *JAMA*, **262**, 2125–30.

254. Cuono, C., Langdon, R., and McGuire, J. (1986). Use of cultured epidermal autografts and dermal allografts as skin replacement after burn injury. *Lancet*, **1**, 1123–4.

255. Cuono, C. B., Langdon, R., Birchall, N., Bartelbort, S., and McGuire, J. (1987). Composite autologous-allogenic skin replacement: development and clinical application. *Plast. Reconstr. Surg.*, **80**, 626–35.

256. Langdon, R. C., Cuono, C. B., Birchall, N., Madri, J. A., Kuklinska, E., McGuire, J., and Moellmann, G. E. (1988). Reconstitution of structure and cell function in human skin grafts derived from cryopreserved allogeneic dermis and autologous cultured keratinocytes. *J. Invest. Dermatol.*, **91**, 478–85.

257. Kangesu, L., Green, C., Navsaria, H., and Leigh, I. M. (1991). The role of dermis in the take of autologous keratinocyte grafts.

258. Kangesu, I., Wausaria, N. A., Monek, S., Fryer, P. R., Leigh, I. M., Green, C. J. (1993). Keratodermal grafts: the importance of dermis for the in viro growth of cultured reratinocytes. *Brit. J. Plastic Surg.*, **46**, 401–9.

12

Clinical trials and statistics
D. J. LEAPER and G. D. MULDER

Controlled clinical trials

Introduction

The rapid increase in attention focused on wound repair during the past two to three decades has paralleled an increased demand for clinical trials examining efficacy and safety of new wound care devices, pharmaceuticals, and other products. Fierce competition has necessitated the implementation of clinical trials which need to be completed with a large patient population in a relatively short time frame. Subsequently, the quality of science and research have been compromised to some extent for the sake of obtaining, questionably valid, published results. Poorly designed and controlled studies yield biased and often unusable data. Study results may purport to show great benefits of a product which, in reality, is of little clinical value, when compared to already available, less expensive, and equally or more effective materials.

Well controlled studies require careful design. This involves appropriate patient population selection, stratification, evaluation of medical, mental, and nutritional status, and appropriate collection of clinical and laboratory demographic variables (entry) and follow-up (compliance). Wounds need to be stratified and selected according to aetiology, duration, and level of healing, as determined for example, by the extent of granulation and re-epithelialization. Other considerations in a well designed clinical trial include, but are not limited to, control and standardization of treatment of underlying pathophysiology, establishment of guidelines for wound assessment (evaluation of healing and definitions of healing), consideration and definition of efficacy, reasonable inclusion and exclusion criteria, and comparison of treatment modality with other popularly used modalities.

This chapter presents guidelines and basic considerations needed for designing a controlled trial of acceptable scientific quality using the chronic leg ulcer as a template. Protocol design may then be revised according to specific study and treatment modality needs.

Patient selection and stratification

Proper selection of patients is of equal importance to appropriate wound choice. Factors relevant to patient selection are listed in Table 12.1.

Age is known to affect the repair process and is a consideration when studying wound repair in the surgical and acute wound setting. One cannot exclude the elderly when examining pressure ulcers, as they tend to occur most frequently in this population (1–4). A generally accepted age range for most other studies is from 18 (usual age of consent) to 80.

Ambulation should be carefully monitored in trials with pressure, venous, and diabetic ulcers and equalized as much as possible in patients within each category. Mobility will have significant effects on pressure distribution in wheelchair and

Table 12.1 Factors relevant to patient selection

Patient selection criteria	Wound aetiology
Age	Aetiology/pathophysiology
Mobility	Duration
Mental status	Level of healing
Residence	
Nutritional status	
Compliance level	
General medical status	

Table 12.2 Complicating factors which may delay wound healing

Medications
Bacterial flora
Chemo/radiation therapy
Vascular status
Nutritional status
Patient medical status
Ambulatory status
Control of underlying pathophysiology
Necrotic eschar/debris

bed-bound patients. Diabetic weight-bearing patients, who are ambulatory, must all be placed in similar footwear or pressure-reducing devices to reduce pressure in an equivalent fashion in all patients. Shoe selection is a major factor influencing treatment outcome in diabetic studies (5–7).

Mobility in the venous patient will affect both calf and pump function. The most beneficial form of compression which can reasonably be utilized must be applied uniformly to all patients enrolled.

Mental status, though considered when determining the patients ability to sign the informed consent, is an important determinant of compliance. Candid questioning may reveal a reluctance to participate in a controlled randomized trial. Negative expectations could also affect study results when patients begin to miss appointments. Patients missing more than two consecutive visits are best dropped from a trial. Patients who are not fully informed of the definition of 'randomized', 'blinded', and 'control treatment' may become upset when, once enrolled, they discover they are receiving an inactive placebo.

Patient population may be placed into one of four categories:

(1) nursing home (or secondary care facility),

(2) hospitalized (inpatient care),

(3) outpatient presenting to a clinic for treatment, and

(4) outpatient being cared for in the home.

When possible, entering patients who are all in the same setting will ensure better control of administered care. Limiting the patients to one setting further permits the use of the same clinical investigators or investigative assistants. Variability in subjective judgements and documentation are thereby kept to a minimum.

Hospital and nursing home environments, with a regular staff, are preferable to outpatients or the community, where there is less control. When using an outpatient clinic, attempts must be made to ensure that the patient is seen by the same clinician for subsequent visits. Forms or cards may be given to patients for home use to record any change or deviation from the treatment protocol.

Compliance

Individual compliance is easily determined when reviewing a patient's past clinical history. Has the patient been in previous studies? How did they perform? Does the patient consistently make appointments? Is there a family member who can ensure that the patient will attend clinics? Common sense on the part of the investigator will significantly reduce the total number of non-evaluable patients in any given study.

General medical status

The overall medical status of a patient will affect study outcome. The importance of specific concurrent medical diseases vary with the type of protocol being implemented. Wound studies focus on factors influencing granulation, re-epithelialization, and wound closure. A list of these considerations (which is not exhaustive) is given in Table 12.2. Each of the items in the list may negatively influence wound closure. The detrimental effects on wound care of each of these factors have been addressed previously (8–10).

Nutritional level

Albumin, protein, and overall nutritional status of a patient may also impede wound closure, thereby affecting study outcome (8–10). A protocol including a malnourished population (e.g. elderly, bedridden, critically ill) must ensure that nutritional status is equivalent in treatment and control groups. The exception to the latter are studies focusing on correcting nutritional deficiencies.

Study design

The format of a wound healing protocol will be determined by the device, material, or drug to be studied. While a basic format can be suggested for all studies (see Table 12.3, which again is not exhaustive), exclusion/inclusion criteria and laboratory tests vary with the safety and efficacy end points. Patient entry, study visits, and follow-up are also dictated by the latter consideration.

A 'lead-in' phase prior to randomization into a treatment group may be applied to both drug and device periods. The lead-in period allows for a standardization of wound care and treatment which results in a separation of wounds into 'responders' and 'non-responders' (7) Wounds which did not respond prior to enrolment may have done so subsequent to poor care. Enrolment into a study providing high standards of care could result in rapid wound closure thus creating bias towards the treatment into which the wound was randomized.

Table 12.3 General laboratory considerations

Blood tests (helps establish baseline and final patient status)
　　Full blood count
　　Multiple analysis – urea and electrolytes; liver function tests
　　Coagulation screen
　　Blood plasma levels for biologicals and cutigens
　　Glycosylated haemoglobin/fasting blood sugar for diabetics

Vascular examination
　　Plethysmography and Doppler index (ABPI)

Histology
　　For identification of receptors, analysis of tissue
　　Quality/components in healing tissue

Cultures (for microbial studies)
　　Aerobic/anaerobic
　　Quantitative/qualitative

Neurological examination
　　Diabetic patients

X-rays
　　When concerned with osteomyelitis
　　With oncogenic materials

Nutrition
　　All patients, especially elderly

Skin perfusion (transcutaneous tissue oxygen electrode, oximetry)
　　For vascular lesions

A lead-in period frequently yields a high attrition rate prior to enrolment yet results in more accurate indications of protocol success once the remaining patients are entered into the study.

Wound assessment

A list of considerations when assessing a wound are listed in Table 12.4. Clinical report forms evaluating wound parameters facilitate data analysis when they are simple, concise, and computer 'friendly'. Whcnever possible, numerical values should be assigned to the evaluation of parameters (e.g. linear analogue scale assessment – LASA – from 0–10). A standardized clinical report form for chronic ulcer evaluation is given in Table 12.5 as an example. The protocol designer should avoid too many choices and descriptions for subjective evaluations. Frequently confusing evaluations include type and amount of exudate, granulation, and re-epithelialization. Descriptions of wound colour (erythema, hyper pigmentation, and peri-ulcer changes, etc.) can be lengthy, misleading and variable depending on the clinician's judgement. Assignment of a numerical value may help to reduce lengthy descriptions and decrease the subjective margin.

Frequency of wound assessment will be dictated by the device/drug being used. A weekly evaluation usually suffices for most device studies even though the study material may require more frequent application. Drug studies more commonly require bi or tri-weekly evaluation.

Wound measurement techniques are influential in providing efficacy data. A reproducible means of measuring wound circumference, area, and depth (when applicable) is needed. Limited techniques are currently available (11). Acetate trac-

Table 12.4 Wound assessment considerations

Stage of wound
Microbial colonization (swab harvest)
Chronicity (duration)
Wound size
Wound environment
Wound aetiology
Amount of granulation and re-epithelialization

Table 12.5 Wound evaluation form

　　　　　　　　　　　　　　　Protocol No＿＿＿＿＿＿＿
　　　　　　　　　　　　　　　Patient No＿＿＿＿＿＿＿

Patient name: ＿＿＿＿＿＿＿＿＿＿＿＿＿＿
Date of examination: ＿＿＿＿＿＿＿＿＿＿＿

Size of wound:
　　Height (cm)
　　Width (cm)
　　Depth (mm)

Stage of ulcer:
　　I
　　II
　　III

Exudate description:
　　Serous
　　Serosanguinous
　　Sanguinous
　　Purulent

Odour:
　　None
　　Mild
　　Strong

Maceration:
　　No
　　Yes (%)

Re-epithelialization:
　　No
　　Yes (%)

Granulation:
　　No
　　Yes (%)

Necrotic tissue:
　　None
　　Low
　　Medium
　　High
　　% of surface

Eschar:
　　No
　　Yes (%)

Erythema:
　　Mild
　　Medium
　　Severe

ings and photographs analysed by computer planimetry are acceptable and extensively used. It is recommended that both tracings and photos are used as the combination provides a 'back-up' in case one of the two measurements is lost. Photography is best when the same film is used (not Polaroid) with a set focal length camera which allows a reproducible distance from the wound each time a picture is taken. Amateur cameras or use of different types of camera for the same study should be avoided. Inclusion and exclusion criteria are based on safety, efficacy, and effects on wound repair. General criteria include those considerations influencing healing. Margins must be allowed for laboratory values which vary from site to site. Medication doses must be considered when listing medications (e.g. steroids and non-steroidal anti-inflammatory drugs) which may impede closure.

Concomitant diseases need not be exclusion criteria unless they have a direct effect on the wounds being studied. There is currently no evidence that a patient with controlled diabetes needs to be excluded from a study involving upper body pressure ulcers. Neither does a patient with venous disease need to be excluded from a study of diabetic foot ulcers, as long as the treatment lesions are determined not to be venous.

Arterial values should be reproducible and accurate. Ankle: brachial indices (ABPI) or Doppler indices are often used as indications of arterial occlusion (12–14). These are frequently elevated secondary to vessel calcification (15) and are not recommended as exclusion criteria. Plethysmography and Tcp_{O_2} are more accurate indices (16).

Alginate moulds can be applied to full thickness wounds to measure volume. These may be inaccurate depending on the method of applying and weighing the mould material. Currently available techniques for volume measurement are either inaccurate or time consuming. A crude method of volume measurement using the Braden scale (17) will provide sufficient data on volume reduction. Precise measurements of volume reduction are of minor importance when compared unit gross reduction in volume over the entire study period.

Perhaps the greatest obstacle in wound repair studies is the determination of the end point of the study, which may range from efficacy, as determined by percentage closure, to complete healing. The most efficacious products would appear to be those that promote complete wound closure while having the lowest risk of recurrent skin breakdown. Clinical studies and patient studies rarely allow such luxuries.

Financing studies may be a problem. Also, extending studies to over 12 weeks further decreases patient willingness to return to the clinic on a regular basis, particularly when little progress is seen by the individual.

The investigator may be left to rely on significant differences between control and treatment results without attaining complete wound healing. The ideal end point, closure, may be the goal of a study yet it does not determine which product is optimal for wound closure.

The ideal protocol would be a three-armed, randomized study, testing the product being investigated, a standard placebo/control, and the best currently available product. Wound studies most frequently have gauze (dry or wet) as a standard control, but gauze, while being a standard, may be much less effective than newer products already available. So test materials may surpass placebo in efficacy yet be inferior to other available products.

The length of a study can best be calculated by estimating the mean time to closure for the wound of particular aetiology. Such calculations are generally inaccurate, but guidelines may be obtained by taking the mean wound size and determining, through a review of clinical data, the expected time for such a wound to heal under optimal treatment and circumstances.

Wound selection

A primary factor in determining product function is wound aetiology. It is imperative that the individuals designing a protocol be familiar with wound pathophysiology in order to prevent the oversight of underlying medical problems delaying closure. Numerous publications are available to assist the investigator (18–22). Indiscriminate inclusion of wounds of different aetiology introduces increasingly difficult to control variables and makes stratification more difficult. The many considerations for wound stratification are listed in Table 12.6.

Wound debridement deserves particular attention. All attempts must be made to change a wound from chronic to acute status. Excessive fibrotic and necrotic tissue as well as all debris should be removed from the wound. Surgical debridement has been shown to be optimal in providing a clean wound bed (23). Natural growth and wound factors may be introduced through fresh bleeding into the debrided wound. Debris and necrotic tissue colonized by pathogenic organisms may also be reduced by aggressive debridement. However, caution is necessary when attempting to create a clean wound in patients with vascular compromise, to avoid increasing the wound size.

Chronicity of wounds (time that an ulcer has been present, for example) may influence study results. Wounds which have been present for less than one month may not be suitable for chronic wound studies unless first placed in a lead-in phase as described earlier. Wounds that have been present for greater

Table 12.6 Considerations for wound stratification

	Wound aetiology		
	Diabetic	Venous	Pressure
Type of diabetes	X		
Compression (extremities)		X	
Neurological disease	X		
Vascular status	X	X	X
Compliance	X	X	X
Ambulatory status (mobility)	X	X	X
Wound stage	X	X	X
Wound duration	X	X	X
Control of pathophysiology	X	X	X
Nutritional status	X	X	X
Use of pressure relieving/ reducing devices	X	X	X
Duration of ulcer	X	X	X

Table 12.7 Suggested size range of ulcers for wound studies

Wound aetiology	Size/cm^2
Diabetic	1.0×1.0 to 6.0×6.0
Venous	2.0×2.0 to 8.0×8.0
Pressure	2.0×2.0 to 10.0×10.0

than one year should be included only after ruling out any major underlying or previously undetected factor which has delayed closure.

Wound size (area/volume) varies greatly with patient presentations. Extremely small and large wounds should be excluded. Table 12.7 lists a suggested range for the three major chronic wounds.

Wound stage can be divided into partial or full thickness wounds. Inclusion of both types of wounds in the same protocol requires entry of a much larger number of patients to prevent bias from occurring towards either treatment or control modalities.

Animal studies

It is beyond the scope of this chapter to discuss the design, role, and importance of animal studies in wound repair. The need of such studies to provide insight into pathways of healing is undisputed. However, one must not neglect the shortcomings of animal models in providing an environment where the complex medical status of a patient can be reproduced. Examinations and biopsies of patients' tissues are a means of providing information on wound histocytopathology which otherwise may be unobtainable. Collection of useful quantitative data may necessitate more aggressive and invasive techniques. Biopsies are a means of gathering information on cellular activities, growth factor response, histological changes, repair regulation, and receptor site activities. These may be obtained without increasing patient risk. The majority of wounds can be safely biopsied by using a 3 or 4 mm punch technique. Data can be combined with animal studies thus providing a more complete picture of the repair process.

Protocol success

The designing of a protocol, as discussed in the preceding text, selection of experienced investigators, careful study control and monitoring, and patient selection and stratification will all be determinants to implementing an academically and scientifically credible study.

Ineffective products result from poorly designed studies. It is necessary to design protocols to go beyond defining product success, which attempt to explain and define those reasons for success and failure. Only through an understanding of the mechanisms which inhibit and stimulate acute and chronic wound closure will successful treatments be developed.

This section provides a stimulus for the development of credible protocols. Wounds, particularly chronic ones, are not incurable, we simply have yet to find the cure. Meticulous and precise attention to design will allow us to produce more effective wound treatment products.

Statistics and audit

Any individual who is involved in patient management should have a grasp of the meaning of probability and be able to assess for themselves the validity of any figures presented to them which purport to improve care. Put more simply, claims made must be scrutinized objectively in order to decide whether practise should change – is treatment A better than treatment B? Equally, individuals should be able to set up their own study or at least, in principle, if they wish to test a hypothesis in the knowledge that their research plans are valid and have a change of showing that a difference can be shown, if it exists at all.

It is conventional to adopt the null hypothesis in research procedures where it is assumed that a test group of data (treatment A) does not differ from a parent group (treatment B). If the probability of a difference occurring by chance is less than 5 in 100 (0.05) then a statistically significant difference is possible and the null hypothesis may be rejected. There is nothing magical about this level of significance. A probability of $p < 0.001$ simply means that a difference can be expected to have arisen by chance less than once in a thousand times. In such circumstances it is conventionally assumed that a true difference exists. However, we should be careful not to make the type I error (α) to reject the null hypothesis wrongly – more simply, accepting that there is a biological difference simply because there is a statistically significant difference. Similarly, the type II error (β) is made when a null hypothesis is not rejected when it should be – just because there is no statistical difference one assumes there is no biological significance. The power of a statistical test therefore is 1-β; the smaller the value of β then the more likely a study is to show a result. These factors must be considered when determining the likelihood of a result from a research trial, together with the number of measurements needed. The Feinstein formula allows these values to be set before a trial or study begins:

$$\frac{(2.80)^2}{(P_1 - P_2)}\left[P_1(100 - P_1) + P_2(100 - P_2)\right]$$

where P_1 is the percentage of events in a parent group (say B) and P_2 that in the test group (A). This gives an α value of 0.05 – a statistically significant difference at the level of 5 per cent and a β value of 0.20 – an 80 per cent power of showing a difference. The number derived by the formula gives the number of events or patients which should be in each arm of the study. The constant 2.80 needs to be adjusted if a higher level of statistical difference or greater power is desired.

Randomization of patients is based on sampling techniques which ensure that patients are truly representative of each group. Usually random number tables or computer generated random numbers are used. There are tests to check for randomness, but these are rarely seen to have been used in practise in trial reports or publications.

Presentation of data

Trial data must be presented in a manner which allows examination of inferences or conclusions by the readers themselves. Tables and graphs really are subsidiary aids to the text and should make results more clear. Data presentation should be complete and comparability of demographic data in particular needs to be given. It is also conventional to express data in appropriate units, ideally Système International (SI), to avoid ambiguity. Three types of data are described below.

1. Nominal data define classes (such as sex) and are mutually exclusive.

2. Ordinal data are semiquantitative and commonly used in biological data sets. These data can be ranked and are usually expressed as a median (the middle value of data ranked from smallest to largest) with the range of data (which may be skewed – non-parametric) spread about the median.

3. Interval data are measured on a continuous scale and are quantitative. There is a Gaussian or equal dispersion about the mean (derived by dividing the total of the added measurements by the number of observations). These are parametric data, usually with larger numbers of observations, and the dispersion about the mean is indicated as standard deviations or errors, or more correctly as confidence intervals, which include 95 per cent of all observations (standard deviation $\times$ 1.96).

Statistical tests

Statistical tests that are used in the comparison of interval data, particularly when there are large numbers, are the parametric group. The most commonly used test is the 't' statistic. When there is a need to compare several mean values and their dispersion, the analysis of variance (ANOVA) is used. Most of these tests, together with deviation of means and confidence intervals, are found in standard computer statistical packages. Those who wish to understand the theory and to work the appropriate formulas 'by hand' can find them in standard statistical textbooks.

For ordinal data, particularly when there are small numbers of measurements, the more simple ranking tests may be used and are more appropriate. Examples include the Wilcoxon, Mann-Whitney, and X^2 and Fisher tests. Again, these can be found in software packages, but the tests are easy to undertake with a hand calculator.

More sophisticated tests need a computer for analysis. These include correlation and regression analysis. In studies of survival after comparative treatments there are the more sophisticated log rank survival analyses, and to extend regression analysis, independent variables can be determined for logistic, stepwise analysis. It is beyond the scope of this chapter to describe these further, but again they are becoming standard fare on computer statistical software.

Specificity and sensitivity

These terms have become standard methods with which to express the usefulness of a new investigation, particularly

Table 12.8 Calculation of specificity and sensitivity

Observed numbers	Expected numbers		
	Yes	No	
Yes	a	b	n_3
No	c	d	n_4
	n_1	n_2	N

a is the number of true positives; b is the number of false positives; c is the number of false negatives; d is the number of true negatives.
N is the total number of observations.
n_1 is the sum of $a + c$; n_2 is the sum of $b + d$; n_3 is the sum of $a + b$; n_4 is the sum of $c + d$.
Accuracy is expressed as $(a + d)/N$.
Sensitivity is expressed as a/n_1 (indicating the false negatives); specificity is expressed as d/n_2 (indicating the false postives).
The predictive value of a positive test is a/n_3; the predictive value of a negative test is d/n_4.

screening, although they can be adopted for many uses. Calculation of specificity and sensitivity is made easy by constructing a 2×2 contingency table (Table 12.8).

Audit

Audit of some form as been undertaken in medicine since records began, but has become formalized and measurable in recent decades. The aim of audit is to evaluate care objectively in order to improve its standard or maintain its standard. Medical audit is based on confidential peer review of medical care. Morbidity and mortality meetings alone are no longer considered to be adequate; audit should include the adequacy of records and include focused or criterion-based audit of aspects of medical care which are perceived to be inadequate. Clinical audit involves evaluation of total care given to patients and is multidisciplinary. Most hospital trusts in the UK now give support staff for this activity. The revisiting of audit topics allows the 'closing of the loop' to ensure maintenance of standards. From audit should come education, improvement of knowledge, and research; serendipity often leads to important new findings.

Audit is based on structure, process, and outcome. Audit of structure should examine, for example, our resources in efficiency and effectiveness in these days of increasing costs of medical care. Audit of process involves the diagnosis and management of patients, together with compliance with laid down policies of care.

This includes the accurate collection of data, using the Office of Population Census and Survey (OPCS) and International Classification of Disease (ICD) guidelines, as well as measurement of performance indicators and good code of practice. Audit of outcome evaluates morbidity and mortality and, more accurately, quality of life (QALYs), and aspects of care such as patients' satisfaction on quality controls.

References

1. Constantian, M. B. (1980). *Pressure ulcers: principles and techniques of management*, p. 15. Little Brown and Co, Boston.

2. Krasner, D. (1990). *Pressure ulcers and overview in chronic wound care*, pp. 75–6. Health Management Publications Inc., King of Prussia, Pennsylvania.

3. Allman, R. M. (1989). Pressure ulcers among the elderly. *New England Journal of Medicine*, **320**, 850–3.

4. Kaminski, J. R., Mitchell, V., Pinchcofsky-Devin, *et al.* Nutritional management of decubitus ulcers in the elderly. *Decubitus*, **2**, 20–2.

5. Levin, M. E. and O'Neal, L. W. (1988). The diabetic foot: medical management of Foot ulcers. *Clinical Materials*, **8**, 273–7.

6. Malone, J. M., Snyder, M., Anderson, G., *et al.* (1989) Prevention of amputation diabetic educations. *Am. J. Surg.*, **158**, 520–4.

7. Pecoraro, R. E., Ahroni, J. E., Boyko, E. J., and Stensel, V. L. (1991). Chronology and determinants of tissue repair in diabetic lower extremity ulcers. *Diabetes*, **40**, 1305–12.

8. Lipschitz, D. A. (1982). Protein calorie malnutrition in the hospitalized elderly. *Primary Care*, **9**, 531–43.

9. Chernoff, R., Mitchell, C. O., and Lipschitz, D. A. (1984). Assessment of the nutritional status of the geriatric patient. *Geriatric Medicine Today*, 3, 129–41.

10. Levenson, S. M. and Seifter, E. (1997). Dysnutrition, wound healing and resistance to infection. *Clinics of Plastic Surgery*, **4**, 375.

11. Gilman, T. H. (1990). Parameter for measurement of wound closure. *Wounds*, **2**, 95–101.

12. Wagner, F. W. (1981). The dysvascular foot: a system for diagnosis and treatment. *Foot and Ankle*, **2**, 64–122.

13. Bare, G. E. and Pomagjel, M. J. (1981). Toe blood pressure by photoplethysmography. An index of healing in forefoot amputations. *Surgery*, **89**, 569–74.

14. Gibbons, G. W., Wheelock, F. C. Jr, Sienegieda C., *et al.* (1979). Non-invasive calification prediction of amputation level in diabetic patients. *Arch. Surg.*, **114**, 1253–7.

15. Abramson, D. I. (1985). *Circulatory problems in podiatry*, pp. 67–8. Karger, New York.

16. Fronek, A. (1988). *Non-invasive diagnostics in vascular disease*, pp. 11–27, 282–9. McGraw-Hill, New York.

17. Mash, N. J. (1990). Standards and protocols for pressure ulcer care. In *Chronic wound care*, (ed. D. Krasner), pp. 89–93. Health Management Publications Inc, King of Prussia, Pennsylvania.

18. Mulder G. and Glugla M. (1990). The diabetic foot, medical management of foot ulcers. In *Chronic wound care*, (ed. D. Krasner), pp. 223–39. Health Management Publications Inc, King of Prussia, Pennsylvania.

19. Mulder, G. (1990). Factors complicating wound repair. In *Wound healing: alternatives in management*, (ed. L. C. Kloth, J. M. McCulloch, and J. A. Feedar), pp. 43–51. F A Davis Company, Philadelphia, Pennsylvania.

20. Mulder, G. D. and Albert, S. F. (1990). Skin problems associated with pressure. In *Geriatric medicine*, (ed. R. W. Schrier), pp. 149–55. W B Saunders, Philadelphia, Pennsylvania.

21. Ryan, T. J. (1987). *The management of leg ulcers*. Oxford University Press, Oxford.

22. Bader, D. L. (1990). *Pressure sores: clinical practice and scientific approach*. MacMillan, London.

23. Knighton, D. R., Fiegel, V. D., Doucette M. M., Fylling, C. P., and Cerra, F. B. (1989). The use of topically applied platelet growth factors in chronic non-healing wounds: a review. *Wounds*, 71–7.

Further reading

Altmann, D. C. (1991). *Practical statistics for medical research*. Chapman and Hall, London.

Armitage, P. and Berry, G. (1987). *Statistical methods in medical research*, (2nd edn). Blackwell, Oxford.

Dudley, H. A. (1993). Statistics. In *Clinical surgery in general*, (ed. R. M. Kirk, A. O. Mansfield, and J. Cochrane), RCS course manual. Churchill Livingstone, Edinburgh.

Ellis, B. W. and Simpson, J. (1993). Audit. In *Clinical surgery in general*, (ed. R. M. Kirk, A. O. Mansfield, and J. Cochrane), RCS course manual. Churchill Livingstone, Edinburgh.

Feinstein, A. R. (1977). *Clinical biostatistics*, C V Mosby, St Louis.

Pollock, A. (1987). Clinical audit. Clinical trials. Statistics. In *Surgical infections*. Edward Arnold, London.

Pollock, A. and Evans, M. (1993). *Surgical audit*, (2nd edn). Butterworth Heinemann, Oxford.

Mathie, R. T., Taylor, K. M., and Calnan, J. S. (1989). *Principles of surgical research*. Butterworth, London.

Rose, G. and Barker, D. J. P. (1981). *Epidemiology for the uninitiated*. British Medical Association, London.

Siegel, S. (1956). *Non parametric statistics for the behavioural sciences*. McGraw-Hill, Tokyo.

Swinscow, D. (1976). *Statistics from square one*. British Medical Association, London.

Swinscow, T. D. S. (1985). Present numerical results. In *How to do it*, (2nd edn). British Medical Association, London.

Wulff, H. E. (1981). *Rational diagnosis and treatment*. Blackwell, Oxford.

13

The future of wound healing

K. G. HARDING

It is only in recent years that interest in the biology and management of wounds has been sustained for a significant period to enable a much better understanding of the subject to be developed. In 1805, in the *Edinburgh Medical and Surgical Journal*, the treatment of leg ulcers was generally 'looked upon as an inferior branch of practice; an unpleasant and inglorious task, where much labour must be bestowed and little honour gained (1). The sentiments of that statement held true until fairly recently but even in 1994 Jeffcote spoke of the complexities of healing diabetic foot ulcers and recognized the 'feeling of critical ignorance of the processes involved in wound healing' (2). Both of these examples illustrate the low profile and lack of attention devoted to this important clinical problem and show the need for much greater attention and knowledge to be sought in this subject.

The recognition that wounds are caused by very diverse agents and pathologies and affect people of all ages is essential for all countries and health care systems in trying to plan for the future. Changing demographics in many western countries are associated with an exponential increase in the proportion of elderly patients in such societies. With advances in surgical and anaesthetic techniques these patients are increasingly subjected to complex operative procedures and surviving, but their risk of difficulties in wound healing increases. Similarly, there are increasing numbers of patients with pressure ulcers, leg ulcers, and diabetic foot ulcers in ageing populations, with attendant increased difficulties in management and healing.

Not only are western societies plagued by this epidemic of wounded patients but recently 'emerging' societies also face equally important, but often different, challenges. In China, for example, burns remain a very common condition and the fall in the numbers of patients with such wounds seen in the USA and Europe has not occurred in China due to a lack of industrial and domestic legislation to reduce risk. In other countries, rational and appropriate wound care may be too expensive. Potential for changing these situations requires not biological and clinical science but environmental and governmental intervention.

Wounds occur in a large proportion of our population but patients with complications of healing consume huge amounts of health care resources. In the UK it is estimated that the management of poorly healing wounds costs the government around one billion (a thousand million) pounds per year but, because of the difficulty in collecting accurate data on patients seen in all aspects of the health care system at present, we can only provide estimates. The results of epidemiological and economic research may help to provide much more accurate information in the future.

Many health care systems are now trying to provide the best quality and most cost-effective health care. In the UK a reduction in the number of patients developing pressure ulcers was one of the ten targets identified in a *Health of the nation* document, and the *St Vincent Declaration* stated that reduction of amputation in patients suffering from diabetes was a major goal of that initiative. These, and many other recent developments, have enabled wounds and the study of wound healing to receive a much higher profile in health care, and provide a potential platform for the subject to become one of the most important areas of investment and health gain in the next century.

In addition to this improved image the range of clinical treatments continues to increase dramatically. Most of the modern wound dressing materials have been developed following Winter's work in the 1960s, when he identified the benefit of a moist environment for healing superficial thickness wounds in a pig model. Since that time a wide range of materials have been developed and although no consistent improvement in healing times has been shown, particularly in chronic wounds, these materials carry obvious benefits to patients, carers, and health care professionals. Development of more sensitive and practical end-points of wound treatment are required to ensure such innovations have a measurable value in the future.

It has to be recognized that wound care does not only require a wound contact material but agents such as bandages, stockings, beds, and shoes are equally important in the overall management of patients with wound problems. Much greater investment in research to evaluate their efficacy is required.

It is interesting to note that despite advances in surgical techniques and increasing use of prophylactic antibiotics, wound infection still occurs in around 5–10 per cent of surgical procedures. Further development of appropriate diagnostic tests and effective antimicrobial agents are clearly required if we are to ensure cost-effective use of resources and rapid healing for all patients.

One of the greatest barriers to developing effective new

treatments has been the lack of a detailed ('complete') understanding of the normal process of healing and the deviations from normality seen in patients with wounds that do not heal. In the past there has been a dependence on cell culture and animal models. Whilst these undoubtedly are of benefit, they do not necessarily reflect the *in vivo* situation accurately. A full understanding of the complexities of healing is required and research work is now emerging which is giving a much clearer understanding.

Unfortunately, wound healing research is currently still in its formative years, and there has been great interest and perhaps too much faith placed in the possible value of molecular factors in healing (e.g. topical growth factor therapy). These experimental results have not been proven when tested in clinical trials, it is not simply the case that wounds fail to heal because of a lack of production of a specific growth factor and there is little evidence that such molecules remain active when placed on a wound surface.

Recently some attention has been paid, not to molecules which stimulate synthesis of new proteins, but to modifying the profile of degradative enzymes thought to be important to healing. However attractive a unifying theory of failure to heal may appear, a simple solution to the complex problem of healing may never arrive.

The importance of skin grafting for surgical wounds has been recognized for many years but new developments, including the use of autografts for chronic wounds, have some appeal. More interesting perhaps is the use of allografts, either of epidermal or dermal cells, in the treatment of such wounds, but again, there are considerable gaps in both basic research and clinical application of such 'living skin equivalents'.

Exciting new work on fetal tissue suggests that the changes which occur after birth may be modified not only to assist in healing but also to control the amount of scar tissue present when a wound has closed.

Integration of the strategies that improve wound prevention, wound treatment, and scar formation will occur over the next decade and it is only by such an approach that major improvements in patient care will occur.

Finally, the other challenge that will require attention in the future is how and who will provide wound care for patients. Should all doctors and all nurses be able to provide the increasingly complex treatments to all patients? Should plastic surgeons or dermatologists be the designated experts in wound care? Should wound care continue to be provided by nurses who are able to offer care to patients either alone or in combination with other specialties? The answers to these and many other questions remain to be addressed, but it is clear that, with the increasing awareness of the importance and complexity of this subject, many individuals who care for patients or are involved in scientific research will have the potential for being involved in wound healing in some capacity or another. Hopefully, the contents of this book have stimulated peoples interest and will encourage them to devote some time and attention to this newly emerging specialty and area of interest.

References

1. The Enquirer on the Treatment of Ulcerated Leg; Edinburgh Medicine and Surgery. Vol. 1, pp. 187–93.
2. Jeffcote, W. (1994). *Practical diabetes*, **11**, 4167.

Index